Ba

KT-431-563

070 202 6824

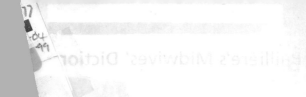

For Baillière Tindall:

Senior Commissioning Editor: Sarena Wolfaard
Project Development Manager: Mairi McCubbin
Project Manager: Pat Miller
Designer: Judith Wright

Baillière's Midwives' Dictionary

TENTH EDITION

Denise Tiran

MSc, RGN, RM, ADM, PGCEA
Principal Lecturer,
Midwifery/Complementary Medicine,
School of Health and Social Care,
University of Greenwich,
London, UK

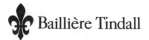

Baillière Tindall

EDINBURGH LONDON NEW YORK OXFORD PHILADELPHIA ST LOUIS SYDNEY TORONTO 2003

BAILLIÈRE TINDALL
An imprint of Elsevier Limited

First edition 1951   Eighth edition 1992
Sixth edition 1976   Ninth edition 1997
Seventh edition 1983   Tenth edition 2003
                            Reprinted 2004

ISBN 0 7020 2682 4

British Library Cataloguing in Publication Data
A catalogue record for this book is available from the British Library

Library of Congress Cataloging in Publication Data
A catalog record for this book is available from the Library of Congress

Note
Medical knowledge is constantly changing. Standard safety precautions must be
followed, but as new research and clinical experience broaden our knowledge,
changes in treatment and drug therapy may become necessary or appropriate.
Readers are advised to check the most current product information provided by
the manufacturer of each drug to be administered to verify the recommended
dose, the method and duration of administration, and contraindications. It is the
responsibility of the practitioner, relying on experience and knowledge of the
patient, to determine dosages and the best treatment for each individual patient.
Neither the Publisher nor the author assumes any liability for any injury and/or
damage to persons or property arising from this publication.
The Publisher

ELSEVIER   your source for books,
                  journals and multimedia
                  in the health sciences
www.elsevierhealth.com

The
publisher's
policy is to use
**paper manufactured
from sustainable forests**

Printed in China
C/02

Contents

Preface

Whilst completing this revision of the Dictionary, I read, in the *Midwives' Journal*, that Vera da Cruz had died, at the age of 92. Miss da Cruz was a renowned midwife and tutor, Vice President of the Royal College of Midwives, examiner for the Central Midwives' Board and author. She wrote *Baillière's Midwives' Dictionary*, which was first published in 1951, as well as a revision of *Mayes' Handbook of Midwifery*, later to become known as *Mayes' Midwifery*. I am therefore immensely proud to be part of the continuing tradition of midwifery by being invited, once again, to update the Dictionary for a contemporary generation of midwives.

In the 51 years since the first edition of the Dictionary, midwifery practice and education have changed, almost beyond recognition. The midwifery profession, now in its second century, has evolved to have a much broader remit, with health education and more women's and family health issues being incorporated into generic practice, and the development of a range of specialist roles. Technological advances have facilitated more successful pregnancies, which would not hitherto have been possible. There is a greater emphasis on evidence-based practice, as well as on interdisciplinary collaboration. Huge changes in the National Health Service have also taken place, and midwives are expected to have increased knowledge and understanding of quality assurance and risk management requirements and processes.

As a result, all of these factors have meant major reforms in midwifery pre- and post-registration education, now at both diploma and degree level, with some practitioners progressing to Masters and doctorate level studies. The need to relate theory to practice has become an integral part of the midwife's role. These developments have consequently expanded our professional language, not only of the terms specific to midwifery, obstetrics and paediatrics, but also of more generic terms. The increased depth of debate on all subjects related to the practice of midwifery has led to the publication of many new specialist textbooks, available to buy or to borrow from professional libraries.

Baillière's Midwives' Dictionary has always been considered to be essential reading for pupil and student midwives, and I hope it will continue to provide an indispensable quick-reference guide for both midwifery students and for more experienced practitioners.

London, 2003   Denise Tiran

Acknowledgements

I would like to thank everyone at Elsevier Science for the invitation to revise the Dictionary. Once again, the unflagging help and support from friends and colleagues in the School of Health and Social Care at the University of Greenwich, and especially at Queen Mary's Hospital, Sidcup, Kent, has been outstanding. I am grateful to Dr Richard Mainwaring Burton, Consultant Microbiologist at Queen Mary's Hospital, Sidcup, for his contribution to Appendix 2, on Normal Blood and Urine Values and Tests.

Finally, as ever, my greatest thanks go to my son, Adam, now 13, for letting me have priority in using the new computer, and for his help in unravelling the complexities of computer technology!

Acknowledgements

A

abdomen the cavity between the diaphragm and the pelvis, lined by peritoneum and containing the stomach, intestines, liver, gallbladder, spleen and pancreas; and, lying behind the peritoneum, the kidneys, suprarenal glands and ureters. The urinary bladder and the uterus become abdominal organs when distended (*see* Figure). *Pendulous a.* a condition in which the anterior part of the abdominal wall hangs down over the pubis.

abdominal concerning the abdomen.

abdominal enlargement enlargement of the abdomen during pregnancy is progressive due to uterine enlargement; visible externally from about 16th week of pregnancy. Undue enlargement of the abdomen may be caused by twins, polyhydramnios, fibroids in the wall of the uterus, or an abnormal development of the ovum (hydatidiform mole).

abdominal examination systematic examination of the abdomen by inspection, palpation and auscultation. The purpose is to determine the equality of the uterine size with the calculated period of gestation and, when relevant, to decide the lie, presentation and position of the fetus and whether the widest presenting transverse diameter is engaged. Inspection is made for shape, size, scars, striae gravidarum, skin tension, contour and fetal movements. Palpation (feeling) should be carried out gently and systematically. The

Abdomen

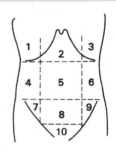

1, Right hypochondrium;
2, epigastrium; 3, left hypochondrium; 4, right lumbar region; 5, umbilical region; 6, left lumbar region; 7, right iliac fossa; 8, hypogastrium; 9, left iliac fossa; 10, pubic.

uterus is palpable abdominally by the 12th week and increases in size at a regular rate. Auscultation (listening) is carried out with a stethoscope (monaural or binaural) or with an electronic monitor. Its object is to hear and count the fetal heart sounds. Other sounds, such as the uterine SOUFFLE, may be heard. Postnatally, daily examination, by inspection and palpation, is performed to determine that uterine

INVOLUTION is occurring, that the uterus is regaining its non-pregnant size and position, and to elicit deviations from normal such as constipation or urinary retention.

abdominal pregnancy ECTOPIC GESTATION in which the fertilized ovum embeds in the abdominal cavity.

abdominal striae See STRIAE GRAVIDARUM.

abdominal wall the structures covering the abdominal organs, namely skin, fat, fascia, muscles and peritoneum.

abduct to draw away from an axis or the median plane.

abduction the act of drawing away from the centre; the state of being away from the centre.

aberrant wandering or deviating from the normal site or course.

ABO blood groups blood groups are classified by the presence or absence of agglutinogens A, B, A and B (AB) or none (O). The serum may contain antibodies, agglutinins anti-A, anti-B, both or neither. Blood given in transfusion must not contain the same antibodies as the recipient's blood group (e.g. a group A person must not receive group B blood which contains anti-A agglutinins) or a fatal reaction will occur. Group AB people have no agglutinin or antibody in the serum so can receive blood from any group, i.e. they are *universal recipients*; group O people have no agglutinogens so their blood can be given to anyone i.e. they are *universal donors*. See also RHESUS FACTOR.

ABO incompatibility occurs in about one in 200 pregnancies where the maternal blood group is O, the serum containing anti-A and anti-B antibodies. If the fetus is therefore group A, B or AB, an antibody differing immunologically from normal

ABO blood groups	
Red blood cell agglutinogen	Serum agglutinin or antibody
A	anti-B
B	anti-A
AB	no antibodies
O	anti-A and anti-B

anti-A and anti-B may cross the placenta and cause haemolysis in the neonate, even in a first baby. Jaundice appears within 24 hours of birth but is usually mild. The bilirubin level rises very rapidly but anaemia is less obvious. The COOMBS' TEST is usually negative, unlike in Rhesus incompatibility. The jaundice is treated with phototherapy or, in severe cases, by exchange transfusion. See also ABO BLOOD GROUPS and RHESUS FACTOR.

abort to bring to a premature end, especially a pregnancy. To check the course of a disease.

abortifacient any means used to cause abortion.

abortion expulsion from the uterus of the products of conception before the 24th week of pregnancy, the fetus not being born alive. *Therapeutic a.* a term often used to describe an induced abortion in accordance with the provisions laid down in the Abortion Act 1967. Before 12 weeks' gestation, this is usually performed by vacuum extraction or dilatation and curettage. Later, drugs such as prostaglandins are used. *Spontaneous a.* may be due to a blighted ovum, such as HYDATIDIFORM or VESICULAR MOLE, or a CARNEOUS MOLE, which may result in a MISSED ABORTION. ECTOPIC GESTATION also usually results in miscarriage. Abortion may be COMPLETE or INCOMPLETE. Complications include haemorrhage and sepsis, and treatment is aimed primarily at preventing these. Some women suffer HABITUAL ABORTION See also THREATENED ABORTION and INEVITABLE ABORTION.

abrachia congenital absence of arms.

abreaction the reliving of an experience in such a way that previously repressed emotions associated with it are released.

abruptio tearing asunder. *A. placentae* or *placental abruption* is where the placenta is partially or completely torn from its site, usually in the upper uterine segment, after the 24th week of pregnancy. See PLACENTA.

abscess a localized accumulation of pus in a space or cavity. *Bartholin's u.* in Bartholin's gland near the orifice of the vagina; *breast a.* in the breast; *pelvic a.* in the pouch of Douglas.

abuse misuse, maltreatment, or excessive use. See CHILD ABUSE. *Drug a.* use of illegal drugs or misuse of prescribed drugs.

accelerated labour See AUGMENTATION OF LABOUR.

accessory extra or supplementary. *A. auricles* are commonly found immediately anterior to the ear.

accidental antepartum haemorrhage now more often called haemorrhage from placental abruption or ABRUPTIO PLACENTAE.

accouchement childbirth.

accoucheur (F. accoucheuse) a person who conducts a birth.

accountable liable to be held responsible for a course of action.

accreditation process of evaluation of an institution or individual for the purpose of obtaining official recognition of standards set against agreed criteria, e.g. education.

accreta morbid attachment. *Placenta a.* a placenta attached to the uterine

muscle due to a deficiency of decidua basalis.

acetabulum a cup-shaped socket in the pelvic innominate bone, into which fits the head of the femur.

acetoacetic acid a product of abnormal fat metabolism, occurring in diabetic and dehydrated mothers.

acetone a by-product of acetoacetic acid. Acetone is one of the ketone bodies produced in abnormal amounts in uncontrolled diabetes and metabolic acidosis. Acetone has a characteristic smell which may be noticed in the mother's breath or urine.

acetonuria ketones in the urine.

acetylcholine chemical transmitter released by some nerve endings at the synapse between one neuron and the next, or between a nerve ending and the effector organ it supplies. These nerves are cholinergic, e.g. parasympathetic nerves and lower motor neurons to skeletal muscles. Acetylcholine is rapidly destroyed by cholinesterase.

achlorhydria absence of hydrochloric acid from the gastric juice; associated with conditions such as pernicious anaemia and stomach cancer.

achondroplasia failure to form cartilage. An inherited type of dwarfism characterized by marked shortening of the long bones. The achondroplastic dwarf has a large head, a normal trunk and very short limbs. Mentality is normal. The great majority of cases occur as a result of a new MUTATION and the gene is an autosomal dominant.

aciclovir an antiviral agent used to treat herpes simplex. Given orally or by intravenous infusion in doses of 200 mg five times daily or 5 mg/kg over 1 hour, repeated 8 hourly.

acid a substance which, when combined with an alkali, will form a salt.

Any acid substance will turn blue litmus red. *Hydrochloric a.* a colourless compound of hydrogen and chlorine. In 0.2% solution it is present in gastric juice and can cause MENDELSON'S SYNDROME if inhaled. Acids play a vital role in the chemical processes that are normally part of the functions of the cells and tissues of the body. A stable balance between acid and bases in the body is essential to life. *See also* ACID–BASE BALANCE.

acid–base balance a state of equilibrium between acidity and alkalinity of the body fluids; also called hydrogen ion (H^+) balance. The positively charged hydrogen ion (H^+) is the active constituent of all acids.

Most of the body's metabolic processes produce acids as their end products, but a somewhat alkaline body fluid is required as a medium for vital cellular activities. Therefore chemical exchanges of hydrogen ions must take place continuously in order to maintain a state of equilibrium. An optimal pH (hydrogen ion concentration) between 7.35 and 7.45 must be maintained; otherwise, the enzyme systems and other biochemical and metabolic activities will not function normally.

acidaemia an alteration, due to an accumulation of acids, in the reaction (pH) of the blood, which is normally slightly alkaline. It may occur in hyperemesis gravidarum and diabetes mellitus. If untreated, it will lead to coma and death. It can occur in labour if the woman is dehydrated and tissue perfusion is poor. The fetus or baby may suffer from acidaemia due to HYPOXIA.

acidosis a pathológical condition resulting from accumulation of acid or depletion of the alkaline reserve (bicarbonate content) in the blood

and body tissues, and characterized by increase in hydrogen ion concentration (decrease in pH to below 7.30). adj. *acidotic*. *Metabolic a.* acidosis resulting from accumulation in the blood of ketoacids (derived from fat metabolism) at the expense of bicarbonate, thus diminishing the body's ability to neutralize acids. Occurs in diabetic ketoacidosis, lactic acidosis and failure of renal tubules to reabsorb bicarbonate. *Respiratory a.* acidosis resulting from ventilatory impairment and subsequent retention of carbon dioxide. Carbon dioxide accumulates in the blood and unites with water to form carbonic acid. Occurs with severe birth asphyxia and other respiratory conditions affecting the newborn. In the mother occurs with either an acute obstruction of the airways or a chronic condition involving the organs of respiration. *See also* ACIDAEMIA.

acinus a minute hollow structure, lined by secreting cells and having a duct. The acini in the breast secrete milk. Sometimes called alveoli. pl. *acini*.

acquired immune deficiency syndrome (AIDS) severe progressive disease caused by the HUMAN IMMUNODEFICIENCY VIRUS and manifesting as fever, weight loss, diarrhoea and lymphadenopathy. Opportunistic infections such as cytomegalovirus, herpes simplex, *Mycobacterium tuberculosis* and *Pneumocystis carinii* will eventually lead to death, as will tumours such as lymphomas and Kaposi's sarcoma. *See also* HUMAN IMMUNODEFICIENCY VIRUS.

acromegaly a chronic disease in which the bones and tissues of the hands, feet and face are enlarged. It results from over-function of the pituitary gland resulting in hypersecretion of growth hormone and is often caused by a pituitary tumour.

acromion a process of the scapula, which forms the point of the shoulder.

acrosome the cap-like membrane-bounded structure covering the anterior portion of the head of the spermatozoon; it contains enzymes involved in penetration of the ovum.

active management of labour obstetric intervention to prevent prolonged labour and its complications. Delay in the first stage of labour may be diagnosed from the PARTOGRAM. Labour which is not progressing satisfactorily may be accelerated by artificial rupture of the membranes and/or an oxytocic infusion. The midwife is responsible for monitoring progress and carrying out medical instructions for the care of these women. *Active management of the third stage of labour* involves the administration of an oxytocic injection (e.g. Syntometrine 1 ml) to facilitate placental separation. This is given with the crowning of the head or the birth of the anterior shoulder and takes effect in 2.5 minutes. This is followed by manual delivery of the placenta and membranes, e.g. by CONTROLLED CORD TRACTION.

active transport the movement of ions or molecules across the cell membranes and epithelial layers, usually against a concentration gradient, resulting directly from the expenditure of metabolic energy. For example, under normal circumstances more potassium ions are present within the cell and more sodium ions extracellularly. The process of maintaining these normal differences in electrolytic composition between the intracellular fluids is active transport. The process differs from simple diffusion or osmosis in that it requires the expenditure of metabolic energy.

acupressure a system of complementary medicine in which pressure is applied to various points on the body to stimulate the innate self-healing capacity of the individual. Acupressure has been used very successfully to treat gestational sickness and can be effective in relieving pain in labour. *See also* ACUPUNCTURE.

acupuncture a system of Chinese complementary medicine based on the principle that the body has energy lines, or meridians, running through it from top to toe. When someone is in optimum health of body, mind and spirit, the energy flowing along the meridians is in equilibrium; ill health or physical or psychological stresses such as pregnancy cause the energy flow to become unbalanced. Application of fine needles to specific acupuncture points along the meridians can rebalance the energy flow and assist in returning the person to full health. Acupuncture has been used to treat a variety of disorders of pregnancy, relieve pain in labour and for caesarean section anaesthesia.

acute developing rapidly and running a short course. The reverse of chronic.

acute fatty atrophy (acute yellow atrophy) a rare complication of pregnancy characterized by rapid progressive atrophy of the liver, where there is massive fatty necrosis. The mortality rate is above 80%.

acute inversion of the uterus turning inside out of the uterus. A rare, serious complication of labour, caused by mismanagement of the third stage of labour, or occasionally occurring spontaneously. The condition is diagnosed by sudden profound shock occurring in the mother accompanied by severe abdominal pain, bleeding if the placenta is wholly or partially separated, palpation of a concave-shaped fundus in the abdomen, or no uterus felt at all if the inversion is complete, palpation of the uterus in the cervix or vagina; the uterus may be visible at the vulva. The midwife should raise the foot of the bed to relieve tension and alleviate shock and call urgently for the obstetrician. An attempt is made to replace the uterus by applying pressure to the lower segment near the cervix and working upwards to the fundus. If replacement of a totally inverted uterus is not possible it should be gently placed inside the vagina to reduce traction on the fallopian tubes and ovaries. Severe shock must be treated by replacing fluids and blood and a narcotic analgesic is administered. A general anaesthetic can then be given to enable manual replacement of the uterus, or the hydrostatic method may be used. If all attempts fail a hysterectomy will need to be performed.

acute renal failure a sudden severe interruption of kidney function. It is usually the complication of another disorder such as haemorrhage or shock and is reversible. OLIGURIA (diminished secretion of urine) is the hallmark of the condition and other symptoms are related to fluid and electrolyte imbalances, anaemia, hypertension and uraemia. Dialysis will be required to monitor fluid and electrolyte imbalances until kidney function improves.

adactylia, adactyly congenital absence of the fingers or toes.

adaptation the ability to overcome difficulties and to adjust oneself to changing circumstances. Neuroses and psychoses are often associated with failures of adaptation.

addict a person exhibiting addiction.

addiction physiological or psychological dependence on some agent, e.g. alcohol or drug, with a tendency to increase its use.

adduct to draw towards a centre or median line.

adduction the art of adducting; the state of being adducted.

adherent placenta a placenta which is firmly attached to the wall of the uterus, and which fails to separate during the third stage of labour. *See* PLACENTA; PLACENTA ACCRETA; PLACENTA PERCRETA.

adhesion union between two surfaces normally separated: usually the result of inflammation when fibrous tissue forms; e.g. peritonitis may cause adhesions between organs; a possible cause of intestinal obstruction, or of sterility through occlusion of the lumen of the fallopian tubes.

adipose tissue *See* TISSUE.

adnexa appendages. *Uterine a.* the ovaries and fallopian tubes.

adolescence the period of development from puberty to the cessation of physical growth.

adoption the legal procedure by which a child is transferred from its natural parents to adopting parents. The child's welfare is paramount and the Adoption Acts 1976 and 1978 (Scotland), with amendments in the 1989 Children Act, detail clearly how and when an adoption can take place and who can adopt. Local authorities offer advice, social work support and may act as an adoption agency, and there are also private and charitable organizations which must be registered with the local authority.

adrenal pertaining to the adrenal or suprarenal glands, two complex endocrine glands, situated one at the upper pole of each kidney.

adrenaline (epinephrine) one of several hormones secreted by the medulla of the adrenal or suprarenal gland. Its function is to aid in the regulation of the sympathetic branch of the autonomic nervous system. Adrenaline is a powerful vasopressor which increases blood pressure, heart rate, cardiac output and the release of glucose from the liver.

A pathological increase in adrenaline secretion is very rare and is due to a tumour of the adrenal medulla (PHAEOCHROMOCYTOMA). It causes acute hypertension. Removal of the tumour cures the condition. In cases of severe hypertension in pregnancy a 24-hour collection of urine may be required to measure the level of VANILLYLMANDELIC ACID (VMA), an excretory product of the catecholamines, which is raised in cases of phaeochromocytoma.

Adrenaline can also be produced synthetically.

adrenocorticotrophic hormone (ACTH) a hormone of the anterior lobe of the pituitary gland, which stimulates the adrenal cortex.

aerobe an organism requiring air or free oxygen to sustain life.

aerobic requiring air or free oxygen in order to grow and multiply.

aetiology the science of causes, e.g. of disease.

afebrile without fever.

affective pertaining to emotional tone or feeling. *A. disorder* any mental disorder characterized by a disturbance of mood accompanied by either manic or depressive symptoms or both. Major affective disorders are those in which the full syndrome of a manic or depressive episode is present: bipolar disorder (manic-depressive illness) and major depression. Other affective disorders include cyclothymic disorder and dysthymic disorder (depressive neurosis), which have less severe mood fluctuations.

afferent towards the centre. *A. nerve* a sensory nerve fibre carrying impulses from the periphery to the central nervous system.

affiliation order a court order made to compel a father to make regular payments towards his child's maintenance.

afibrinogenaemia absence of fibrinogen in the blood; more usually HYPOFIBRINOGENAEMIA. Acquired hypofibrinogenaemia is usually secondary to DISSEMINATED INTRAVASCULAR COAGULATION (DIC).

afterbirth a lay term for the placenta and membranes expelled from the uterus after the birth of the fetus.

aftercoming head the fetal head (coming after the trunk) in a breech delivery. *See* BREECH.

afterpains painful uterine contractions occurring after labour. They are common, especially in multiparous women, in the early puerperium and are frequently felt during breastfeeding. Severe and persistent afterpains would raise the suspicion that blood clot, membrane or a fragment of placenta might be retained in the uterus.

agenesis absence of an organ due to non-appearance of its primordium in the embryo.

agglutination aggregation of separate particles into clumps or masses. 1. the clumping together of red blood corpuscles in serum. This may occur in the body if incompatible cells are transfused. Agglutination of sensitized red blood cells by urine reveals the presence of chorionic gonadotrophin in a pregnancy test. 2. the clumping together of platelets owing to the action of platelet agglutinins. 3. the clumping of bacteria when brought into contact with specific immune serum.

agglutinin a substance which reacts with an AGGLUTINOGEN and causes agglutination to occur.

agglutinogen a substance which stimulates a specific agglutinin to cause agglutination.

agnathia failure of development of the jaw.

air the atmosphere surrounding the earth, mainly composed of two gases: oxygen (approximately 21%) and nitrogen (approximately 79%).

air hunger deep, sighing respiration which occurs when the body's oxygen supply is depleted as in severe haemorrhage or shock.

airway 1. the passage by which air enters the lungs. 2. a mechanical device used for securing unobstructed respiration during general anaesthesia or other occasions when the patient is not ventilating or exchanging gases properly.

ala a wing, e.g. the sacral ala. pl. *alae.*

alba, albicans white.

albumin any protein that is soluble in water and moderately concentrated salt solutions and is coagulable by heat. *Serum a.* a plasma protein formed principally in the liver. Albumin is responsible for much of the colloidal osmotic pressure of the blood, and thus is a very important factor in regulating the exchange of water between the plasma and the interstitial compartment (space between the cells). A drop in the amount of albumin in the plasma leads to an increase in the flow of water from the capillaries into the interstitial department. This results in an increase in tissue fluid which, if severe, becomes apparent as oedema. Albumin also serves as a transport protein carrying substances such as fatty acids, bilirubin, many drugs and some hormones.

albuminuria the presence in the urine of albumin, usually serum albumin. It occurs in renal disease, severe cardiac disease and in some complications of pregnancy.

alcohol women should be advised to restrict alcohol intake during pregnancy, especially in the first trimester. High alcohol consumption can lead to low birthweight babies, neonatal feeding and sleeping problems and/or fully developed FETAL ALCOHOL SYNDROME.

Aldomet *See* METHYLDOPA.

aldosterone one of the hormones of the adrenal cortex, the principal biological activity of which is the regulation of the electrolyte and water balance by promoting the retention of sodium (and, therefore, of water) and the excretion of potassium; the retention of water induces an increase in plasma volume and an increase in blood pressure. Its secretion is stimulated by angiotensin II.

Alexander technique a method of psycho-physical re-education by which people learn better use of themselves, involving postural realignment and the use of various physical and psychological relaxation methods. Followers of the Alexander technique normally require a series of 20 to 30 lessons, but the technique can be used to relieve problems in pregnancy such as persistent backache.

alimentary pertaining to nutrition. *A. tract* the passage through which the food passes from mouth to anus.

alkalaemia increased alkalinity or pH of the blood, caused either by an overdose or accumulation of alkaline substances or by an excessive loss of acids, e.g. by vomiting.

alkali a substance capable of uniting with an acid to form a salt. Alkalis turn red litmus blue. In the body, alkalis form carbonates and combine with fatty acids to form soaps. Alkalis play a vital role in maintaining the normal functioning of the body chemistry. *See also* ACID–BASE BALANCE *and* BASE. *A. reserve* the ability of the combined buffer systems of the blood to neutralize acid. The pH of the blood is normally slightly on the alkaline side, between 7.35 and 7.45. Since the principal buffer in the blood is bicarbonate, the alkali reserve essentially is represented by the plasma bicarbonate concentration. However, haemoglobin, phosphates and other bases also act as buffers. A lowered alkali reserve means a state of acidosis; an increased reserve indicates alkalosis. Alkali reserve is measured by the combining power of carbon dioxide, which is the amount of carbon dioxide that can be bound as bicarbonate by the blood.

alkaloids organic nitrogenous substances which from the active principle of certain drugs, e.g. morphine, atropine and strychnine.

alkalosis a pathological condition resulting from accumulation of base or from loss of acid without comparable loss of base in the body fluids, and characterized by decrease in hydrogen ion concentration (increase in pH). Alkalosis is the opposite of ACIDOSIS.

allantois membranous sac projecting from ventral surface of embryo, which eventually helps to form the placenta.

allele one of two or more alternative forms of a gene at the same site in a chromosome, which will determine alternative characters in inheritance.

alpha-adrenergic mechanism autonomic nerve pathway mechanism through which excitatory responses occur as a result of the release of adrenergic substances such as adrenaline (epinephrine) and noradrenaline (norepinephrine).

alpha-fetoprotein (AFP) a plasma protein produced by the fetal liver, yolk sac and gastrointestinal tract. It is present in amniotic fluid and maternal serum and is usually measured in maternal serum prenatally between 16 and 18 weeks. A raised level at that time may be indicative of wrong gestational age, multiple pregnancy, neural tube defect, fetal death or, rarely, Turner's syndrome. A low level could be due to wrong gestational age or Down's syndrome. Further investigations in cases of raised AFP include a repeat serum AFP test, ultrasound scan to confirm gestation, amniocentesis to estimate the AFP level in the amniotic fluid. Levels may vary with maternal age, weight, diabetes mellitus, cigarette smoking and race. The midwife is responsible for careful counselling of the expectant parents before and after the test. *See also* BART'S TEST, LEEDS TEST.

alternative medicine a form of medicine which is different from conventional health care; it is an holistic system of care which recognizes the inter-relationship between body, mind and spirit. More commonly termed COMPLEMENTARY MEDICINE, although the word 'alternative' implies that these are forms of health care which may be used instead of conventional care.

alveolus any hollowed out structure, e.g. a tooth socket, an air sac in the lungs, or an acinus as in the breasts. pl. *alveoli.*

ambient surrounding or prevailing.

ambivalence the property of having equal power in two directions or on both sides at the same time. In psychiatry, having equally strong opposing emotions, such as love and hate for the same person.

ambulatory walking.

amelia a developmental anomaly with absence of the limbs.

amenorrhoea absence of menstruation. *Primary a.* absence of menstruation in a post-pubertal woman who has never menstruated. *Secondary a.* cessation of menstrual periods in a woman who has previously menstruated. The commonest cause is pregnancy, but it may also occur following a change of work, climate or environment, or it may be a symptom of disease.

amino acids organic substances derived from proteins, and essential to human nutrition.

aminophylline an alkaloid from camellia, which relaxes plain muscle spasm of the bronchioles and coronary arteries. It may be given by mouth, intravenously or as a suppository, and is useful in treating asthma and heart failure.

ammonia alkaline gas formed by the decomposition of proteins, amino acids and other nitrogen-containing substances. Converted to urea in the liver.

amnesia loss of memory, especially inability to recall past events or words.

Amnihook a device for performing an AMNIOTOMY.

amniocentesis puncture of the amniotic sac, usually through the abdominal wall and uterus, to obtain a sample of amniotic fluid on which the following tests may be carried out: the LECITHIN/SPHINGOMYELIN RATIO, CHROMOSOME ANALYSIS, estimation of concentrations of BILIRUBIN and ALPHA-FETOPROTEIN, and DNA analysis for fetal sexing and to detect certain gene-carrying conditions such as Duchenne muscular dystrophy, sickle cell disease and thalassaemia. It may also be carried out to relieve extreme discomfort in cases of severe polyhydramnios. A needle is inserted into the amniotic sac via the abdominal wall, with the aid of ultrasound to localize the placental site and thereby avoid puncturing it. A small amount of amniotic fluid is withdrawn by syringe and sent for analysis. Mothers who are Rhesus negative should be given a reduced dose of anti-D immunoglobulin after the procedure to prevent them making antibodies.

amnion the innermost membrane enveloping the fetus and enclosing the liquor amnii. *A. nodosum* a nodular condition of the fetal surface of the amnion, observed in oligohydramnios, which may be associated with absence of kidneys in the fetus.

amnioscope an endoscope used for AMNIOSCOPY.

amnioscopy 1. inspection of the amniotic sac, amniotic fluid and fetus by direct visualization using an endoscope passed through the abdominal and uterine walls. 2. visualization of the intact amniotic membranes and fluid *per vaginam* in late-pregnancy when there is some cervical dilatation or during labour by means of an amnioscope to detect meconium-stained liquor and oligohydramnios.

amniotic fluid the fluid contained in the amniotic sac, also called liquor amnii. This fluid surrounds and is swallowed by the fetus. It is secreted from the cells of the amnion, transudate from fetal vessels in the cord and placenta and from maternal vessels in the decidua. The amount varies from 500 to 1500 ml at term.

Amniotic fluid is normally clear and straw-coloured, and is composed of 99% water and 1% solids, which include protein, carbohydrate, lipids and phospholipids, electrolytes, urea, uric acid and creatinine, pigments, enzymes and placental hormones. In addition it contains desquamated cells, lanugo, vernix caseosa and increasing amounts of urine from the fetus. The fluid allows the fetus to move freely and equalizes pressure, acts as a shock absorber, equalizes the temperature and provides some nutritive substances for the fetus. Excess amniotic fluid is called POLYHYDRAMNIOS and an abnormally small amount is referred to as OLIGOHYDRAMNIOS.

amniotic fluid embolism the entry of liquor amnii, which contains vernix and other solids, into the maternal circulation via the sinuses of the placental site. A rare cause of collapse in labour or of HYPOFIBRINOGENAEMIA.

amniotic sac the bag of membranes, the amnion or fetal membrane which contains the fetus, suspended in amniotic fluid.

amniotomy surgical rupture of the amniotic sac for induction of labour. The mother is placed in the lithotomy or dorsal position and the midwife or obstetrician performs an examination *per vaginam*. The forewaters are ruptured by passing an instrument through the cervix and piercing the membranes, whilst taking care not to damage the fetal presenting part. Straight or curved Kocher's forceps may be used or a specially designed AMNIHOOK. The procedure is performed by the doctor for induction of labour, but may be performed by a midwife to accelerate labour. It may also be necessary to rupture the membranes so that the amniotic fluid can be observed, or to prevent the risk of cord prolapse when the cord is presenting below the fetal part. Rarely, a hindwater rupture may be performed. *See also* Appendix 4.

amoxicillin a penicillin analogue similar in action to ampicillin but more efficiently absorbed from the gastro-intestinal tract and therefore requiring less frequent dosage and not as likely to cause diarrhoea. Given orally, 250 mg three times daily.

ampicillin a broad-spectrum penicillin of synthetic origin which is active against many of the Gram-negative pathogens, in addition to the usual Gram-positive ones that are affected by penicillin. May be given orally, 250–500 mg four times daily, or intramuscularly or intravenously, 0.5–1 g. Useful in treating listeriosis in the neonate.

ampulla the dilated end of a canal, e.g. of a fallopian tube.

amyl nitrite a vasodilator given by inhalation for angina pectoris and to relieve the muscular spasm in CONSTRICTION RING.

anaemia a reduction in the number of red blood cells, or in the amount of haemoglobin present in them. Anaemia may result from haemorrhage, excessive breakdown of red blood cells or failure to manufacture them. Iron deficiency anaemia is the most common type, probably related to poor nutrition, and is aggravated in early pregnancy due to the physiological haemodilution which occurs. Routine iron therapy is not given to all women but those who have a low serum ferritin may require iron supplementation. Severely anaemic women may need intramuscular or intravenous iron or, rarely, a blood transfusion to prevent additional problems occurring in labour, such as morbidity associated with major haemorrhage. Sometimes women whose anaemia fails to respond to iron therapy are found to have MEGALOBLASTIC ANAEMIA which is due to folic acid deficiency.

anaerobe a micro-organism which requires no free oxygen for its existence, e.g. *Clostridium welchii*.

anaesthesia a state in which the whole body (*general anaesthesia*) or part of it (*local* or *regional anaesthesia*) is insensible to pain, feeling or sensation. It is induced to permit the performance of surgery or other painful procedures.

anaesthetic an agent which induces anaesthesia. A general anaesthetic renders the patient unconscious; a local anaesthetic induces anaesthesia of a particular part of the body.

anal pertaining to the anus.

analgesia insensibility to pain.

analgesic an agent capable of inducing analgesia. A pain-relieving drug.

anaphylaxis an unusual or exaggerated allergic reaction (often within seconds) of an organism to foreign protein or other substances. adj. *anaphylactic*. Substances most likely to produce anaphylaxis include drugs, particularly antibiotics, local anaesthetics, and codeine; drugs prepared from animals such as insulin, adrenocorticotrophic hormone, and enzymes; diagnostic agents such as iodinated X-ray contrast media; biological fluids used to provide immunity, such as vaccines, antitoxins, and gamma globulin; protein foods, the venom of bees, wasps, and hornets; and pollens, moulds and animal dander.

Symptoms, caused by the release of histamines, include bronchospasm, peripheral vasodilation and increased capillary permeability, together with constriction of the bronchioles and bronchi.

Immediate treatment in cases of severe anaphylaxis is the administration of adrenaline which causes bronchodilatation, reduces laryngeal spasm and elevates the blood pressure. Steroid therapy is initiated to counteract the effects of histamine by decreasing capillary permeability. Additional measures include the administration of intravenous fluids and plasma to restore intravascular fluid volume. Pressor agents, such as dopamine, noradrenaline and isoprenaline, are given to increase and maintain the blood pressure.

anastomosis a communication between two vessels or other structures, either natural or established operatively.

androgens any steroid hormone that promotes male characteristics. The two main androgens are androsterone and testosterone. adj. *androgenic*. The androgenic hormones are manufactured mainly by the testes under stimulation from the PITUITARY GLAND. They are responsible for the growth of the penis and scrotum and for the secondary sexual characteristics, such as the growth of hair on the face and a deep voice. They also stimulate the growth of muscles and bones throughout the body, and thus account in part for the greater strength and size of men as compared with women.

android male-like, masculine. *A. pelvis* see PELVIS.

anencephaly a gross congenital malformation in which the cranial vault and the cerebral hemispheres fail to develop. Causes primary face presentation.

angina pectoris severe pain and constriction in the chest, often radiating down the left arm, caused by inadequate blood flow to the heart.

angiography radiography of vessels of the body after introduction into them of a suitable contrast medium.

angioma a tumour composed of blood vessels, e.g. a naevus on the skin.

angiotensin a vasoconstrictor principle formed in the blood when RENIN is released from the kidney. By its vasopressor action it raises blood pressure and diminishes fluid loss in the kidney by restricting blood flow.

angular pregnancy implantation of the fertilized ovum in the angle where the fallopian tube enters the uterus.

ankylosis abnormal fixation or union of the bones forming an articulation, resulting in a stiff joint. Ankylosis of the sacrococcygeal joint is a rare cause of difficulty during delivery.

anococcygeal pertaining to the anus and coccyx. The anococcygeal body or raphe is a mass of muscular and fibrous tissue between the anus and the coccyx; part of the insertion of the levatores ani muscles.

anode a positive electrode to which negative ions are attracted. adj. *anodal.*

anodyne an agent which relieves pain.

anomaly marked deviation from normal.

anorexia loss of appetite for food. *A. nervosa* complete lack of appetite with extreme emaciation. Conception is rare in women with this disorder as ovulation usually ceases.

anovular absence of ovulation.

anoxia the state of being deprived of OXYGEN. *See also* ASPHYXIA.

anoxic relating to or affected with anoxia.

antacid a substance neutralizing acid, e.g. magnesium trisilicate.

ante- prefix meaning 'before'.

anteflexion bending forwards, e.g. of the body of the uterus on the cervix.

antenatal before birth. *A. care* care provided by midwives and obstetricians during pregnancy to ensure that the fetal and maternal health are satisfactory. Deviations from normal can be detected and treated early. The mother can be prepared for labour and parenthood and health education can be offered. A detailed history and baseline observations and investigations are obtained at the first antenatal appointment. Subsequent appointments involve monitoring the progress of pregnancy and the health of mother and fetus.

antepartum before parturition i.e. birth. *A. haemorrhage* bleeding from the genital tract at any time after the 24th week of pregnancy until the baby is born. Causes are PLACENTA PRAEVIA; ABRUPTIO placental or incidental causes e.g. cervical polyps or erosion, vaginitis or, rarely, carcinoma of the cervix. The midwife's responsibilities are to call a doctor; maintain records of observations; administer analgesia; to take blood for cross-matching; and to provide support. An internal examination should *never* be performed.

anterior before; in front of.

anteroposterior from front to back.

anteversion turning forwards, e.g. of the uterus in relation to the vagina.

anthropoid man-like, e.g. anthropoid apes, man-like apes. *A. pelvis see* PELVIS.

anti- prefix meaning 'against', 'opposite'.

antibiotic pertaining to antibiosis, therefore destructive to life. Antibiotic drugs are drugs derived from living micro-organisms, which destroy or inhibit the growth of pathogenic bacteria.

13

antibodies specific substances formed in the body which counteract the effects of antigens or bacterial toxins. Antibodies, the effectors of the immune response, can be transferred passively from one individual to another as, for example, the transfer of maternal antibody across the placental barrier to the fetus, which has not yet developed a mature immune system. The developmental process of antibody production is usually completed a few months after birth.

anticoagulant an agent which prevents or delays the clotting of blood, e.g. heparin.

anticonvulsant a drug which prevents fits or convulsions, e.g. phenobarbital.

anti-D gamma globulin a sterile solution of globulin derived from human blood plasma containing antibody to the erythrocyte factor Rh D. Rhesus negative mothers should be given anti-D within 72 hours of delivery or miscarriage of a Rhesus positive baby to prevent them making antibodies to the Rhesus factor, which could cause haemolytic disease of a Rhesus positive fetus/baby in a subsequent pregnancy. It is also given following invasive procedures such as amniocentesis.

antidepressant effective against depressive illness. A drug used for relief of symptoms of depression.

antidiuretic 1. pertaining to or causing suppression of rate of urine formation. 2. an agent that causes suppression of urine formation. *A. hormone (ADH)* vasopressin; a hormone that suppresses the secretion of urine. It has a specific effect on the epithelial cells of the renal tubules, stimulating the reabsorption of water independently of solids, and resulting in concentration of urine. Secreted by the hypothalamus, but stored and released by the posterior lobe of the PITUITARY GLAND, it also has vasopressor activity.

antidote an agent which counteracts the effect of poison.

antiemetic drug that prevents or alleviates nausea and vomiting.

antigen any substance which, on introduction into the body, brings about immunity by stimulating antibody production.

antihistamine a term used to describe a group of drugs that block the tissue receptors for histamine. They are used in the treatment of various allergic conditions. They may be used in the treatment of hyperemesis gravidarum.

antihypertensive effective against hypertension. An agent that reduces high blood pressure. Some, such as methyldopa (Aldomet), act on alpha-adrenergic mechanisms in the central or sympathetic nervous system to reduce peripheral vascular resistance. Vasodilators act directly on the arterioles to produce the same effect. Beta-blockers, such as propranolol (Inderal), act at beta-adrenergic receptors in the heart and kidneys to reduce cardiac output and renin secretion.

antiseptics agents used to prevent sepsis, i.e. infection.

antiserum a serum derived from the blood of an animal or human being with a disease and possessed of properties that are antagonistic to the bacteria producing the disease. pl. *antisera*.

antispasmodic relieving spasm.

antithrombin any naturally occurring or therapeutically administered substance that neutralizes the action of thrombin and thus limits or restricts blood coagulation.

antithromboplastin any agent or substance that prevents or interferes with the interaction of blood clotting factors as they generate prothrombinase (thromboplastin).

antitoxin an antibody produced to neutralize a bacterial toxin. Serum from immunized animals containing the specific antitoxin is used in the prevention and treatment of DIPHTHERIA and TETANUS.

anuresis retention of urine in the bladder.

anuria failure of the kidneys to secrete urine. It may complicate severe concealed haemorrhage from abruptio placentae, eclampsia and septic abortion, and lead to bilateral cortical necrosis of the kidney.

anus the extremity of the alimentary canal, through which the faeces are discharged. *Imperforate a.* one which, owing to congenital defect, is not patent.

Anusol rectal cream or suppositories used to relieve pain associated with haemorrhoids.

aorta the large artery proceeding from the left ventricle of the heart. *Abdominal a.* that part of the vessel in the abdomen. *Arch of the a.* the curve of the tube over the heart. *Thoracic a.* that part which passes through the chest.

aperient a drug which produces an action of the bowels.

Apert's syndrome a congenital abnormality in which there is fusion at birth of all the cranial sutures in addition to syndactyly (webbed fingers).

Apgar score a scoring system devised by Dr Virginia Apgar to assess the condition of a baby during its first few minutes of life so that severe asphyxia neonatorum can be diagnosed and treated at once. *See also* ASPHYXIA NEONATORUM *and* Appendix 1.

aphtha the whitish spots caused by the fungus *Candida albicans*. THRUSH. pl. *aphthae.*

aphthous vulvitis infestation of the vulva with thrush (*Candida albicans*).

APL principle the anterior pituitary-like hormone of the placenta, chorionic gonadotrophin.

aplastic relating to any structure with incomplete or defective development.

apnoea absence of breathing. Apnoeic periods occur in the respiration of newborn infants in whom the respiratory centre is immature or depressed. *A. monitors* are designed to give an audible signal when a certain period of apnoea has occurred.

aponeurosis a flat sheet of fibrous connective tissue attaching muscle to bone or other tissues.

apoplexy sudden failure of cerebral function due to haemorrhage from, or thrombosis of, a cerebral vessel. It is characterized by coma, stertorous breathing and a varying degree of paralysis.

appendicitis inflammation of the vermiform appendix. Uncommon and much more dangerous in pregnancy since the appendix is drawn up in the abdomen and the inflammatory process can spread more readily.

appendix vermiformis the vermiform appendix. A worm-like tube with a blind end, projecting from the caecum in the right iliac region.

Apresoline *See* HYDRALAZINE.

aquanatal exercises a form of ante- and postnatal exercises in water enabling women to tone muscles, keep fit and meet other expectant and new mothers, and offered in some areas as an additional option for preparation for labour. The classes are usually conducted in a local public swimming pool by an experienced aquanatal teacher with a midwife in attendance if the teacher is not a midwife or health visitor.

aqueduct a canal for the passage of fluid. The *a. of Sylvius* is a canal leading from the third to the fourth ventricle of the brain. One of the causes of hydrocephalus is stenosis of this aqueduct. An obstruction of the absorption of cerebrospinal fluid occurs after meningitis or subarachnoid haemorrhage.

arachnoid the web-like membrane which is the middle covering of the brain between the dura mater and the pia mater. In the subarachnoid space beneath it, the cerebrospinal fluid circulates.

arbor vitae literally, the tree of life. 1. the tree-like appearance of white matter in the cerebellum. 2. the appearance of the folds of columnar epithelium lining the cervix uteri.

arborescent branching like a tree.

arcuate arched, bow-shaped. The arcuate ligament is a strong ligament stretching across the subpubic arch of the pelvis.

arcus tendineus a thickening, generally known as the 'white line' in the pelvic fascia, which gives origin to part of the levator ani.

areola the pigmented area which surrounds the nipple. It darkens during pregnancy and is termed the primary areola, with a secondary areola developing later around its perimeter. The lacteal sinuses lie under this area of the breast.

arnica a homoeopathic remedy used to prevent and treat bruising, shock and trauma. It is useful in the early puerperium to ease perineal discomfort. One arnica tablet should be taken within an hour of delivery, then one tablet three times daily for three days, then stop. Arnica cream is useful for bruised buttocks but

should not be applied over open wounds such as the episiotomy line.

aromatherapy a complementary therapy involving the use of highly concentrated essential oils extracted from plants. Chemical constituents within the oils give them their therapeutic properties, but can also cause adverse reactions. Essential oils can be administered by massage, in the bath, by inhalation, in compresses, douches, pessaries and creams. They should rarely be applied neat to the skin nor administered gastrointestinally, unless under expert supervision. There are many essential oils contraindicated during pregnancy and childbirth as they may cause fetal malformations, miscarriage or undesirable systemic effects such as hypertension, and it is wise to avoid the use of all essential oils during the first trimester. Certain oils are also contraindicated for use on children. Midwives should be appropriately trained to utilize aromatherapy in their practice or to advise mothers about its use.

artefact an artificially produced lesion.

arteriography radiography of an artery or arterial system after injection of a contrast medium into the blood stream.

arteriole a small artery.

arteriosclerosis a hardening and thickening of the artery walls. Atheromatous plaques are deposited on the inner surface so that ischaemia of the organ or tissues occurs. It causes high blood pressure and precedes the degeneration of internal organs associated with old age or chronic disease.

artery a vessel which carries blood from the heart to some other part of the body.

arthritis inflammation affecting a joint.

artificial feeding 1. feeding via orifices other than the mouth, e.g. gastrostomy, jejunal, nasal, oesophageal and rectal feeding. In preterm or sick babies, one of these routes may be employed. 2. in reference to the feeding of infants, giving food other than human milk.

artificial insemination a means of achieving conception by mechanically inserting viable semen into the vagina; this may be either semen produced by the partner (AIH – artificial insemination by husband) or semen from a known or more usually an unknown donor (AID – artificial insemination by donor). In the first instance the partner may legally adopt the baby, whereas in the latter the donor has no legal rights over the child, nor responsibility for his or her upbringing. In order for the procedure to be considered the woman must be fit and menstruating regularly.

artificial respiration maintenance of respiration by any artificial means. As a first aid measure, mouth to mouth (or mouth to mouth and nose in babies) can be used, once the airways have been cleared of mucus and other debris. The administration of oxygen, and mechanical methods of maintaining respiration may be necessary in severe cases. *See also* Appendix 7.

artificial rupture of membranes (ARM) an aseptic procedure performed *per vaginam* to induce or to accelerate the progress of labour.

A-scan ULTRASOUND display used for measuring size and thickness accurately. It is used particularly for fetal CEPHALOMETRY. *See also* ULTRASOUND.

ascites an accumulation of free fluid in the peritoneal cavity. The condition is rarely seen in pregnancy. In the fetus or neonate, ascites is associated with HYDROPS FETALIS.

aseptic free from pathogenic bacteria.

asexual without sexual organs.

asphyxia suffocation. *A. neonatorum* is failure of the child to breathe at birth. There is a deficiency of oxygen in the blood and an increase in carbon dioxide in the blood and tissues. *See also* APGAR SCORE, Appendix 1.

aspiration the withdrawing of fluid or air from a cavity by suction. *Meconium a.* fetal inhalation of meconium stained liquor. The hypoxic fetus passes meconium into the liquor. Premature inhalation prior to, or immediately following delivery draws the meconium-stained liquor into the lungs where it causes chemical pneumonitis and plugging of the airways. The obstruction produces areas of consolidation and underaeration, as well as hyperinflation, contributing to the potentially pathological condition meconium aspiration syndrome. Preventative measures include careful suction under direct vision and intubation by an experienced paediatrician at birth, if possible before the baby breathes. *Chorionic villus a.* a sample of the chorionic villi is aspirated by a syringe or suction pump towards the end of the first trimester of pregnancy. The procedure is carried out under ultrasound guidance either *per vaginam* or transabdominally. The sample of villi obtained may be examined for DNA analysis chromosomal analysis or for the diagnosis of some inborn errors of metabolism. *Vacuum a.* removal of the uterine contents by application of a vacuum through a hollow curette or a cannula introduced into the uterus – a method of termination of early pregnancy.

aspirator any apparatus for withdrawing air or fluid from a cavity of the body.

assessment critical analysis and judgement of the status or quality of a particular condition, situation or subject. The initial stage in a process approach to midwifery care, followed by planning, implementation and evaluation of care.

assimilation the process whereby food is changed into body tissue.

assimilation pelvis a variation from the normal development of the sacrum. (*a*) In a high assimilation pelvis the last lumbar vertebra has become fused into the sacrum. The pelvis is deep, and there may be funnelling and associated difficulty in labour. (*b*) In a low assimilation pelvis the first sacral vertebra takes the characteristics of a lumbar vertebra. Thus the pelvis is shallow and the condition does not affect labour.

asthma a disease marked by recurrent attacks of paroxysmal dyspnoea, with wheezing, cough and sense of suffocation. Varying foreign proteins cause these spasms of the smooth muscle of the bronchioles in allergic people.

Astrup machine an apparatus for ascertaining the pH value of the blood.

asymmetry inequality in size or shape of two normally similar structures, or of two halves of a structure normally the same. An asymmetrical pelvis is a pelvis in which one side is distorted as a result of disease, injury or congenital maldevelopment.

asynclitism a parietal presentation of the fetal head in which the transversely placed sagittal suture lies close to the symphysis pubis or sacrum; the sideways rocking mechanism of fetal descent during labour, in a flat pelvis. In anterior asyn-clitism the anterior parietal bone moves down behind the symphysis pubis until the parietal eminence enters the brim. The movement is then reversed and the head rocks back until the posterior parietal bone passes the sacral promontory. In posterior asynclitism the movements are reversed, the posterior parietal bone negotiating the sacral promontory before the anterior parietal bone passes behind the symphysis pubis. *See* SYNCLITISM.

'at risk' register a register of children considered to be at risk of NON-ACCIDENTAL INJURY (NAI) or abuse. *See also* OBSERVATION REGISTER.

atelectasis incomplete expansion of the lung. *Primary a.* present from the moment of birth. *Secondary a.* this may occur owing to aspiration of meconium, infected liquor, vaginal discharge or, more rarely, maternal blood. The failure of all or part of the lungs to expand; it results from respiratory obstruction or weakness of the respiratory muscles at birth, especially in the preterm baby.

athetosis a condition marked by involuntary movements of the limbs. Seen in children who have suffered intracranial birth trauma or kernicterus.

atlas the 1st cervical vertebra, articulating with the occipital bone of the skull.

atonic pertaining to atony. *A. uterus* uterus lacking efficient muscle tone, either during labour or in the early puerperium.

atony lack of muscle tone.

atresia absence of the opening of a natural canal, e.g. of the oesophagus or vagina; usually a congenital malformation.

atrial pertaining to the atrium. *A. fibrillation* a cardiac arrhythmia marked by rapid randomized contractions of the atrial myocardium, causing a totally irregular, often rapid, ventricular rate. *A. septal defect* a congenital heart defect in which there is persistent patency of the atrial septum, owing to failure of closure of the foramen ovale.

atrium a chamber of the heart, formerly called 'auricle'. pl. *atria*.

atrophy wasting of any part of the body, due to degeneration of the cells from disuse, lack of nourishment or of nerve supply.

atropine the active principle of belladonna. An alkaloid which depresses salivation and the secretions of the respiratory tract, relaxes muscular spasm, accelerates the heart rate and dilates the pupil. It is employed before the administration of general anaesthesia.

attitude the relation of the fetal parts – head, spine and limbs – to each other. The fetal attitude is normally one of flexion but may be deflexed or extended when the position of the occiput is not anterior.

atypical varying from the normal pattern.

audit a means of evaluating care, management and organization to ensure quality and cost-effectiveness. Clinical audit is usually a cyclical event in which every aspect of health care can be examined and, if necessary, changes made to improve relevant aspects.

auditory concerning the hearing sense. *A. response cradle* a device used to screen infants for impairment of hearing. A set of headphones is used to play noises to the baby and a computer analyses the baby's movements in response to the sounds.

augment to increase, enhance or accelerate. *Augmentation of labour* acceleration of a labour which has been diagnosed as not progressing

adequately. This may be done by performing AMNIOTOMY or by the intravenous administration of an oxytocic drug such as Syntometrine.

aura the premonition which often precedes an epileptic fit but not an eclamptic fit. *See* ECLAMPSIA.

aural pertaining to the ear.

auricle 1. the external portion of the ear. 2. former term for either of the two atria or upper chambers of the heart.

auscultation a method of examining the internal organs by listening to the sounds which they give out. Auscultation of the FETAL HEART SOUNDS is performed during pregnancy and labour, using a Pinard's stethoscope, Doppler ultrasound or cardiotocography.

autistic withdrawn. A term describing a child who has great difficulty in making personal relationships.

autoclave a strongly built and hermetically sealed apparatus which uses steam at high pressure to sterilize equipment.

autogenous generated within the body and not acquired from external sources.

autoimmune disease disease due to immunological action of an individual's own cells or antibodies on components of the body.

autoinfection self-infection, i.e. transferred from one part of the body to another by fingers, towels, etc.

autolysis self-digestion. The breakdown of tissue in the involution of the uterus which occurs in the puerperium. The surplus muscle is broken down into simple substances which are absorbed by the blood stream and excreted in the urine.

autonomic self-governing. *A. nervous system* the sympathetic and parasympathetic systems which control involuntary muscle.

autonomy self-governing, independent. Professional autonomy of the midwife means that she is personally responsible for her own actions but that she is legally permitted to oversee the total care of women with normal pregnancies and labours.

autopsy post-mortem examination.

autosome any chromosome other than the X or Y sex chromosomes.

avascular not vascular. Bloodless.

avitaminosis a state due to vitamin deficiency.

axilla the armpit.

axillary pertaining to the axilla. *A. tail of Spence* a process of mammary tissue extending to the axilla.

axis 1. an imaginary line passing through the centre of a body. 2. the second cervical vertebra.

axis of the birth canal an imaginary line representing the course taken by the fetus in its passage through the birth canal, downwards and backwards through the pelvic brim and the major part of the cavity; then, at the level of the ischial spines, turning through a right angle to proceed downwards and forwards. *See also* PELVIS.

axis of the pelvis an imaginary line passing at right angles through the centres of all the planes of the bony pelvis.

axis traction forceps obstetric forceps designed to allow traction to be applied in the line of the pelvic axis when the head is above the level of the pelvic outlet. Axis traction is rarely used now.

azoospermia absence of spermatozoa in semen.

B

Babinski's reflex or sign stroking the sole of the foot triggers a reflex in which the large toe bends upwards instead of downwards. Seen in neonates as a normal reflex; flexion develops later once the infant learns to walk.

Baby Friendly Initiative (BFI) part of a global campaign by the World Health Organization and the United Nations Children's Fund to ensure that all mothers are facilitated in breastfeeding to enable them to benefit from the health and social advantages. *Ten Steps to Successful Breastfeeding* introduced by WHO and UNICEF offer health professionals an inexpensive, effective means by which to promote breastfeeding, with an award incentive. A Global award is given for a hospital which has implemented all 10 steps and has a 75% breastfeeding rate; the UK Standard is awarded as above but where the breastfeeding rate is 50–75%; and a Certificate of Commitment is given where a hospital is working towards the 10 steps.

Ten steps to successful breastfeeding

- Breastfeeding policy available which is communicated to all staff.
- All healthcare staff trained to implement the policy.
- All pregnant mothers informed of the benefits and management of breastfeeding.
- Mothers assisted to commence breastfeeding within half an hour of delivery.

- Education of mothers re breastfeeding and maintenance of lactation even if they are separated from their babies.
- Neonates to be given nothing other than breast milk unless medically necessary.
- 24-hour rooming in.
- On demand breastfeeding.
- No teats or pacifiers to be given to breastfeeding babies.
- Establishment of breastfeeding support groups.

Bach Flower remedies a system of complementary medicine, devised by Dr Edward Bach and based on homoeopathic principles, flower remedies can be used to treat emotional and psychological disorders. There are 38 flower remedies plus RESCUE REMEDY. *See also* HOMOEOPATHY.

bacille Calmette–Guérin (BCG) a vaccine used for inoculation against tuberculosis. It should be given during the first week of life to the infants of tuberculous mothers.

bacilluria the presence of bacilli in the urine.

bacillus a general term for any rod-shaped organism. They are mostly Gram-negative except for *Koch's b.* and *Döderlein's b.* which are Gram-positive (*see* GRAM STAIN). pl. *bacilli*.

backache in pregnancy is usually due to an exaggerated lordosis resulting from progesterone and relaxin levels. Postural correction and, occasionally, wearing a lumbar support may help. Severe cases should be referred to a physiotherapist, osteopath, chiropractor or Alexander technique teacher.

backward displacement of the uterus *See* RETROVERSION of the uterus.

bacteraemia the presence of bacteria in the blood.

bacteraemic shock *See* ENDOTOXIC SHOCK.

bacteria microscopic unicellular organisms, universally distributed. When a part of the normal flora (commensals) they may be beneficial to health, e.g. DÖDERLEIN'S BACILLUS. Pathogenic bacteria are those which, on entering tissues, can cause disease. Bacteria are classified into two major groups, Gram-positive and Gram-negative, based on their reaction to the Gram stain. Other important characteristics used in the classification of bacteria are their form and structure, metabolic reactions, and their requirements for atmospheric oxygen. Aerobes require oxygen and anaerobes only grow in the absence of oxygen. Facultative anaerobes adapt to either environment. Bacteria can cause disease by producing *toxins*, by causing inflammation or the formation of granulomas, or by inducing a hypersensitivity reaction. *Exotoxins* are extremely potent poisons produced by some Gram-positive bacteria. *Endotoxins* cause hypotension, fever, DIC and shock. Other toxins include haemolysins and leukocidins which destroy red and white blood cells, kinases which lyse blood clots and enzymes which attack tissue.

bacteriological examination microscopic examination of body fluids or tissue to identify bacteria.

bacteriology the science of the study of bacteria.

bacteriophage a virus which infects bacteria.

bacteriostatic able to prevent the multiplication of bacteria.

bacteriuria bacteria in the urine, usually only considered of significance if there are 100 000 organisms per ml. Five per cent of all pregnant women have asymptomatic bacteriuria, some of whom will develop pyelonephritis in pregnancy if untreated.

bag of membranes the amnion and chorion which contain the liquor amnii surrounding the fetus; sometimes called the bag of waters or the amniotic sac.

ballottement bouncing. Tapping a structure which lies in fluid, such as the fetus in the amniotic sac, in such a way that it rebounds against the examining fingers. *Internal b.* is elicited by inserting two fingers into the vagina at about 16 to 18 weeks of pregnancy and tapping the fetus, causing it to float away and quickly return to the examining fingers. *External b.* can be elicited when making an examination *per abdomen* when the head is not engaged, the fetal head is given a sharp tap on one side, floats away and is then felt to return against the examining fingers.

Bandl's ring the extreme thickening of the RETRACTION RING of normal labour, which occurs when labour is obstructed. A Bandl's ring is palpable as a transverse ridge across the abdomen, and is a sign of imminent rupture of the uterus.

barbiturates a large group of hypnotic drugs which are derivatives of barbituric acid. They should be avoided, except when required as anticonvulsants, as dependence and tolerance occur readily.

Barlow's test a test to diagnose congenital dislocation of the hip (CDH) in the newborn. It is a modification of Ortolani's test. The baby lies on his/her back with his/her feet pointing towards the examiner. The examiner grasps each leg with knees and hips flexed, placing middle fingers of each hand over the greater trochanter and the thumb of each hand on the inner aspect of the thigh. The thighs are then abducted and the middle finger of each hand pushes the greater trochanter forward. If the hip is dislocated the femoral head will be felt to 'clunk' as it enters the acetabulum. If no 'clunk' is felt the hip is not dislocated. In cases of CDH the femoral head can be displaced backwards out of the acetabulum by exerting slight pressure when the hips are flexed and adducted (Barlow's sign).

Barr body a small dark-staining body seen in the nucleus of normal female cells, often obtained from a smear of the buccal cavity and examined microscopically.

barrier contraception mechanical barrier to prevent sperm from entering cervical canal, e.g. diaphragm.

barrier nursing precautions taken by staff to prevent infection from one mother spreading to other mothers and/or staff. This normally involves caring for the mother and/or baby in a separate room or cubicle. Staff wear gowns, and frequently gloves, masks, goggles and overshoes when carrying out care. *Reverse barrier nursing* barrier nursing, using the same methods, but which is carried out with the aim of protecting the patient from external infection, for example, after organ transplantation.

bartholinitis inflammation of one or both of BARTHOLIN'S GLANDS producing an abscess or cyst.

Bartholin's glands two glands situated in the labia majora, with ducts opening in the vagina, just external to the hymen; they produce the secretion which lubricates the vulva.

Bart's test antenatal screening test, originally developed from work at St Bartholomew's Hospital (Bart's) in London, which aims to identify which women are at a higher risk of having a baby with Down's syndrome or an open neural tube defect. These women would then be offered a diagnostic test such as amniocentesis. The blood test can be performed any time between 15 and 22 weeks' gestation, but normally between 16 and 18 weeks, confirmed by ultrasound. The blood is analysed for serum alpha-fetoprotein levels, which are known to be low in Down's syndrome, free alpha and beta human chorionic gonadotrophin levels, which are raised in Down's syndrome, and unconjugated oestriols, which may be low when there is an affected fetus. Maternal age is

Bart's test: Interpretation of risk factors	
Maternal age	Risk of screen-positive result for Down's syndrome
Below 25	1:45
25–29	1:30
30–34	1:15
35–39	1:5
40–44	1:2
Over 45	More than 1:2

taken into consideration due to the increased incidence of Down's syndrome in older mothers, and each woman's risk factors are calculated individually. Risk factors higher than 1:300 for Down's syndrome are high and are called a screen positive result. The result is also screen positive if the alpha-fetoprotein level is more than two and a half times higher than the median level. Risk factors of below 1:300 are screen negative.

basal metabolic rate this is the minimum heat produced by a person who is resting, and who has fasted 18 hours. The method used enables the amount of oxygen consumed to be measured, and the result obtained is expressed as a percentage above or below what is normal for anyone of the person's age, height and weight. In pregnancy the rate is increased by about 30%.

base 1. the lowest part or foundation of anything. *B. of the fetal skull* consists of 2 temporal, 1 ethmoid and 1 sphenoid bone, and part of the OCCIPUT, firmly fused together. 2. the main ingredient of a compound. 3. the non-acid part of a salt; a substance that combines with acids to form salts. In the chemical processes of the body, bases are essential to the maintenance of the normal ACID–BASE BALANCE. Excessive concentration of bases in the body fluids leads to ALKALOSIS, therefore the pH rises.

basophil a leucocyte which has an affinity for basic dyes.

battledore placenta a placenta in which the umbilical cord is attached to the margin instead of the centre. *See also* PLACENTA.

Bell's palsy facial paralysis due to oedema of facial nerve. Occasionally occurs in pregnancy but is usually temporary.

Battledore Placenta

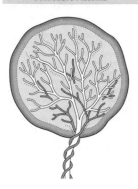

Benedict's qualitative reagent a solution containing sodium carbonate, sodium citrate and copper sulphate, used as a test for the detection of glucose and other reducing substances in urine or stools.

benzodiazepine any of a group of drugs having similar molecular structure. The group includes the sedative-hypnotics chlordiazepoxide, diazepam, oxazepam, flurazepam, and clorazepate, which are anti-anxiety agents; and the anticonvulsant clonazepam. Prolonged use of these drugs often causes dependence.

bereavement loss, usually of a loved one, through death or separation, but may apply to loss of previous good health, wealth or position. Produces psychological reaction with 'stages' of anger, denial, disbelief, finally, acceptance.

beta- second letter in the Greek alphabet, B; used to denote the second position in a classification system. **B. adrenergic receptors** specific sites effector cells that respond to adrenaline. **B. blocker** a drug that blocks the action of adrenaline at beta-adrenergic receptors on cells of effector organs, e.g. antihypertensive drugs. When used in late pregnancy, they may cause neonatal hypoglycaemia and bradycardia. **B. haemolytic streptococcus** a virulent streptococcus capable of haemolysing erythrocytes. The beta haemolytic streptococci are divided into serotype groups designated by letters, e.g. Group A. Cause of serious infections in the neonate.

betamethasone sodium phosphate a synthetic glucosteroid, the most active of the anti-inflammatory steroids. It may be administered to a mother who is likely to deliver a baby under 34 weeks' gestation. It decreases the risk of respiratory distress syndrome (RDS) by inducing an increase in the lecithin level in the infant. Given intramuscularly, 24 mg in divided doses.

bi- prefix meaning 'two'.

bicarbonate a salt of carbonic acid (H_2CO_3) in which one hydrogen atom has been replaced by a base, e.g. sodium bicarbonate, $NaHCO_3$. It is usually used to correct ACIDAEMIA.

bicornuate having two horns. **B. uterus** a congenital malformation in which there is a partial or complete vertical division of the body of the uterus. Normal pregnancy and labour is possible but it may be associated with persistent malpresentation and retained placenta.

bidet a low narrow basin on a stand with running water used for washing the perineum and external genitalia.

bifid cleft into two parts or branches. In SPINA BIFIDA the spinous processes

of one or more vertebrae fail to unite and remain divided, or cleft.

bifurcation a forking or separating into two branches. Occasionally the uterus may have a bifurcation as a result of abnormal fetal development. This may lead to an inability to carry a pregnancy successfully to term.

bilateral pertaining to both sides.

bile a dark green substance secreted by the liver cells, stored in the gallbladder and passed into the intestine, where it assists digestion by emulsifying fats, and activating lipase. **B. ducts** the ducts through which the bile passes from the liver and gallbladder to the intestine. **B. pigments** BILIRUBIN and BILIVERDIN.

biliary pertaining to the bile duct.

bilirubin a bright yellow-orange bile pigment, resulting from the breakdown of haemoglobin. It is fat-soluble and unconjugated until it is rendered water-soluble, i.e. conjugated by the liver, when it is excreted as stercobilin in the faeces. If this process fails at any point, bilirubin passes into the skin and sclera, and JAUNDICE or ICTERUS results.

bilirubinometer an instrument for measuring the serum bilirubin concentration.

biliverdin green bile pigment, oxidized form of bilirubin.

Billings' method a method of family planning. The woman and her partner are taught to recognize the changes in the cervical mucus which occur 3 to 4 days before ovulation in order that they may avoid intercourse around that time. The mucus increases in amount and becomes thinner in consistency to facilitate the passage of the spermatozoa through the cervix. This method of family planning when used in conjunction with other natural methods such as monitoring the body temperature is known as the sympto-thermal method.

bimanual using both hands. *B. examination* examination, usually of the pelvic cavity, in which one hand is on the abdomen, the other with one finger in the rectum, or one or two fingers in the vagina.

bimanual compression of the uterus a manoeuvre to arrest severe postpartum haemorrhage after delivery of the placenta when the uterus is atonic. The right hand is introduced into the vagina and closed to form a fist, which is pressed into the anterior vaginal fornix. The left hand, on the abdominal wall, pulls the uterus forwards, so that the anterior and posterior walls are pressed firmly together. This enables direct pressure to be applied to the placental site to stop the bleeding.

binovular developing from two ova. In binovular twin pregnancy two complete gestation sacs, each with fetus, placenta, chorion and amnion, develop in the uterus together. Also termed *dizygotic, dichorionic* or *fraternal* twins. The infants may be of the same or different sexes and like or unlike each other in appearance, in the same way as any siblings who are not twins. About five times as common as uniovular twins.

biochemistry chemistry of living matter.

biological pregnancy tests pregnancy tests based on the effect of pregnancy hormones on living animals; now mainly superseded by immunological tests, e.g. Gravindex.

biophysical profile a non-invasive test of fetal well-being using ultrasound to measure fetal heart rate, fetal tone, somatic movements, breathing movements and amniotic fluid volume. Each factor is scored to

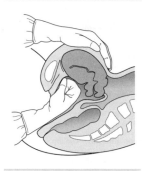

Bimanual Compression of the Uterus

obtain a total biophysical score, which is an accurate predictor of fetal death in high risk pregnancies. The score may be affected by gestation, maternal illness, therapeutic medication, substance abuse or fetal abnormality.

biopsy observation of living matter. Removal of tissue from the body for microscopic examination and diagnosis.

biorhythm any cyclic biological event, e.g. menstrual cycle, sleep pattern, affecting daily life.

biparietal diameter between the parietal eminences of the fetal skull; traditional measurement is 9.5 cm in a normal baby at term. It may be determined by ultrasonic cephalometry from 9 weeks' gestation using an A-scan. Serial measurement of the biparietal diameter in pregnancy is used to assess fetal maturity and growth. The fetal head is said to be engaged when the biparietal diameter, which is the widest transverse diameter of the skull, has passed through the brim of the maternal pelvis; this indicates that delivery by the vaginal route should be possible. Crowning occurs when the biparietal diameter distends the vulva during delivery and the head no longer recedes during contractions.

biparous giving birth to two infants at the same time, i.e. twins.

bipolar relating to two poles or ends, and used in reference to the fetus and the parturient uterus.

birth canal the bony and soft tissue structures through which the fetus must pass in order to be born. *See* PELVIS.

birth certificate a statement issued by the registrar for births, marriages and deaths for the district in which the child was born. It certifies details of parentage, name and sex of child, and date and place of birth. This certificate must be obtained by the parents, or failing them, anyone present at the delivery, within 42 days of birth in England (21 days in Scotland). It gives legal status to the child and is necessary before the child can receive Child Benefit. A birth certificate is issued to any child born alive, irrespective of the period of gestation. A stillbirth certificate is issued for babies of 24 weeks maturity or longer who did not breathe or show other signs of life after complete expulsion from the mother.

birth control the prevention or avoidance of conception.

birth injury trauma to the child sustained during birth. *See* HAEMORRHAGE, CEPHALHAEMATOMA *and* ERB'S PARALYSIS.

birth mark a congenital blemish or spot on the skin, usually visible at birth or soon after. *See also* NAEVUS.

birth, notification of a person present, or in attendance, at the birth or

within 6 hours afterwards, must notify the Director of Public Health within 36 hours (Public Health Act, 1936). This responsibility is accepted by the midwife when in attendance.

birth plan a plan prepared by the expectant mother, usually in conjunction with her partner and midwife, which records her preferences for care during and after labour.

birth rate the number of births during one year per 1000 total estimated mid-year population (crude birth rate), per 1000 estimated mid-year female population (refined birth rate), or per 1000 estimated mid-year female population of child-bearing age (true birth rate), that is between the ages of 15 and 45.

birth, registration of either parent must register the birth within 42 days at the registrar's office in the district in which the birth took place (21 days in Scotland). Failure to do so incurs a fine. The responsibility rests with the midwife if the parents default.

birth stool a stool on which a mother sits to give birth.

birth weight the weight of a baby immediately following delivery. Accuracy is important because it forms a baseline for assessing future development and is also used for national statistics. The average birth weight in the UK for a healthy baby born at term is currently 3.5 kg.

birthing chair a chair on which a woman gives birth. Some are electronically operated, thus can be tilted back quickly and easily as required. They combine the advantages of the upright position with good visibility and access for the midwife during delivery. Disadvantages are a higher mean blood loss and an increased incidence of postpartum haemorrhage. To reduce these problems it is recommended that the chair be tilted to 40° to the vertical immediately before delivery and throughout the third stage of labour. Some delivery beds can now be converted into a chair.

birthing room usually refers to a room for normal labour and delivery which is furnished in a comfortable and home-like fashion.

bisacodyl oral aperient or suppository used to combat constipation.

bisacromial diameter a diameter measured between the acromion processes on the shoulder blades. The fetal measurement is about 12 cm.

bisexual hermaphrodite. Having gonads of both sexes.

Bishop's score a method of assessing the favourability of the cervix, prior to induction of labour.

bitemporal a diameter measured between the most distant points of the coronal suture; on the fetal skull it measures 8.2 cm.

bitrochanteric diameter a diameter measured between the greater trochanters of the femora; it measures 10 cm on the fetus, and is the diameter to engage in breech presentation.

bladder the reservoir for urine, of obstetrical importance owing to its position in front of the uterus and vagina. Pressure on the bladder from the enlarging uterus, or the presenting part, once engaged near term, may cause frequency of micturition. A retroverted uterus may incarcerate the bladder, leading to urinary retention between 12 and 20 weeks of pregnancy. Bladder distension during labour may inhibit uterine action and may lead to delay or haemorrhage.

blastocyst a very early pregnancy about a week after conception. The outer layer, the trophoblast, develops into the placenta and the chorion, and the inner cell mass, a mass of cells projecting into the cavity, develops into the fetus and the amnion.

blastoderm germinal cells of the embryo consisting of three layers – ectoderm, mesoderm, endoderm.

bleeding time the time required for a small inflicted wound to cease bleeding. The normal time is 3–4 minutes.

Bishop's score				
Criteria	Score			
Cervix	0	1	2	3
Dilation (cm)	Closed	1–2	3–4	5+
Length (cm)	3	2	1	0
Consistency	Firm	Medium	Soft	
Position	Posterior	Central	Anterior	
Head				
Station (in cm)				
above ischial spines	−3	−2	−1	0

Score 5 or below: in a primigravida this is *unfavourable*. Action. Ripeness of the cervix is encouraged by the insertion of prostaglandin E_2 (Prostin E_2) in the form of a vaginal pessary on the evening prior to induction.
Score 6 or more: indicates a favourable cervix for induction.

blighted ovum abnormal ovum.

BLISS (Baby Life Support Systems) a charitable organization which raises money for equipment for babies requiring special and intensive care in neonatal units.

blister a collection of serum between the epidermis and the true skin. The appearance of watery blisters on the body of an infant within the first 3 weeks of life may be a sign of PEMPHIGUS NEONATORUM.

block 1. an obstruction or stoppage. 2. regional anaesthesia. *Epidural b.* anaesthesia produced by injection of local anaesthetic between the vertebral spines and beneath the ligamentum flavum into the extradural space. It is widely used for the relief of pain in labour. *Paracervical b.* anaesthesia of the inferior hypogastric plexus and ganglia produced by injection of the local anaesthetic into the lateral fornices of the vagina. *Pudendal b.* anaesthesia produced by blocking the pudendal nerves, accomplished by injection of local anaesthetic into the tuberosity of the ischium. See also EPIDURAL ANALGESIA, PARACERVICAL BLOCK, PUDENDAL BLOCK.

blood the fluid that circulates through the heart and blood vessels, supplying oxygen and nutritive material to all parts of the body, and carrying off waste products, etc. It has an essential role in the maintenance of fluid balance. Blood is composed of two parts: 1. plasma, the fluid portion, and 2. formed elements, the blood cells and platelets suspended in the fluid. *Plasma* accounts for about 55% of the total volume of the blood. It consists of about 92% water, 7% proteins and less than 1% inorganic salts, organic substances other than proteins, dissolved gases, hormones, antibodies and enzymes. Plasma from which fibrinogen has been removed is called serum. *Blood cells and platelets* comprise the other 45% of the total volume of blood. They include erythrocytes (red blood cells), leucocytes (white blood cells) and platelets (thrombocytes). There are 35×10^{12} red blood cells in the average adult and they carry oxygen from the lungs to the tissues via the haemoglobin. Leucocytes are the body's primary defence against infections. They are longer than red blood cells and normally the blood has about 8×10^9 white blood cells per litre. When infection is present their numbers are greatly increased. Platelets initiate blood clotting and are concerned in contraction of a clot. When they encounter a leak in a blood vessel, they adhere to the edges of the injured tissue and create a matrix on which the clot forms. There are about $350–500 \times 10^9$ platelets in the blood. *Fresh b.* is useful in cases of active sepsis or haemolytic disease, or to replace blood lost through haemorrhage. *Stored b.* is kept for up to 3 weeks at 4°C and is useful for all emergency cases of haemorrhage.

blood clotting coagulation. See CLOTTING.

blood count See Appendix 2.

blood gas analysis laboratory studies of arterial and venous blood for the purpose of measuring oxygen and carbon dioxide levels and pressure or tension, and hydrogen ion concentration (pH). Analyses of blood gases provide the following information: Pao_2 – partial pressure (P) of oxygen (O_2) in the arterial blood (a); SaO_2 – percentage of available haemoglobin that is saturated (Sa) with oxygen (O_2); $Paco_2$ – partial pressure (P) of carbon dioxide (CO_2) in arterial blood (a); pH – an expression of the extent to which the blood is alkaline or acidic; HCO_3 – the level of plasma bicarbonate; an indicator of the metabolic acid–base status.

blood grouping *See* ABO BLOOD GROUPS.

blood pressure the pressure or force which the blood exerts against the walls of the blood vessels. Though there is some pressure in all blood vessels, the term is generally used in reference to the arterial blood pressure. This pressure is determined by several interrelated factors, including the pumping action of the heart, the resistance to the flow of blood in the arterioles, the elasticity of the walls of the main arteries, the blood volume and extracellular fluid volume, and the blood's viscosity, or thickness. The blood pressure is measured in the brachial artery by means of a sphygmomanometer. Two levels are recorded: a systolic pressure, which is the maximum pressure during contraction of the ventricles; and a diastolic pressure, which is the pressure in the vessel when the ventricles are at rest. The midwife should assess the mother's blood pressure at every antenatal appointment and refer to the obstetrician if the systolic pressure rises above 130 mmHg, or the diastolic pressure rises above 90 mmHg, or where the diastolic pressure rises more than 15 mmHg above the first trimester baseline reading.

blood products a group of products derived from blood. Most units of blood are issued for transfusion as packed red cells; the supernatant fluid (plasma) contains platelets, white cells, coagulation factors and plasma proteins, including immunoglobulin. Blood products may be issued for immediate use, e.g. red cells, platelets, frozen down in their natural state for later use, e.g. fresh frozen plasma (FFP), or pooled and concentrated to achieve therapeutic levels, e.g. factor VIII concentrate for the treatment of haemophilia.

blood sugar the concentration of sugar in the blood. The commonest measurement is for glucose and this is recorded in millimoles per litre (mmol/l). Adult non-pregnant values are between 3.3 and 5.3 mmol/l, and pregnant values between 3.3 and 6.1 mmol/l. Neonatal concentrations may be much lower: 2.2–5.3 mmol/l. *See also* HYPOGLYCAEMIA.

blood transfusion the introduction of blood from a donor to the circulation of a recipient.

blood urea the proportion of urea in the blood. Normally it is between 2.5 and 5.8 mmol/l (15–35 mg/100 ml). In pregnancy the level is lowered to between 2.3 and 5.0 mmol/l (14–30 mg/100 ml).

blood volume the total quantity of blood in the body. The regulation of blood volume in the circulatory system is affected by the intrinsic mechanism for fluid exchange at the capillary membranes and by hormonal influences and nervous reflexes that affect the excretion of fluids by the kidneys. A rapid decrease in the blood volume, as in haemorrhage, greatly reduces the cardiac output and creates a condition called SHOCK or circulatory shock. Conversely, an increase in blood volume, as when there is retention of water and salt in the body because of renal failure, results in an increase in cardiac output. The eventual outcome of this situation is increased arterial blood pressure. Assessment of blood volume can be done through the use of intravascular catheters such as the CENTRAL VENOUS PRESSURE catheter, which measures pressure in the right atrium, and the Swan–Ganz catheter, which measures pressure on both sides of the heart.

body mass index (BMI) weight in kilograms divided by height (metres) squared. BMI 20–25 is normal; below 20 is underweight; over 25 is overweight.

bone marrow a substance found in the hollow cavities of bones. *Red b. m.* in trunk and skull bones only, forms all red and white cells except some lymphocytes. *Yellow fatty b. m.* is present in the long bones of adults and is not normally concerned with blood formation.

booking term given to the initial appointment with the midwife of a pregnant woman wishing to arrange to receive antenatal and labour care. The appointment may be held in the mother's home, at the general practitioner's surgery or health centre or in the hospital antenatal clinic. The midwife records details of the mother's personal and family medical, surgical, obstetric and social history and undertakes baseline observations of weight, urinalysis and blood pressure; blood tests are sent to the laboratory. There is an opportunity for the mother and midwife together to plan the most appropriate care for pregnancy, labour and the puerperium, to develop a relationship and to discuss any issues of concern.

borborygmus the rumbling sound produced by flatus in the intestine.

bougie a flexible instrument made of plastic or gum-elastic and used to dilate a stricture, as in the oesophagus or urethra or vagina.

bowel the intestine. *B. sounds* sounds caused by the propulsion of the intestinal contents through the lower alimentary tract. The absence of bowel sounds is symptomatic of greatly decreased or totally absent peristaltic movement. This can occur in such conditions as paralytic ileus and advanced intestinal obstruction which may occur following abdominal surgery such as caesarean section.

Bowman's capsule the commencement of the kidney nephron, which surrounds a tuft of renal capillaries – the *glomerulus*. Filtration takes place from the blood into the TUBULE; called also glomerular capsule.

Boyle's anaesthetic machine a continuous-flow anaesthetic machine which supplies oxygen and nitrous oxide together with cyclopropane, halothane and other anaesthetic agents as required.

brachial relating to the arm. *B. artery* the continuation of the axial artery along the inner side of the upper arm. *B. plexus* a nerve plexus situated just above the clavicle and in the root of the neck. It is formed by anterior primary rami of the Vth, VIth, VIIth and VIIIth cervical spinal and 1st thoracic nerves. The plexus may be damaged during birth by forcible widening of the angle between the head and shoulders during a breech delivery or a vertex presentation with shoulder dystocia. ERB'S PARALYSIS or KLUMPKE'S PARALYSIS may result.

brachydactylia abnormally short fingers.

bradycardia an abnormally slow heart beat as shown by slowing of the pulse rate to less than 60 per minute or, in the case of the fetus, to a heart rate of less than 100 beats per minute.

bradykinin peptide formed by degradation of protein by enzymes. Powerful vasodilator which also causes contraction of smooth muscle.

brain the highly specialized area of the central nervous system contained within the cranium. *See also* FALX CEREBRI *and* TENTORIUM CEREBELLI.

brain death irreversible coma.

brain scanning an imaging technique used to detect abnormalities of the brain, e.g. intraventricular haemorrhage in the newborn.

bran husk of grain, high in roughage and B vitamins. Frequently recommended for alleviation of constipation during pregnancy but women must also be encouraged to at least double their fluid intake.

Brandt–Andrews manoeuvre a method of delivering the membranes and placenta after their descent into the vagina. One hand lifts the contracted uterus away from the placenta, while the other hand applies counter-tension on the cord. This method has now been superseded by controlled cord traction.

brassiere pregnant women should be encouraged to wear a well-fitting, supportive brassiere with wide shoulder straps. Postnatally, front-opening brassieres which are large enough for the lactating breasts should be advised.

Braxton Hicks contractions painless, irregular uterine contractions occurring during pregnancy, so called after the obstetrician of that name who first described them. As pregnancy advances they gradually increase in intensity and frequency and become more rhythmic during the third trimester; they improve blood flow to the placenta and fetus; are often mistaken for true labour; and sometimes referred to as 'false labour'.

breast the mammary glands, normally two in number, are situated on the anterior chest wall over the second to the sixth ribs and separated from the chest wall by a layer of loose connective tissue. *See* diagram.

breast pump a suction apparatus, used to withdraw milk from the

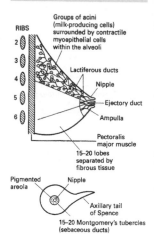

Anatomy of the Breast

Groups of acini (milk-producing cells) surrounded by contractile myoepithelial cells within the alveoli

RIBS
2
3
4
5
6

Lactiferous ducts
Nipple
Ejectory duct
Ampulla
Pectoralis major muscle
15–20 lobes separated by fibrous tissue

Pigmented areola
Nipple
Axillary tail of Spence
15–20 Montgomery's tubercles (sebaceous ducts)

breast. The vacuum can be created by hand pressure on a rubber bulb, or by an electrical pump.

breech the buttocks. *B. presentation* a longitudinal lie of the fetus in which the buttocks present in the lower pole of the uterus. Causes may be pelvic, uterine, fetal or incidental. The incidence of breech presentation at term is approximately 2.5%. Diagnosis can be made abdominally by palpating the fetal head in the fundus, vaginally by feeling the buttocks, anal orifice, genitalia or feet, but confirmation using ultrasound may be necessary. Attempts to change the presentation by using EXTERNAL VERSION or MOXIBUSTION are sometimes made.

Types of Breech Presentation

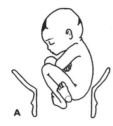

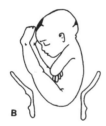

A, With flexed legs; B, with extended legs.

The main dangers during delivery are to the fetus, and include intracranial haemorrhage, hypoxia, fractures, dislocations and soft tissue injuries. The second stage of labour involves performing an episiotomy before the anterior buttock is delivered to minimize compression later on the fetal head. The feet are guided over the perineum, a loop of cord is pulled down to prevent traction on the umbilicus. If the arms are flexed, the shoulders are delivered with the next contraction; extended arms are delivered using LÖVSET'S MANOEUVRE. Once the trunk and shoulders are born, the baby is allowed to hang by his/her own weight (BURNS–MARSHALL TECHNIQUE) for about one minute, to aid flexion and descent of the head. When the hair line appears at the vulva the baby is held firmly by the ankles and the trunk is raised in a wide arc up and over the mother's abdomen. The MAURICEAU–SMELLIE–VEIT MANOEUVRE is used when the head is extended and fails to descend.

bregma the anterior fontanelle, a kite-shaped membranous area in the head of the fetus and infant at the junction of the frontal, coronal and sagittal sutures. *See also* FETAL SKULL.

brim of the pelvis the pelvic inlet. *See* PELVIS.

British Pharmacopoeia (BP) the official publication containing the list of drugs and other medicinal substances in use in the United Kingdom. The book gives details of how these substances are obtained or prepared, and their dosages and methods of administration. It is compiled under the auspices of the General Medical Council and is regularly revised and brought up to date.

broad ligaments two folds of peritoneum, continuous with that of the uterus, and extending to the sides of the pelvis. They contain the fallopian tubes, the parametrium, the ovarian blood and lymph vessels and the nerves of the uterus and, in their bases, the ureters.

bromethol a basal anaesthetic.

bromocriptine a dopamine agonist, a derivative of ergot alkaloids used to inhibit prolactin secretion. It may be used to suppress lactation. Given orally, 2.5 mg on day 1, then 2.5 mg twice daily for 14 days.

33

bronchopulmonary dysplasia a chronic respiratory condition occurring in babies who have been ventilated for long periods or have needed prolonged oxygen therapy. It results in serious disruption of lung growth. Examination of radiographs and lung specimens reveals patches of collapse and fibrosis. Following ventilation these babies usually require supplementary oxygen for several weeks or even months to keep the arterial oxygen tension above 55 kPa.

bronchus one of the main branches of the trachea. pl. *bronchi*.

brow presentation a cephalic presentation in which the attitude of the head is midway between flexion and extension. Since the mentovertical diameter of 13.0–13.75 cm presents, and this diameter is greater than any of those of the average pelvis, brow presentation is a possible cause of obstructed labour. Causes may be an android pelvis, with a consequent occipitoposterior position of the fetal head impacting in the sacrocotyloid diameter of the pelvis and resulting in extension of the head, or abnormality of the fetal head such as hydrocephaly or anencephaly. It occurs only about once in every 1000–1500 labours. Diagnosis is made by palpating a very high head abdominally, or failure to palpate the head vaginally, although occasionally the bregma and orbital ridges can be felt on vaginal examination. Where the mother has access to hospital treatment caesarean section will be performed to prevent complications. If this is not feasible, it may be possible by vaginal manipulation to flex the head so that the vertex presents, or to extend it further into a face presentation and then apply forceps. Internal podalic version and

Brow Presentation

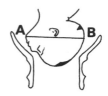

A–B, Mentovertical diameter 13.5 cm.

breech delivery may also sometimes be attempted.

brown fat a thermogenic type of adipose tissue containing a dark pigment, and arising during embryonic life in specific areas such as between the shoulder blades, behind the sternum, in the neck and around the kidneys and suprarenal glands. It is utilized by the newborn for the production of heat as required.

Brushfield's spots grey or yellow spots sometimes observed in the irises of the eyes of children with Down's syndrome.

B-scan ULTRASOUND display which produces a two-dimensional cross-sectioned picture of internal anatomy. Used to locate the position of the fetal skull prior to cephalometry, for placentography and diagnosis of abnormal conditions, e.g. hydatidiform mole, pelvic tumours and intrauterine death.

buccal smear scrapings from the buccal mucosa which are examined microscopically to study BARR BODIES.

buffer a chemical substance which, when present in a solution, helps to resist a change in pH. *Bicarbonate b.* this is the principal buffering system in the blood and involves the bicarbonate ions and carbon dioxide.

bulbocavernosus muscles two of the perineal muscles which surround the vaginal introitus and have a weak sphincter-like action.

bulla a blister. pl. *bullae*.

bupivacaine hydrochloride (Marcain) a local analgesic drug used for epidural, intrathecal and paracervical analgesia. Duration of action 2–4 hours. Dose – 0.25%, 0.5%, 0.75%. May cause blood pressure to fall.

Burns–Marshall technique one method for delivering the head during a breech delivery. Once the trunk is delivered, the baby hangs by his/her own weight for a minute to aid flexion and descent of the head. When the hair line appears at the vulva the head is at the outlet. The head is delivered by raising the trunk (holding the baby by the ankles and exerting slight traction) and carried through a wide arc up and over the mother's abdomen. The perineum is retracted exposing the baby's nose and mouth, permitting the airway to be cleared and oxygen to be given. The birth of the head is completed very slowly, usually with the aid of obstetric forceps applied to the after-coming head.

C

caecum 1. the first or proximal part of the large intestine, forming a dilated pouch distal to the ileum and proximal to the colon, and giving off the vermiform appendix. 2. any blind pouch.

caesarean section an obstetric operation whereby the fetus is extracted from the uterus through an incision made in the abdominal and uterine walls following the 24th week of pregnancy. *Lower segment caesarean section* (LSCS) involves a horizontal incision in the lower uterine segment. The possibility of rupture of the uterus during a subsequent labour is greatly reduced when a LSCS is performed. *Classical caesarean section* involves a vertical incision in the body of the uterus, the scar of which is more likely to rupture in subsequent pregnancies. Indications for caesarean section include cephalopelvic disproportion; grade III or IV placenta praevia; placental abruption in order to deliver a live fetus; fetal distress in the first stage; failure to progress, especially where there are malpresentations or malpositions; serious maternal medical conditions; preterm delivery when the extrauterine environment is deemed to be safer for the fetus than the intrauterine environment.

The midwife's role is one of preoperative preparation and postoperative care and observations; she may also be required to act as an assistant to the anaesthetist or to attend the mother throughout the operation if anaesthesia is via an epidural; to act as the scrub nurse or 'runner' in theatre; or to receive the baby and provide immediate resuscitative care to the infant. *See also* Appendix 3 (Figure 7).

calcaneum, calcaneus the bone of the foot which forms the heel.

calcification the deposit of lime in any tissue. Calcification may be present in the mature and postmature placenta.

calcium a chemical element. Symbol Ca. It is the most abundant mineral in the body. In combination with phosphorus it forms calcium phosphate, the dense, hard material of the bones and teeth. It is an important cation (a positively charged ion) in intra- and extracellular fluid and is essential to the normal clotting of the blood, the maintenance of a normal heart beat, and the initiation of neuromuscular and metabolic activities. In pregnancy, a diet rich in calcium is required and can be obtained from milk, cheese and green vegetables; it may be given in vitamin form. Vitamin D is essential for its absorption. Tetany resulting from hypocalcaemia, may occur in newborn babies.

calculus a stone which may be formed in the gallbladder, bile duct, kidney or ureter.

Caldwell–Moloy classification the classification of female pelves as gynaecoid, android, anthropoid and platypelloid.

calipers compasses for measuring diameters and curved surfaces, e.g. the fetal skull.

callus 1. the tissue which grows round fractured ends of bone and develops into new bone to repair the injury. 2. localized hyperplasia of the horny layer of the epidermis due to pressure or friction.

calorie a unit of heat, the amount needed to raise 1 g of water through 1°C. A calorie (kilocalorie) equals 1000 cal and is the amount of heat needed to raise 1 kg of water through 1°C. This unit is used to measure body heat and energy needs in food; 1 g of carbohydrate or protein gives 4 kcal and 1 g of fat gives 9 kcal. During pregnancy and lactation the mother needs about 2500 kcal/day. A full-term infant needs 110 kcal/kg body weight/day after the fourth day of life. The SI counterpart of this unit is the JOULE (J), which equals 4.2 cal.

cancer a general term to describe malignant growths. *See* CARCINOMA.

Candida a genus of yeast-like fungi that are commonly part of the normal flora of the mouth, skin, intestinal tract and vagina, but can cause a variety of infections. *See also* CANDIDIASIS. *C. albicans* the usual pathogen in human infection.

candidiasis mucous membrane infected with *Candida albicans*. Affects particularly the vagina, skin, mouth or nails, but may invade the bronchi and lungs and can become systemic.

Canesten *See* CLOTRIMAZOLE.

cannula a tube for insertion into a cavity or blood vessel; during insertion its lumen is usually occupied by a trocar.

capillary hair-like. 1. minute vessels connecting arterioles and venules, the walls of which act as a semipermeable membrane for interchange

Caput Succedaneum

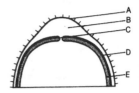

A, Skin; B, subcutaneous tissue; C, aponeurosis; D, periosteum; E, bone.

of various substances between the blood and tissue fluid. 2. minute vessels of the lymphatic system.

caput head. *C. succedaneum* an oedematous swelling formed on the fetal head by pressure from the dilating cervical os which, after rupture of the forewaters, restricts the venous return in the superficial tissues. It is present before delivery but disperses within a few hours. Other characteristic features are that it pits on pressure, can cross suture lines when present on the scalp and is found over the face or buttocks if these are the presenting parts. Bruising may also be a feature. *See also* CEPHALHAEMATOMA.

carbimazole an antithyroid drug used in the treatment of thyrotoxicosis. May cause fetal hypothyroidism.

carbohydrate food composed of carbon, hydrogen and oxygen (CHO). The sugar, starch and cellulose foods which provide heat and energy; 1 g of carbohydrate yields 17 kJ (4 kcal). Carbohydrates may be stored in the body as glycogen for future use or, if eaten in excessive amounts, as fats.

carbon dioxide (CO_2) a gas present in minute quantities in the atmosphere and formed in the body tissues by the oxidation of carbon and excreted by the lungs; used with oxygen to stimulate respiration. It is usually measured as P_{CO_2}.

carbon monoxide (CO) a colourless, odourless, tasteless gas, formed by burning carbon or organic fuels with a scant supply of oxygen; inhalation causes central nervous system damage and asphyxiation.

carbonate a salt of carbonic acid.

carcinogenic causing carcinoma.

carcinoma cancer. A malignant epithelial tumour which may develop in any part of the body.

cardia 1. the cardiac opening. 2. the cardiac part of the stomach; that part of the stomach surrounding the oesophagogastric junction, distinguished by the presence of cardiac glands.

cardiac pertaining to the heart. *C. arrest* sudden and often unexpected stoppage of effective heart action. Emergency cardiac care and cardiopulmonary resuscitation (CPR) are the only hopes of survival for the affected person. *C. disease in pregnancy* was formerly caused by mitral stenosis resulting from rheumatic fever or chorea in childhood, but today in the United Kingdom is more likely to be due to congenital heart disease. Cardiac disease often worsens during pregnancy so careful monitoring is essential; some may need long-term antenatal admission to hospital. Labour is often short, and care is aimed at preventing problems associated with over-exertion and cardiac overload; forceps delivery or caesarean section may be advocated. The third stage of labour is the most hazardous for the mother due to the increase in blood volume as a result of strong uterine contractions. Oxytocic drugs can exacerbate this so the midwife should always consult the obstetrician regarding the administration of oxytocics for any woman with heart disease.

cardinal of first importance.

cardinal ligaments also known as the transverse cervical or Mackenrodt's ligaments. Two thickened bands of parametrium which stretch from the cervix uteri to the lateral walls of the pelvis, and help to support the uterus.

cardiogram a graphic representation of the heart's action made by the electrocardiograph.

cardiotocography (CTG) a graphical correlation between fetal heart rate patterns and uterine contractions in labour. Also a non-stress test for fetal well-being in pregnancy.

cardiovascular relating to the heart and blood vessels.

caries decay or necrosis of bone. *Dental c.* decay of teeth.

carneous mole a mass of blood clot surrounding a dead embryo, and retained by the uterus. Also termed blood mole, fleshy mole, missed abortion. *See* TUBAL MOLE.

carotene a deep yellow pigment which is converted into vitamin A by the liver.

carotid bodies small neurovascular structures lying in the bifurcation of the right and left carotid arteries, containing chemoreceptors that monitor oxygen content in blood and help to regulate respiration.

carpal tunnel syndrome tingling and numbness in the hand resulting from pressure on the median nerve as it passes through the carpal tunnel at the wrist. This condition may occur in pregnancy, since local oedema increases the pressure. It is often worse at night but may be relieved by sleeping with the hands splinted. The condition usually resolves spontaneously after delivery. Severe cases may be treated successfully with osteopathy.

carpopedal spasm muscular spasm of the hands and feet in TETANY.

carrier a person who carries in the body pathogenic organisms, but has no symptoms of disease. Such a person may transmit poliomyelitis or typhoid fever. Haemolytic streptococci from the throat of a carrier could be transmitted to the genital tract of a recently delivered woman. In genetics it is an apparently normal individual who carries a RECESSIVE or SEX-LINKED GENE. *C. oil* an oil, such as grapeseed or sweet almond, in which essential oils used in aromatherapy are diluted and applied to the skin in massage or added to the bath water.

cartilage a specialized, fibrous connective tissue present in adults, and forming most of the temporary skeleton in the embryo, providing a model in which most of the bones develop, and constituting an important part of the organism's growth mechanism.

caruncle, caruncula a small fleshy eminence, often abnormal. pl. *carunculae. Carunculae myrtiformes* small elevations of mucous membrane around the vaginal orifice; the remnants of the ruptured hymen.

case conference a meeting of professionals involved in the care of a particular person (often a child), to agree patterns of action and to monitor progress.

case mix database computerized record system which combines all the data received from patient administration systems and operational systems to provide a comprehensive set of information about all the treatment and services received by each patient or client during an episode of care. The information helps to develop normal care profiles for different groups, to analyse and compare different treatment regimes, to produce comparative costings for different treatments etc. It may also be used as part of the medical audit process.

casein one of the proteins of milk. The casein of cows' milk is less digestible, and present in larger quantities, than that of human milk.

caseinogen the precursor of casein. Caseinogen is converted into casein by the renin of the gastric juice in babies.

caseload midwifery a system of care in which each midwife is responsible for a group of women, i.e. a caseload. This results in better communication and continuity of care for the women and improved job satisfaction for the midwife.

cast a structure moulded in a hollow organ and retaining the shape of the cavity of the organ, when shed, e.g. a decidual cast shed from the uterus in tubal pregnancy, or casts from the renal tubules found in the urine in kidney disease.

castration the removal of the male testicles or the female ovaries.

catamenia menstruation.

cataract an opacity of the crystalline lens or its capsule which impairs vision. Congenital cataract is sometimes seen in newborn babies. It may be a familial condition or it may occur in babies of women who have contracted RUBELLA in early pregnancy. It also may be associated with GALACTOSAEMIA.

catecholamine any of a group of sympathomimetic amines (including dopamine, adrenaline, and noradrenaline), the aromatic portion of whose molecule is catechol. The catecholamines play an important role in the body's physiological response to stress. Their release at the sympathetic nerve endings increases the rate and force of muscular contractions of the heart, thereby increasing cardiac output, constricts peripheral blood vessels, resulting in elevated blood pressure; elevates blood glucose levels by hepatic and skeletal muscle glycogenesis; and promotes an increase in blood lipids by increasing the catabolism of fats.

catgut suture material made from the gut of sheep; used mainly for buried sutures as it is absorbed by the body.

catheter a tube made of polythene, rubber, gum-elastic or silver, and perforated near its blind end. Introduced into various hollow organs, vessels or canals for the purpose of CATHETERIZATION.

catheterization the introduction of a catheter to introduce or withdraw fluid or to measure fluid pressure, e.g. bladder, cardiac or umbilical catheterization.

cathode a negative electrode.

cation an ion carrying a positive electric charge. Examples are sodium (Na), copper (Cu).

cauda equina literally, horse's tail. The nerves into which the spinal cord divides at its termination in the lumbar region.

caudal block regional analgesia achieved by the introduction of the agent through the sacral hiatus. It is less reliable than entering the epidural space by the lumbar route. *See* EPIDURAL ANALGESIA.

caul the amnion, which occasionally does not rupture, but envelops the infant's head at birth. It should be ruptured as quickly as possible to establish a clear airway.

caulophyllum a homoeopathic remedy which may be used, in certain women, to induce or accelerate labour. *See also* HOMOEOPATHY.

cautery a hot instrument or a chemical agent used to destroy tissue by burning it. Sometimes used in the treatment of cervical erosion.

cavity of the pelvis the hollow within the pelvic walls, bounded by the pelvic brim (or inlet) above and the outlet below.

-cele suffix meaning 'a tumour', e.g. meningocele, a swelling consisting of a protrusion of meninges.

cell the structural unit of which all multi-celled organisms are made. It consists of a nucleus with central nucleolus, and CHROMOSOMES. The surrounding cytoplasm is semifluid and contains mitochondria, RIBOSOMES and other bodies. The whole is contained within the cell membrane. All living cells arise from other cells, either by division of one cell to make two, as in MITOSIS and MEIOSIS, or by fusion of two cells to make one, as in the union of the sperm and ovum to make the zygote in sexual reproduction. The cells of the body differentiate during development into many specialized types with specific tasks to perform. Cells are organized into tissues and tissues into organs.

cellulitis a diffuse inflammatory process within solid tissues, characterized by oedema, redness, pain and interference with function. It may be caused by infection with streptococci, staphylococci, or other organisms. Cellulitis usually occurs in the loose tissues beneath the skin, but may also occur in tissues beneath mucous membranes, or around muscle bundles or surrounding organs. Pelvic cellulitis involves tissues surrounding the uterus and is called parametritis. It may occur as a complication of septic abortion or following labour, if infection has been introduced into the genital tract.

cellulose a carbohydrate; the outer covering of vegetable cells, i.e. vegetable fibres. Not digestible in the alimentary tract of humans, but gives bulk, and as 'roughage' stimulates peristalsis.

Celsius an internationally recognized unit of temperature. Water freezes at 0° and boils at 100°. These units were called 'Centigrade' in the UK but this is not used in SYSTÈME INTERNATIONAL D'UNITÉS (SI units), as in some countries it is a measurement of angle.

census enumeration of a population. The national census was first introduced in England and Wales in 1801 and has since been repeated every 10 years (except 1941). It usually records name, address, sex, occupation, marital status and other social information.

Centigrade *See* CELSIUS.

centile *See* PERCENTILE.

centimetre the one-hundredth part of a metre.

central nervous system the brain and spinal cord.

central venous pressure (CVP) the pressure of blood in the right atrium. It indicates the balance between the cardiac output and the venous return. Measurement of central venous pressure is made possible by the insertion of a catheter through the median cubital vein to the superior vena cava. The distal end of the catheter is attached to a manometer on which can be read the amount of pressure being exerted by the blood inside the right atrium. The manometer is positioned at the bedside so that the zero point is at the level of the right atrium. Each time the mother's position is changed the zero point on the manometer must be reset. It is invaluable to ensure adequate fluid replacement without overloading the circulation when the amount of

Cephalhaematoma

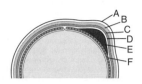

A, Skin; B, subcutaneous tissue; C, aponeurosis; D, periosteum; E, blood under periosteum; F, bone.

blood lost cannot be accurately estimated, e.g. in concealed ABRUPTIO PLACENTAE. The normal range is +5 to +10 cm of saline when the zero point of the scale corresponds to the mid-axillary line.

centrifuge an apparatus which rotates at great speed. It will hold test tubes of blood, urine, etc., and such rotation will precipitate bacteria, cells and other substances.

cephalhaematoma a collection of blood beneath the periosteum of one of the cranial bones. It causes a fluctuant swelling which develops on the head of the newborn child within 48 hours of birth. Very occasionally the cranial bone beneath is found to be fractured. A cephalhaematoma is distinguished from a CAPUT SUCCEDANEUM by the fact that it develops after birth, and is limited to the area of one bone. It takes several weeks to subside, and the mother should be told to expect this. No treatment is necessary unless severe jaundice occurs.

cephalic version conversion to a head presentation. *See* VERSION.

cephalometry measurement of the head. Antenatally this is usually the measurement of the biparietal diameter. The most accurate is by means of ULTRASOUND. It is used to assess fetal maturity and growth. *See also* BIPARIETAL DIAMETER. After birth the head is measured with a tape measure.

cephalopelvic pertaining to the relationship of the fetal head to the maternal pelvis. *C. disproportion* a misfit between the fetal head and the maternal pelvis, diagnosed when the fetal head will not engage in the pelvis after 36 weeks of pregnancy.

cephaloridine an antibiotic derived from CEPHALOSPORIN. It can cross into the fetal circulation via the placenta. May be given orally, intramuscularly or intravenously.

cephalosporin a naturally occurring antibiotic similar chemically to PENICILLIN.

cerclage encircling of a part with a ring or loop, as for correction of an incompetent cervix uteri or fixation of the adjacent ends of a fractured bone.

cerebellum the hindbrain, below the cerebrum and behind the medulla oblongata.

cerebral pertaining to the cerebral hemispheres.

cerebral dysrhythmia a condition in which the brain shows an abnormal pattern of electrical waves on an electroencephalogram (ECG) tracing. It occurs in epilepsy and has been noted in eclampsia, such women tending to have convulsions.

cerebral haemorrhage bleeding from or into one of the cerebral hemispheres.

cerebral palsy a persisting motor disorder which may result from hypoxia *in utero*, asphyxia neonatorum, and periods of apnoea and cyanosis, as may occur in RESPIRATORY DISTRESS SYNDROME, HYPOGLYCAEMIA and other conditions.

cerebrospinal relating to the brain and spinal cord. *C. fluid* the fluid in the ventricles of the brain, secreted by the choroid plexuses and circulating in the subarachnoid space covering the brain, and in the membranes surrounding the spinal cord. It protects the nerves in the brain and spinal cord from jar and injury. An excessive quantity of this fluid is found in HYDROCEPHALUS.

cerebrum the largest part of the brain, occupying the greater portion of the cranium and consisting of the right and left cerebral hemispheres. The centre of the higher functions of the brain.

cervical pertaining to the neck. In obstetrics, pertaining to the cervix uteri or neck of the uterus. *C. cerclage see* SHIRODKAR OPERATION. *C. cytology* the examination of cells from the cervix to detect abnormal changes. *C. incompetence* failure of an injured cervix to hold the pregnancy in the uterus: a cause of abortion after the 12th week of pregnancy, characterized by premature rupture of the membranes and painless expulsion of the fetus.

cervical intraepithelial neoplasia (CIN) classification of types of cervical dysplasia. CIN I is mild, reversible dysplasia; CIN II is moderate dysplasia but is also reversible. CIN III is severe dysplasia and carcinoma *in situ*. The condition is irreversible and requires surgery to prevent the development of invasive carcinoma.

cervicitis infection of the mucous membrane lining the cervix uteri. *Acute c.* occurs in GONORRHOEA. *Chronic c.* usually results from a low-grade infection following slight tearing of the cervix during delivery. The inflamed mucous membrane protrudes through the external os to the vaginal part of the cervix, forming an erosion which bleeds readily. It can be treated by destruction of the infected tissues by cauterization.

cervix a constricted portion or neck. *C. uteri*, the neck of the uterus; it is about 2.5 cm long and opens into the vagina. *Cervical canal* starts at the internal os, which communicates with the body of the uterus and ends at the external os, which opens into the vagina.

chancre the initial lesion of SYPHILIS developing at the site of inoculation.

'Changing Childbirth' Report (1993) a report produced by the Department of Health following a governmental working party, chaired by Baroness Cumberlege, which examined the current state of maternity care. Recommendations were made regarding improvements which should offer the women more accessible, effective and efficient services that respond to women's needs by providing increased choice, control and continuity in the care they receive. It was suggested that each woman should be under the care of a 'LEAD PROFESSIONAL' who could be a midwife, obstetrician or general practitioner.

chemical change this differs from physical change in that a profound alteration in properties results, usually permanently and usually accompanied by use of energy in a new substance, e.g. hydrogen (2 atoms) plus oxygen produces water.

chemical compound any substance produced by chemical change which may then be broken up into its components only by chemical means, unlike a mixture, which can usually be separated mechanically.

chemoreceptor a collection of cells sensitive to alterations in chemicals contacting them. They are found in the carotid body and aortic body. These receptors are responsive to changes in the oxygen, carbon dioxide and hydrogen ion concentration in the blood. When oxygen concentration falls below normal in the arterial blood, the chemoreceptors send impulses to stimulate the respiratory centre so that there will be an increase in alveolar ventilation and consequently, an increase in the intake of oxygen by the lungs.

chemotherapy the treatment of illness by chemical means; that is, by medication. adj. *chemotherapeutic*.

chest the thoracic cavity containing the lungs, heart, trachea, bronchi, oesophagus and large blood vessels and nerves.

chi-squared test a statistical test to determine whether two or more groups of observations differ significantly from one another, i.e. more than would be expected by chance.

chickenpox varicella. Infectious disease of childhood. Incubation period 12–20 days. Slight fever and eruption of transparent skin vesicles which dry up and may leave pits in the skin. Can be severe in neonates.

chignon the large caput succedaneum seen on the head of an infant delivered by ventouse vacuum extraction. *See* VACUUM EXTRACTOR.

child abuse anything which individuals, institutions or processes do or do not do which directly or indirectly harms children or damages their prospects of a safe and healthy development into adulthood. If a child is seen to be in danger of suffering significant harm, from physical, sexual, emotional or neglectful causes, the child may be registered under the Child Protection Register. If a midwife has reasonable cause to suspect the abuse of a child in a family under her care she must take the appropriate action in order to protect the child. *See also* CHILDREN ACT.

child health clinic a centre for well children to attend on a regular basis to ensure normal progress and development. A medical officer and a health visitor are in attendance.

child minder one who is registered with the local authority social services department and who is approved by the department to mind a few children aged from birth to 5 years during the day.

Child Support Agency government agency set up under the Child Support Act 1991 to operate a scheme for child maintenance in cases where the parents of children are living apart. The Agency is responsible for assessing each case where one parent has requested Child Maintenance, reviewing the situation at 2-yearly intervals and, if necessary, collecting the money from the absent parent.

childbirth the act or process of giving birth to a child. Called also parturition. *Natural c.* a term used to describe an approach to labour and delivery whereby the mother and her partner are well prepared and remain in control of events which are allowed to progress naturally, and without intervention. Medical interference, drugs and other stimuli to labour are therefore avoided.

Children Act 1989 this Act brings together the comprehensive law relating to children, defining the rights of children, identifying the responsibilities of parents and detailing procedures for the protection of children. The welfare of children is paramount in all court decisions, which should be made with minimum delay and, where possible, take the child's wishes into account. In family proceedings the court may issue a *contact order* requiring the person with whom the child lives to have access to another named person, or a *residence order* which settles arrangements over where a child lives.

The court can make *care* and *supervision orders* to place a child in the care of a local authority. A *child assessment order* enables the child to remain in his/her normal residence but the adult responsible for him/her must allow access to the child for assessment. An *emergency protection order* is issued to remove a child from potential harm to the care of (usually) the local authority.

chiropody study and care of feet and treatment of foot diseases. More commonly termed podiatry nowadays.

chiropractic a form of complementary medicine, originally developed from osteopathy, but having evolved with a different philosophy. Chiropractic treatment is beneficial for a wide range of sensory, organic, vascular and muscular problems, and involves mobilization and manipulation of joints with the aim of restoring alignment within the spine, and therefore its relationship with the rest of the body. It may be a useful form of treatment for physiological disorders of pregnancy, and has been shown to be effective in treating colic in infants, hyperactivity in children, menstrual and menopausal symptoms in women.

chiropractor a practitioner of *chiropractic*.

Chlamydia a bacterium which is grown only with difficulty. One species causes trachoma in tropical climates. *C. trachomatis* is responsible for at least half the cases of nonspecific urethritis (NSU) in males, and is now more likely than the gonococcus to cause OPHTHALMIA NEONATORUM. It is acquired from the birth canal but the mucopurulent discharge is not seen until 5–10 days after birth.

chloasma mask. The 'pregnancy mask', or pigmentation of the skin of the forehead, nose and cheeks seen quite commonly in pregnancy.

chloral elixir a hypnotic for babies contains 200 mg in 5 ml of solution. Dose: 30 mg/kg body weight for the first 2 weeks of life.

chloral hydrate a hypnotic and sedative with mild action as a pain reliever but used more commonly to induce sleep. It is now rarely used.

chloramphenicol a broad-spectrum antibiotic with specific therapeutic activity against rickettsiae and many different bacteria. Side-effects include serious, even fatal, blood dyscrasias in certain patients. Frequent blood tests are recommended during therapy. Chloromycetin is a proprietary preparation of chloramphenicol.

chlordiazepoxide anti-anxiety drug for short-term use; also used in acute alcohol withdrawal. A member of the benzodiazepine group of drugs.

chlorhexidine a coal-tar derivative which has a wide antibacterial action. It is especially effective against coagulase-positive staphylococci and is extensively used in antibiotic skin cleansers for surgical scrub, preoperative skin preparation and cleansing skin wounds. Hibitane is the proprietary preparation of chlorhexidine.

chloride a salt of chlorine. One of the electrolytes important in helping to maintain the normal balance of the blood necessary to health.

chlorothiazide a diuretic drug that also has an antihypertensive effect. It is used in the treatment of the oedema of congestive heart failure, and in hypertension.

chlorphenamine (chlorpheniramine) maleate a preparation used for the relief of allergy and the emergency treatment of anaphylactic reactions. Piriton.

chlorpromazine a phenothiazine used as an antipsychotic agent and antiemetic. Side-effects include drowsiness and slight hypotension. Largactil.

chlorpropamide drug used in the treatment of diabetes. Contraindicated in pregnancy. May cause neonatal hypoglycaemia.

choanal atresia a membranous or bony obstruction of the posterior nares. As a neonate breathes mainly through the nose, considerable respiratory difficulty occurs at or shortly after birth, leading to cyanosis.

cholecystitis inflammation of the gallbladder.

chondroblast embryonic cell that forms cartilage.

chordee downward curvature of penis caused by congenital anomaly such as hypospadias.

chorditis inflammation of spermatic (or vocal) cords.

chorea St Vitus' dance. A disease, related to rheumatism and probably of bacterial origin, affecting the nervous system. It is characterized by irregular involuntary muscular movements, and can prove very exhausting to the patient. This condition occurring during pregnancy has sometimes been termed chorea gravidarum. It may also be called Sydenham's chorea. It is occasionally seen in young primigravid women with or sometimes without a history of rheumatism and/or chorea in childhood. It is dangerous in so far as the pregnancy throws an additional strain on the already impaired heart.

chorioangioma a collection of fetal blood vessels in WHARTON'S JELLY, forming a tumour on the placenta. It is of little clinical significance, but is, rarely, associated with POLYHYDRAMNIOS.

choriocarcinoma a highly malignant NEOPLASM, usually arising from the trophoblast of a HYDATIDIFORM MOLE. It develops in about 3% of hydatidiform moles and is detected by raised levels of chorionic gonadotrophin in serum or urine and by radioimmunoassay. It is treated by cytotoxic chemotherapy and, if necessary, hysterectomy.

chorioepithelioma the former term for CHORIOCARCINOMA.

chorion the outer of the two membranes enclosing the fetus *in utero*. It is derived from the PLACENTA from the trophoblast. It is opaque and friable in nature and may sometimes be retained after delivery. *C. biopsy* tissue removed from the gestational sac early in pregnancy so that chromosome and other inherited disorders can be identified. Because this can be done as early as 8 weeks' gestation, termination (where recommended and agreed) can be undertaken before 12 weeks, which is not possible with amniocentesis. *C. frondosum* the part of the chorion covered by villi in the early weeks of embryonic development before the placenta is formed. *C. laeve* the non-villous, membranous part of the trophoblast which develops into the chorion.

chorionic gonadotrophin a substance produced from the BLASTOCYST, stimulating the CORPUS LUTEUM to produce oestrogen and progesterone as the pituitary GONADOTROPHINS are decreasing, so ensuring the continuation of the pregnancy. The presence of the human chorionic gonadotrophins (HCG) in a woman's urine is diagnostic of pregnancy. *See also* PREGNANCY TESTS.

chorionic villi minute finger-like projections arising from the TROPHOBLAST and persisting in the chorion frondo-

sum. These have an outer SYNCY-TIOTROPHOBLASTIC layer with multiple nuclei and without cell walls, and an inner CYTOTROPHOBLASTIC layer with cell walls containing single nuclei. Within are fetal capillaries embedded in mesoderm. Oxygenated maternal blood spurts in cascades over the villi in the intervillous spaces, so that oxygen, nutrients, etc., may pass into the fetal circulation and carbon dioxide, etc., may pass out. This exchange becomes easier after 24 weeks of gestation when the cytotrophoblastic cell layer remains only in isolated areas.

choroid plexus vascular fringe-like folds in the pia mater in the third, fourth and lateral ventricles of the brain; concerned with formation of cerebrospinal fluid.

Christmas disease an hereditary haemorrhagic diathesis clinically similar to haemophilia A (classic haemophilia) but due to deficiency of clotting factor IX; called also haemophilia B.

chromatin the substance of the chromosomes, composed of DNA and basic proteins (histones), the material in the nucleus that stains with basic dyes. *Sex c.* Barr body; the persistent mass of the material of the inactivated X chromosome in cells of normal females.

chromatography a technique for analysis of chemical substances. The term literally means colour writing and the technique is used for some investigations, for example, to detect and identify in body fluids certain sugars and amino acids associated with inborn errors of metabolism.

chromosome one of a number of minute thread-like structures contained in the cell nucleus, composed of DEOXYRIBONUCLEIC ACID (DNA) and protein and carrying the genes,

One Pair of Chromosomes Showing Gene Banding

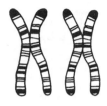

which transmit the inherited characteristics. In the human body the cells carry 46 chromosomes, 22 pairs of autosomes, and the two sex chromosomes (XX or XY), which determine the sex of the organism. *C. analysis* fetal cells obtained by AMNIOCENTESIS or by lymphocytes from a blood sample can be cultured in the laboratory until they divide. Cell division is arrested in mid-metaphase by the drug colchicine. The chromosomes can be stained by one of several techniques that produce a distinct pattern of light and dark bands along the chromosome, and each chromosome can be recognized by its size and banding pattern. The chromosomal characteristics of an individual are referred to as his/her KARYOTYPE. *See also* GENE.

chronic prolonged or permanent, e.g. chronic disease.

cilia fine hair-like processes which grow on the free border of certain epithelial cells. The lining of the fallopian tubes is ciliated epithelium, and the cilia, waving to and fro, produce a current which carries the ovum from the ovarian end of the fallopian tube to the uterus. Sing. *cilium*.

ciliated having cilia.

ciprofloxacin antimicrobial, active against Gram-negative organisms and *Chlamydia* in particular. Should be used with caution during pregnancy and breastfeeding.

circulation movement in a circular course, as of the blood. *Fetal c.* the circulation of blood in the fetus. Before birth the foramen ovale and the ductus arteriosus bypass the lungs, and blood is carried to and from the placenta by the umbilical vessels and the ductus venosus.

circumcision excision of the prepuce. It is performed on healthy Jewish male children on the eighth day of life as a religious ceremony. Medically, it is considered necessary if the urinary meatus of the prepuce is obstructed. The PLASTIBELL is commonly used for circumcision in many hospitals. *Female c.* or female genital mutilation, involves excision of the labia and clitoris and narrowing of the vaginal introitus. Particularly common in areas such as the Sudan. Complications include delay in labour, necrosis of the bladder wall, permanent urinary fistulae or vesicovaginal fistulae.

circumvallate literally, surrounded by a wall. A *c. placenta* has a distinct ridge on the fetal surface, caused by a double fold of chorion near its periphery. This is slightly more likely to separate partially, causing antepartum haemorrhage.

clamp a surgical instrument used to compress any part of the body, e.g. to prevent or arrest haemorrhage. *Hollister c.* a plastic device for occluding the vessels of the umbilical cord. It is applied at birth, about 1–2 cm from the umbilicus, for about 48 hours, after which it is removed.

clavicle the collar bone, articulating with the sternum and the acromion process of the scapula. Fracture of

Cleft Lip

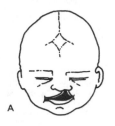

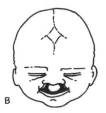

A, Unilateral; B, bilateral.

the fetal clavicle is an uncommon birth injury. It may be due to a traumatic breech delivery or in shoulder dystocia, as with an undetected large baby of a mother with gestational diabetes. Alternatively, it may occur spontaneously during easy birth in the rare condition of congenital OSTEOGENESIS IMPERFECTA. *See also* CLEIDOTOMY.

cleft lip a congenital defect resulting from the failure of fusion, in the embryo, of the median nasal and maxillary processes. It may be uni-lateral or bilateral. It is usually reparable during the first few weeks or months of life.

cleft palate a congenital defect which is often associated with CLEFT LIP. The cleft may be central or on one side of the palate only. The most severe variety is a complete cleft of the palate accompanied by a bilateral cleft lip, in which case there is an unsightly fleshy projection below the nose. Cleft palate interferes with the child's ability to suck, and, later, with speech. Modern operative treatment is very successful.

cleidotomy division, with scissors, of the fetal clavicles, in very rare cases, to facilitate delivery where there is obstruction due to excessive breadth of the shoulders, e.g. in a large ANEN-CEPHALIC fetus.

climacteric the changes in the body occurring at the time of the MENOPAUSE.

clinic a place where patients or clients receive advice and treatment.

clinical pertaining to or founded on actual observation and treatment of patients, as distinguished from theoretical or experimental. *C. trial* assessment of the effectiveness of modes of treatment by carefully following response to therapy in defined patient groups. A controlled clinical trial is one where a comparison is made of one or more active treatments against each other and against placebo. *Double-blind c. trial* comparison of different treatments (active and placebo) in which neither patients nor observers know which patient is receiving treatment until a trial code is decoded after completion of the study. *C. directorate* a system of devolved management within the resource management initiative, in which a clinical specialty such as obstetrics and gynaecology is headed by a director who is usually a medical practitioner and assisted by a senior midwife and a business manager. The directorate is responsible for its own budgeting and use of resources.

clinical governance framework through which NHS organizations are accountable for continuous improvement of quality of services and for safeguarding high standards of care by creating an environment in which excellence will flourish. *See also* NATIONAL INSTITUTE FOR CLINICAL EXCELLENCE *and* NATIONAL SERVICE FRAMEWORKS.

clinical nurse specialist qualified nurse who has acquired advanced knowledge and skills in a specific area of clinical practice.

clinical risk index for babies professional scoring tool used to assess initial neonatal risks and for comparing performance of one neonatal intensive care unit with another.

clinical risk management the means by which adverse events occurring in organizations, usually related to the delivery of patient care, are systematically reviewed in order to seek ways to prevent further incidents.

clinical thermometer an instrument for taking the body temperature, orally, rectally or in the axilla.

clitoridectomy excision of the clitoris.

clitoris a small sensitive organ, consisting of erectile tissue, situated at the anterior junction of the labia minora. It is the homologue of the male penis.

clomethiazole edisilate (Heminevrin) a hypnotic, sedative and anticonvulsant drug with a depressant action on the central nervous system. It is used to treat insomnia, agitation and confusion. It is also used to treat acute withdrawal symptoms in alcoholism and drug addiction, and for the control of sustained epileptic fits and eclampsia.

clomifene citrate a GONADOTROPHIC drug used to stimulate ovulation. A proprietary preparation is Clomid.

clone cells which are genetically identical to each other and have descended by asexual reproduction from the parent cell, to which they are also genetically identical.

clonic of the nature of a jerk. The convulsive stage of a fit is called the clonic stage.

Clostridium an anaerobic Gram-positive spore-bearing bacillus, e.g. that of tetanus or gas gangrene.

clot usually blood cells forming a partially solidified mass in a matrix of fibrin. It may also occur in lymph. The solid part of blood after it escapes from the blood vessels.

clotrimazole (Canesten) an antifungal agent. Pessaries or cream administered vaginally for the treatment of vaginal 'thrush'.

clotting formation of a jelly-like substance from blood shed at the site of an injury to a blood vessel. Occasionally clots form within blood vessels, causing arteriosclerosis, thrombosis or varicose veins. *C. time* time taken for shed blood to clot, usually 5 minutes. *See* COAGULATION.

cloxacillin a semi-synthetic penicillin; its sodium salt is used in treating staphylococcal infections due to penicillinase-producing organisms.

clubfoot *See* TALIPES.

coagulase a substance formed by certain strains of staphylococci (thus termed *coagulase-positive*) causing clotting in plasma. Coagulase-positive staphylococci (e.g. *Staphylococcus aureus*) are considerably more dangerous, especially to newborn babies, than those which are coagulase-negative (e.g. *Staphylococcus albus*).

coagulation formation of a clot. *C. disorders* occur in some cases of severe placental abruption, intra-uterine death, endotoxic shock and, rarely, amniotic fluid embolism. All labile clotting factors are reduced; fibrinogen is low and there is THROMBOCYTOPENIA. Profuse bleeding occurs and the blood fails to clot; available fibrinogen is redirected and leads to DISSEMINATED INTRAVASCULAR COAGULATION. Investigations include cross-matching, full blood count, prothrombin time, clotting time, platelet counts, fibrinogen and fibrinogen degradation products. Treatment will be dependent on the results of these tests.

coarctation of the aorta stricture of the aorta at, or just below, the position of the ductus arteriosus; often diagnosed by absence of femoral pulses.

cocaine hydrochloride a topical anaesthetic applied to mucous membranes. Cocaine is more commonly known now as a drug of abuse; psychological dependence may develop in long-term users. It may be absorbed through mucosal surfaces or smoked as with the highly addictive 'crack'. It is a powerful vasoconstrictor and is associated with spontaneous abortion, maternal hypertension, placental abruption and subsequent stillbirth and small for gestational age babies, possibly as a result of its appetite-suppressing effects which leads to poor maternal weight gain. Arterial thromboses are more common in pregnant cocaine abusers and maternal death may result from cardiac arrhythmias, coronary ischaemia, intracranial aneurysms, cerebral haemorrhage or hypertensive convulsions. Fetal malformations such as intestinal atresia, limb defects and genitourinary disorders may occur and neurological problems may be seen in infancy.

coccus a spherical micro-organism. *See* BACTERIA.

coccydynia persistent pain in the area of the coccyx.

coccygeus one of two muscles arising from the ischial spines and inserted into the lateral borders of the sacrum and coccyx, and forming part of the PELVIC FLOOR. Also called ischiococcygeus.

coccyx the terminal bone of the spinal column, in which four rudimentary vertebrae are fused together.

Cochrane database database of systematic reviews of published research. An international multidisciplinary collaboration of health professionals, consumers and researchers who review randomized controlled clinical trials related to pregnancy and childbirth; other medical specialties also have collaborative review groups to examine relevant research.

Code of Professional Conduct document produced by Nursing and Midwifery Council aiming to inform nurses, midwives and health visitors of the standard of professional conduct required in the exercise of their professional accountability and practice, and to inform the public, other professions and employers of the standard of professional conduct expected of a registered practitioner.

cohort group of people who possess a common characteristic, e.g. same sex or same profession. Used in research to make generalizations derived from quantitative data.

coitus sexual intercourse. Copulation. *C. interruptus* method of contraception where the penis is withdrawn from the vagina before ejaculation of semen.

colic severe spasmodic pain in the abdomen; most common during the first 3 months of life. The infant may pull up his legs, cry loudly, turn red-faced, and expel gas from the anus or belch it up from the stomach. *Biliary c.* colic due to the passage of a gallstone through the bile ducts. *Renal c.* colic caused by the passage of a stone along the ureter. Painful, ineffective, irregular contractions of the uterus are sometimes termed colicky.

coliform resembling *E. coli.* See BACTERIA.

collapse a state of prostration due to circulatory failure *See also* SHOCK.

colloidal solution a suspension in water or other fluid, of molecules of a type which do not readily pass through animal membrane. Examples are blood, plasma, and the various plasma substitutes, which are valuable in the treatment of shock, because they are retained in the circulation.

colon the section of the large intestine extending from the caecum to the rectum.

colostrum the thin, yellow, milky fluid secreted by the breasts from 16 weeks of pregnancy and for 3 to 4 days after birth until lactation is initiated. Colostrum is high in protein, and initially low in lactose; its fat content is equivalent to breast milk. It is an important source of passive antibody.

colour index a measurement of the proportion of haemoglobin in the red blood cells. In normal blood the figure is 1, in iron deficiency anaemia it is less than 1 and in megaloblastic anaemia it is more than 1.

colpo- pertaining to the vagina.

colpocele hernia of either bladder or rectum into vagina.

colpohysterectomy removal of the uterus via the vagina.

colpoperineorrhaphy repair of the pelvic floor, vagina and perineal body, usually undertaken for PROLAPSE.

colporrhaphy repair of the vagina. *Anterior c.* for CYSTOCELE. *Posterior c.* for RECTOCELE.

colposcope a speculum for examining the vagina and cervix by means of a magnifying lens; used for the early detection of malignant changes.

colposcopy examination of vaginal and cervical tissue with a colposcope, usually performed after an abnormal cervical smear result, to detect abnormal epithelium or benign tumours.

colpotomy incision of the vaginal wall. *Posterior c.* incision through the posterior vaginal fornix to the pouch of Douglas to drain a pelvic abscess.

columnar epithelium a type of epithelium containing cylindrical cells.

coma a condition of deep unconsciousness from which it is not possible to rouse the patient. It may have various causes including cerebrovascular accident, diabetes mellitus, alcoholism, eclampsia and uraemia.

comatose in a condition of coma.

commensal an organism which lives on another without harming it. *See also* LACTOBACILLUS ACIDOPHILUS.

commissure a connection. *Posterior c.* a fold of skin connecting the labia minora posteriorly.

Committee on Safety of Medicines (CSM) an organization responsible for controlling the release of new drugs in the UK. Also collects data on adverse reactions to drugs via the yellow card system. This data enables the CSM to issue warnings about serious adverse effects.

Community Health Council an organization which enables the consumer's interests to be represented to those responsible at district level for the National Health Service. Apart from a paid secretary, the members are drawn from local organizations, whose representatives work on a voluntary basis.

compatibility mixing together of two substances without chemical change or loss of power.

compensation in heart disease, the ability of the weakened heart nevertheless to function adequately.

complement that which adds to something or makes up a deficiency.

complementary making up a deficiency. *C. feed* is an artificial feed given to an infant to make up the deficient amount of a breastfeed. Not now recommended for normal healthy babies. cf. SUPPLEMENTARY. *C. medicine* a form of alternative medicine which is outside the mainstream conventional type of health care but which may be used in conjunction with orthodox medicine. These include osteopathy, chiropractic, acupuncture, homoeopathy, herbalism, massage, aromatherapy, reflexology, hypnotherapy and shiatsu and many more.

complete abortion bleeding from the genital tract before the 24th week of pregnancy which results in miscarriage. All the products of conception are expelled and there is no requirement for surgical evacuation of the uterus.

compound presentation presentation of more than one part of the fetus, e.g. head and hand; head and foot; breech, hand and cord. A rare complication of labour.

compression 1. pressing together, as in bimanual compression of the uterus to prevent haemorrhage. 2. in embryology, the shortening or omission of certain developmental stages.

computed tomography (CT) a radiological imaging technique that produces images of 'slices' 1–10 mm thick through the body. Used to diagnose such conditions as subdural haemorrhage, excess fluid or intra-ventricular haemorrhage in preterm infants.

computed axial tomography (CAT) *See* COMPUTED TOMOGRAPHY.

computerized records many health records are now held on computer systems which are required by law to be secure and to maintain confidentiality, usually achieved by limiting access. Most systems currently also provide a paper printout which is stored as a manual record. *See also* DATA PROTECTION ACT.

conception 1. the formation of an idea. 2. the fusion of spermatozoon and ovum to form a viable zygote. The onset of pregnancy.

condom a contraceptive device, a sheath covering the penis, worn during coitus.

condyloma a wart-like growth near the external genitalia or anus, which may occasionally be syphilitic in origin.

cone biopsy removal of a cone-shaped section from the cervix, performed to confirm diagnosis when a cervical smear test result suggests the presence of precancerous cells.

Confidential Enquiry a unique form of audit in which case notes are scrutinized by relevant professionals to identify substandard care and make recommendations for future practice. The triennial Confidential Enquiry into Maternal Deaths and the Confidential Enquiry into Stillbirths and Deaths in Infancy (CESDI) are directly related to maternity care and midwives may be involved in providing appropriate information; the Confidential Enquiry into Perioperative Deaths is also available but is unlikely to involve maternity cases.

congenital born with. Used to describe a condition, generally a malformation, present at birth. Also includes an infection which takes place *in utero*.

Congenital Disabilities (Civil Liabilities) Act 1976 this Act is applicable in England, Wales and Northern Ireland and provides for a child to be entitled to recover damages where the child has suffered as result of a breach in a duty of care owed to the mother or the father unless that breach of duty of care occurred before the child was conceived and either or both parents knew of the occurrence. In Scottish law the same provisions are made. The accuracy and preservation of records is therefore essential.

congenital dislocation of the hip (CDH) a condition arising from abnormal development of the acetabulum, femoral head or surrounding tissues, more commonly if there is a family history, if the fetus has presented by the breech, and in girls. About 1–2% of neonates have dislocated or dislocatable hips, usually found as part of the routine examinations performed by midwives and paediatricians in the first 24 hours of life and confirmed on ultrasound. Treatment is to stabilize the hip in abduction and flexion using a special harness; many dislocatable hips resolve spontaneously while a few children require surgery.

congenital heart defect structural defect of heart or great vessels, or both.

congenital infection infection acquired *in utero*, including rubella, cytomegalovirus, herpes simplex, human immunodeficiency virus, toxoplasmosis.

congestion abnormal accumulation of blood in a part of the body.

congestive pertaining to or associated with congestion. *C. heart failure* a broad term denoting conditions in which the heart's pumping capability is impaired.

conjoined twins *See* TWINS.

conjugate 1. to join or yoke together as, in the liver, bilirubin is combined with albumin by the activity of GLUCURONYL TRANSFERASE to render it water-soluble so that it may be excreted via the gut. *See also* ICTERUS GRAVIS *and* JAUNDICE. 2. a conjugate diameter of the pelvis. *See also* PELVIS.

conjunctiva the mucous membrane lining the inner surface of the eyelids and covering the anterior aspect of the eye.

conjunctivitis inflammation of the conjunctiva. *See* OPHTHALMIA NEONATORUM.

connective tissue tissue which binds together or supports the structures of the body. Adipose tissue, areolar tissue, bone, cartilage, fat, blood and fibrous tissue are all connective tissues.

consanguinity blood relationship.

consent in law, voluntary agreement with an action proposed by another. Consent is an act of reason; the person giving consent must be of sufficient mental capacity and be in possession of all essential information in order to give valid consent. Written informed consent is generally required before many invasive clinical procedures, such as investigations, including amniocentesis and surgery.

constipation a decrease in frequency of defecation, difficulty in defecating or a change in bowel habits from the normal. Common in pregnancy due to the smooth muscle relaxation which occurs as a result of progesterone. Excessive tea consumption, inadequate fluid intake, a diet lacking fibre content or prophylactic iron supplementation may exacerbate the condition. Postnatally, inhibition and a fear of damage to the already bruised area may contribute to poor bowel habits.

constriction ring a localized annular spasm of the uterine muscle at any level but often near the junction of the upper and lower uterine segments. In the first and second stages of labour it may form round the neck of the fetus and in the third stage forms an HOURGLASS CONSTRICTION of the uterus, causing a retained placenta. It may result from the use of oxytocic drugs in a uterus with uncoordinated function, following early rupture of the membranes, and especially if intrauterine manipulation is carried out. Relaxation may occur with inhalation of amyl nitrite but often deep anaesthesia is required.

Consultant in Public Health Medicine following recent changes in the NHS the Consultant in Public Health Medicine has replaced the community physician and is now responsible for functions such as promoting health, preventing disease and fostering cooperation between the health and social services.

contagion communication of disease from one person to another by direct contact.

continuing professional education (CPD) further study after the attainment of basic qualifications. Under the Nursing and Midwifery Council's regulations, all midwives, nurses and health visitors are required to demonstrate periodic updating and refreshment throughout their professional lives, in order to provide contemporary, research based care to patients and clients.

continuity of care term used to describe care given to one woman from booking until discharge to the health visitor, in which good communication from one appointment to the next and between all professionals ensures that there are no omissions or duplications in the care of that mother. Continuity does not necessarily mean that only one professional is in contact with the mother: this would indeed be unrealistic. However, verbal and written communication between professionals should be comprehensive enough to avoid errors and to facilitate the mother's sense of security in the care she is receiving. Various schemes of care exist in an attempt to provide continuity of care. See also CASELOAD MIDWIFERY, CHANGING CHILDBIRTH REPORT, TEAM MIDWIFERY.

continuous inflating pressure (CIP) pressure of water used against a baby's spontaneous breathing in respiratory distress syndrome (RDS). Its purpose is to prevent HYPOXAEMIA, apnoeic attacks or rising levels of carbon dioxide in the blood (Pco_2).

continuous negative pressure (CNP) a rarely used method of treating a neonate with the RESPIRATORY DISTRESS SYNDROME. Sub-atmospheric pressure is applied to the baby's thorax in a body box.

continuous positive airways pressure (CPAP) a technique used to prevent total alveolar collapse on expiration in a baby with RESPIRATORY DISTRESS SYNDROME. Positive pressure of 2–5 cmH$_2$O is applied into the respiratory tract by the nasal or endotracheal route or by face mask. CPAP is used with patients who are breathing spontaneously. When the same principle is used in mechanical ventilation, it is called positive end-expiratory pressure (PEEP).

contraception the prevention of conception. *Barrier methods of c.* for women include occlusive caps such as the diaphragm, vault cap or vimule, and spermicidal cream, foam or jelly should be used with it for extra protection. Men can use a condom or sheath, and there is now a female condom available, although this has been developed more for the protection from transmission of HIV than for prevention of pregnancy. Oral contraceptive pills for women may be a combination of oestrogen and progesterone or progesterone alone; a male contraceptive pill is also being developed. Injectable progestogen is available for women requiring a method as reliable as possible. Intrauterine devices or coils can be inserted into the uterus and can remain *in situ* for several years. 'Natural' methods of family planning include the rhythm method or 'safe period', the temperature method, Billings' method and coitus interruptus or withdrawal. The most reliable method of contraception is sterilization, of either the woman by laparoscopy or laparotomy, or the male by vasectomy.

contraceptive pertaining to contraception. Any means used to prevent conception.

contracted pelvis a pelvis in which any diameter of the brim, cavity or outlet is so shortened as to interfere with the progress of labour.

contraction a temporary shortening of muscle fibre, which returns to its original length during relaxation. Contractions of the uterus during pregnancy are painless and are termed Braxton Hicks contractions, after the obstetrician of that name. During labour they are usually painful and are accompanied by RETRACTION.

controlled cord traction a method of delivering the placenta and membranes, in which, once the placenta is known to have separated, the mid-

wife places the ulnar border of her left hand in the suprapubic region and gently pushes the contracted uterus upwards, while with her right hand she gains a firm hold on the cord and exerts gentle traction, following the curve of Carus. The membranes are eased out slowly and gently to avoid tearing them, which may lead to retained products. If active management of the entire third stage of labour is undertaken (i.e. an oxytocic drug is administered to facilitate separation of the placenta) it is *not* necessary to await signs of separation and descent before attempting controlled cord traction; however, if the placenta has been allowed to separate physiologically it is *imperative* to await these signs to avoid the risks to the mother of haemorrhage or even uterine inversion.

controlled drugs preparation subject to the Misuse of Drugs Act 1971, Misuse of Drugs (Notification of and Supply to Addicts) Regulations, 1973, and the Misuse of Drugs Regulations, 1985, which regulate the prescribing and dispensing of psychoactive drugs, including narcotics, hallucinogens, depressants and stimulants. A midwife requiring pethidine for use in the community applies to the local supervisor of midwives who issues a signed supply order form to enable the midwife to obtain the drug from the approved pharmacist. Unwanted controlled drugs may only be surrendered to an authorized person, i.e. the pharmacist who provided the drug or a medical officer, but not the supervisor of midwives. Destruction of controlled drugs is carried out by the midwife in the presence of an authorized person, i.e. a supervisor of midwives, pharmaceutical officer, regional medical officer, police officer or inspector of the Home Office Drugs Branch.

Controlled drugs obtained by a woman on prescription for home delivery belong, in law, to the woman. Midwives using controlled drugs in a hospital or institutional setting must locally agreed procedures and policies.

controlled trial a research method in which one group of subjects in a trial are not exposed to the experimental treatment or investigation, in an attempt to decrease the possibility of error and increase the possibility that the findings of the study are an accurate reflection of reality.

convulsions violent involuntary contractions of voluntary muscle. In a newborn baby the commonest causes are HYPOXIA, cerebral birth injury and HYPOGLYCAEMIA. In the mother they may be due to eclampsia, epilepsy or hysteria.

Cooley's anaemia an uncommon, severe type of anaemia found mainly in the Mediterranean races. Thalassaemia.

Coombs' test a test for detecting antibody in blood. *Direct C. t.* to detect antibody on red cell surfaces in umbilical cord blood. *Indirect C. t.* to detect free antibody in maternal blood.

copper cuprum. Symbol Cu. An element, minute quantities of which are essential to health.

Copper-7 an INTRAUTERINE CONTRACEPTIVE DEVICE containing copper wire embedded within the plastic shape.

co-proxamol *See* DEXTROPROPOXYPHENE HYDROCHLORIDE.

copulation sexual intercourse. Coitus.

cord *See* UMBILICAL CORD.

cordocentesis percutaneous umbilical blood sampling (PUBS); an invasive antenatal investigation to obtain a sample of fetal blood from the umbilical cord or intrahepatic vein, in the second or third trimester, under ultrasound guidance. It enables diagnosis of a variety of fetal conditions including genetic disorders, karyotyping in structural abnormality or intrauterine growth retardation, infections, haematological or biochemical status, certain chromosomal disorders and for clarification of ambiguous results from amniocentesis or chorionic villus biopsy.

cornea the transparent anterior part of the eyeball situated in front of the lens. It is covered by conjunctiva, and severe conjunctivitis may be associated with a spread of infection to the cornea, causing ulceration, scarring and impairment of vision. *See also* OPHTHALMIA NEONATORUM.

cornu a horn. The junction of uterus and fallopian tube. pl. *cornua*.

coronal suture the suture between the two frontal and the two parietal bones. *See* FETAL SKULL.

coronary encircling. *C. arteries* those which supply the heart. *C. thrombosis see* THROMBOSIS.

corpus body. *C. albicans* white body. The white scar left on the surface of the ovary following the retrogression of a corpus luteum. *C. luteum* literally, yellow body. The structure, first greyish and later yellow, which develops from the Graafian follicle after ovulation. In the menstrual cycle it lasts 12 days before degenerating. If pregnancy occurs it lasts about 14–16 weeks, i.e. until the placenta is formed and fully functioning. *C. uteri* the body of the uterus.

corpuscle a small body or cell, e.g. the blood cell.

corrosive an agent which destroys or eats into other substances.

cortex the outer layers of an organ, e.g. the cerebral hemispheres, kidney, suprarenal gland or ovary.

cortical necrosis irreparable damage to the renal cortex due to severe vasospasm of the arteries supplying the cortex, which can occur following any severe shock, especially after abruptio placentae.

corticoids the name given to a group of hormones secreted by the adrenal cortex.

corticosteroid any of the hormones produced by the ADRENAL cortex; also their synthetic equivalents. Called also adrenocortical hormone and adrenocorticosteroid. All the hormones are steroids having similar chemical structures, but quite different physiological effects. Generally they are divided into *glucocorticoids* (cortisol, or hydrocortisone; and cortisone and corticosterone), *mineralocorticoids* (aldosterone and desoxycorticosterone, and also corticosterone) and androgens.

cortisone one of several hormones known as CORTICOSTEROIDS or STEROIDS, produced from the adrenal cortex. It is anti-allergic and anti-inflammatory and is widely used in allergic states, e.g. asthma, rheumatoid arthritis, severe skin conditions and ulcerative colitis. Hydrocortisone has a similar action. Prednisone and prednisolone are synthetic forms of cortisone and hydrocortisone respectively.

coryza a cold in the head, with headache, watery discharge from the eyes and nasal catarrh.

costal pertaining to the ribs.

cot death See SUDDEN INFANT DEATH SYNDROME.

cotyledon a division or lobe. A lobe of the placenta.

counselling a generic term used to describe a process of consultation and discussion in which one individual, the counsellor, listens and enables the other, the client, to make appropriate decisions. The general aim is to help the client solve problems, increase awareness and promote constructive exploration of difficulties so that the future may be approached more confidently and more constructively.

couvade psychosomatic condition in which the father experiences symptoms of pregnancy and childbirth; common in many societies.

Couvelaire uterus the appearance of the uterus in severe concealed abruptio placentae (accidental haemorrhage), where the high tension in the uterus forces blood between the fibres of the myometrium, giving it a deep purplish-blue bruised appearance.

coxa hip joint. *C. valga* hip deformity in which there is an increase in the angle between the neck and the shaft of the femur. *C. vara* deformity in which there is a decrease in the angle between the neck and the shaft of the femur.

cracked nipple damage to the nipple may occur during breastfeeding if the baby is not fixed on the breast correctly, which puts undue pressure on a part of the nipple and areola and leads to soreness and ultimately bleeding. The condition can be prevented by teaching the mother how to position the baby at the breast correctly. Should damage occur the nipple may be too sore for the mother to continue feeding but mechanical expression of milk should be encouraged to stimulate lactation. Creams containing camomile or the application of moist camomile teabags may ease the discomfort and aid healing.

cramp painful spasmodic muscular contraction, common in pregnancy. It may be associated with vitamin B, calcium or salt deficiency and can be relieved by the intake of appropriate foods. Night cramps may be due to ischaemia of leg muscles and may respond to elevation of the foot of the bed.

cranial relating to the cranium. *C. nerves* the 12 pairs of nerves arising directly from the brain.

cranioclast an instrument rarely used now for crushing the fetal skull.

craniosacral therapy a form of osteopathic treatment in which very gentle manipulation of the cranium attempts to release tensions within the skull which are thought to be the cause of various problems. The therapy has been successfully used to treat babies fractious after difficult forceps or vacuum extraction deliveries, colic and hyperactivity in older infants.

craniostenosis premature closure of the cranial suture lines in an infant, which may require surgery to relieve raised intracranial pressure.

craniotomy the almost obsolete operation of perforation and extraction of the crushed fetal skull to allow vaginal delivery.

cranium the skull.

creatine a non-protein substance synthesized in the body from three amino acids; arginine, glycine (aminoacetic acid), and methionine. Creatine readily combines with phosphate, which is present in muscle, where it serves as the storage form of high-energy phosphate necessary for muscle contraction.

creatinine a nitrogenous compound formed as the end-product of creatine metabolism. It is formed in the muscle in relatively small amounts, passes into the blood and is excreted in the urine. A laboratory test for the creatinine level in the blood may be used as a measurement of kidney function. Since creatinine is normally produced in fairly constant amounts as a result of the breakdown of phosphocreatine and is excreted in the

urine, an elevation in the creatinine level in the blood indicates a disturbance in kidney function or an abnormal muscle-wasting process. To determine the creatinine clearance, urine is collected for 24 hours and the serum creatinine is measured by a venous blood sample. Thus the rate of creatinine excretion per minute can be calculated. This test may be carried out in cases of severe hypertension in pregnancy.

crèche a DAY NURSERY.

Credé's expression a manoeuvre to complete the separation of, and to expel, a partially separated placenta when severe postpartum haemorrhage occurs. It consists in massaging the uterus to make it contract, then squeezing it behind and in front of the fundus in an attempt to force the placenta down into the vagina, from which it is expelled. It is rarely performed, since it is intensely painful and shock-producing.

cretinism congenital thyroid deficiency. It causes arrested physical and mental development with dystrophy of bones and soft tissues. The child has a large head, short limbs, puffy eyes, a thick and protruding tongue, excessively dry skin, lack of coordination and mental handicap. The acquired or adult form of thyroid deficiency is MYXOEDEMA. Administration of thyroid extract, which must be administered for life, can result in normal growth and mental development.

cri du chat syndrome an hereditary congenital syndrome characterized by hypertelorism, microcephaly, severe mental deficiency, and a plaintive cat-like cry; due to the deletion of part of the short arm of chromosome 5.

cricoid ring-shaped. *C. cartilage* a ring-like cartilage forming the lower and back part of the larynx. Pressure on the cricoid cartilage during the induction of general anaesthesia occludes the oesophagus, thereby preventing acid reflux from the stomach. Cricoid pressure is maintained until the endotracheal tube is in position and the anaesthetist has checked that the seal provided by the cuff is effective.

criminal abortion termination of pregnancy performed outside the legal parameters of the 1967 Abortion Act. They are extremely dangerous and are associated with high mortality and morbidity.

cross-matching a procedure vital in blood transfusions and organ transplantation. The donor's erythrocytes or leucocytes are placed in the recipient's serum and vice versa. Absence of agglutination, haemolysis and cytotoxicity indicates that the donor and recipient are blood group compatible or histocompatible.

crown–rump length (CRL) this is measured in the first trimester to assess accurately the age of a fetus by a REAL-TIME SCANNER.

crowning the moment during birth when the suboccipitobregmatic and biparietal diameters of the fetal head are distending the vulval ring, and the head no longer recedes between contractions.

cryosurgery the use of a refrigerated probe to remove abnormal tissue such as a cervical erosion.

cryptomenorrhoea subjective symptoms of menstruation without flow of blood.

culture 1. the propagation of microorganisms or of living tissue cells in special media conducive to their growth. 2. a collective noun for the symbolic and acquired aspects of human society, including convention, custom and language. 3. a singular noun for the customs and

Section of Bony Female Pelvis

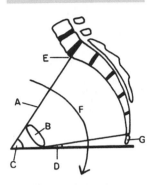

Curve of Carus and angles of inclination; A, plane of pelvic brim; B, symphysis pubis; C, angle of inclination of brim 55°; D, angle of outlet 5°; E, sacral promontory; F, curve of Carus; G, coccyx.

features of an ethnic (racial, religious or social) group.

curette a metal loop, which may be blunt or sharp, used for the removal of unhealthy tissues by scraping, or to obtain biopsy material. *Curettage* an operation, using a curette, which is commonly performed to remove the uterine endometrium.

curve of Carus an arc corresponding to the pelvic axis, being the route which the fetus must take on its passage through the birth canal. *See diagram.*

Cushing's syndrome overactivity of the adrenal cortex resulting in excess glucocorticoids governing carbohydrate metabolism, leading to obesity especially of the face ('moon face') and trunk. Amenorrhoea, hirsutism (*see* HIRSUTE) and weakness also occur.

cutaneous concerning the skin.

cyanocobalamin vitamin B$_{12}$, found in liver, eggs, fish. Essential for formation of erythrocytes and prevention of anaemia. Administered by injection in cases of pernicious anaemia.

cyanosis blueness of the skin and mucous membranes due to a deficiency of oxygen.

cyclopropane a gas used for general anaesthesia.

cyesis pregnancy. *Pseudocyesis* false pregnancy.

cyst a tumour with a membranous capsule and containing fluid. *Chocalate c.* of the ovary is associated with endometriosis. *Corpus luteum* or *luteal c.* is one which develops from the corpus luteum. It occurs in HYDATIDIFORM MOLE. *Dermoid c.* contains skin, hair, teeth, etc., and is due to abnormal development of embryonic tissue. *Multilocular c.* of the ovary is divided into compartments. *Papilliferous c.* of the ovary is lined with papillae which may grow through the cyst wall into the peritoneal cavity, and give rise to ascites. *Pseudomucinous c.* of the ovary contains fluid similar to mucin. In pregnancy the presence of an ovarian cyst should be diagnosed early. It is generally removed about the middle of pregnancy. It might otherwise interfere with the normal course of labour or become malignant.

cystic fibrosis also known as mucoviscidosis or fibrocystic disease of the pancreas. A disease with an autosomal recessive inheritance, in which the mucus-secreting glands of the body secrete an unusually thick tenacious mucus. This causes fibrosis in

Cystocele

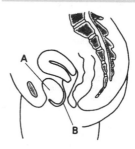

A, Bladder; B, anterior vaginal wall.

the pancreas and MECONIUM ILEUS in the newborn. Later complications are repeated chest infections. The diagnosis is made by the serum immunereactive trypsin (IRT) test. A sweat test, if carried out, shows a raised level of sodium chloride. A raised ALBUMIN level in the meconium may also be significant. One individual in 25 is a genetic CARRIER of the disease and in Britain one individual in 2000 is affected.

cystitis inflammation of the bladder.

cysto- a prefix relating to the bladder.

cystocele a hernia of the bladder into the vagina, as a result of damage to the pelvic floor during childbirth. *See* COLPORRHAPHY.

cystoscope an instrument for inspecting the interior of the bladder.

cystoscopy inspection of the interior of the bladder with a cystoscope.

cystotomy incision of the bladder, e.g. for the removal of calculi.

cyto- pertaining to cells.

cytogenetics a branch of GENETICS mainly concerned with the study of CHROMOSOMES.

cytology the science of the structure and functions of cells. Vaginal and cervical cytology are being applied increasingly in the early detection of abnormalities. In pregnancy, desquamated cells from the vaginal wall suggest hormone changes which reveal placental insufficiency and danger to the fetus. It is possible by cervical cytology to detect very early malignant disease in the genital tract, and, although this is not common in women of childbearing age, routine examination in antenatal, postnatal and family planning clinics has been recommended. Similar routine checks are advisable in gynaecological clinics, especially for women over 35.

cytomegalic inclusion disease an infection due to cytomegalovirus and marked by nuclear inclusion bodies in large infected cells. In the congenital form, there is HEPATO-SPLENOMEGALY with cirrhosis and microcephaly with mental or motor handicap. Acquired infection may cause a clinical state similar to infectious mononucleosis.

cytomegalovirus a virus found in the human salivary gland. Infection *in utero* may, rarely, cause cytomegalic inclusion disease in the newborn. The baby may be small for gestational age, and suffer from JAUNDICE with liver and spleen enlargement and THROMBOCYTOPENIA. MICROCEPHALY may also follow this disease.

cytoplasm all the protoplasm of a cell, excluding the nucleus.

cytotrophoblast the cellular layer of the trophoblast. Langhans' cell layer. It becomes much less obvious after 19–20 weeks of gestation. *See also* CHORIONIC VILLI.

D

dactyl a finger or toe.

dai *See* TRADITIONAL BIRTH ATTENDANT.

Danol a preparation of danazol, an anterior pituitary suppressant.

Data Protection Act 1984 this act, which came into force in 1984, gives people the right to know what information is held about them on computer, including health-related data. The Data Protection (Subject Access Modification) (Health) Order 1987 restricted access to health information which might cause serious physical or mental harm to an individual or reveal the identity of another person. The Act did not apply to manual records and in 1990 the Access to Health Records Act was passed to enable people to have access to any computerized or manual health-related records made after 1991. Patients and clients must apply to gain access to their records; the same exceptions to access as in the original Data Protection Act remain.

database information collected, stored, reviewed and updated; used for evaluation and audit or as a research resource. *See* Appendix 13.

day nursery a centre for the care, during the daytime, of children up to the age of 5 years. Provided by the Social Services Department or by voluntary agencies. Priority is given to children from 'at risk' families and to those with a handicap.

deafness lack or loss, complete or partial, of the sense of hearing. Total deafness is quite rare but partial deafness is common. A great many cases of congenital deafness are caused by infectious diseases, especially viral infections, contracted by the mother during pregnancy. Of these, rubella is the most common.

death the cessation of all physical and chemical processes that occurs in all living organisms or their cellular components. *Brain d.* the diagnosis of clinical brain stem death is governed, in the UK, by a set of guidelines ratified by the Medical Royal Colleges and their Faculties. *Cot d.* sudden infant death syndrome (SIDS). *D. certificate* a certificate issued by the registrar for deaths after receipt of a preliminary certificate completed and signed by an attending doctor, indicating the date and probable cause of death. Only after issue of this certificate, indicating that the death has been registered, can burial or cremation take place. *D. grant* a payment made by social security from the social fund which is payable to low income families only. This payment is recoverable from the estate of the deceased. *D. rate* the number of deaths per stated number of persons (100 or 10 000 or 100 000) in a certain region in a certain time period.

decapitation severing the head from the body. A destructive operation occasionally employed in obstructed labour.

decidua the pregnant endometrium. It is thickened and more vascular, to

Decidua

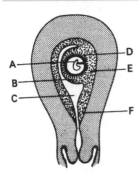

Sixth week of pregnancy.
A, Embryo; B, capsular decidua;
C, uterine cavity; D, chorionic villi;
E, basal decidua; F, true decidua.

receive and provide for the nutrition of the fertilized ovum. It is shed when pregnancy terminates. *D. basalis* the part on which the ovum rests and which covers the maternal surface of the placenta. *D. capsularis* that part covering the ovum as it projects into the uterine cavity. *D. vera* the true lining of the uterus, which for the first 12 weeks of pregnancy is not in contact with the ovum.

decidual cast the expulsion of the decidua intact, in the shape of the uterine cavity, following the death of the ovum in an ectopic pregnancy. *See* ECTOPIC GESTATION.

decompensation inability of the heart to maintain adequate circulation; it is marked by dyspnoea, venous engorgement, cyanosis and oedema.

deep transverse arrest obstruction of the fetal head during the second stage of labour. It results from an occipitoposterior position in the first stage but an attempt by the fetus to turn into an anterior position (long rotation) fails and the head becomes caught between the ischial spines of the pelvic outlet, especially if they are prominent. Kjelland's forceps delivery or manual rotation followed by Wrigley's forceps delivery will be required to release the head from the obstruction. The baby is likely to have excessive moulding and should be observed for signs of intracranial damage.

deep vein thrombosis a blood clot in a vessel which can become life-threatening if it occludes the vessel completely, for example in the coronary arteries causing heart attack, or in the cerebral vessels causing cerebrovascular accident. The thrombosis may also move from its original site to another, causing problems elsewhere, e.g. pulmonary embolism. In the puerperium mothers are at risk of deep vein thrombosis due to the changes in clotting factors occurring at term to prevent excess haemorrhage. Midwives are responsible for daily examination of the mother, including observing the legs for signs of thrombosis.

defecation evacuation of the bowels.

defibrillation termination of atrial or ventricular fibrillation, usually by electric shock.

deficiency disease condition caused by dietary or metabolic deficiency.

deflexion a fetal attitude in which the head is not flexed, or only partially flexed, as may occur in occipitoposterior positions of the vertex.

degeneration a structural change which lowers the vitality of the tissue in which it takes place. *Fatty d.*

63

fat is deposited in tissues. *Red d. See* NECROBIOSIS.

dehiscence a bursting open or rupture. Commonly applied to the rupture of an abdominal wound following surgery; also refers to the rupture of the Graafian follicle at the point of ovulation.

dehydration excessive loss of fluid from the body or failure to take sufficient fluid to balance loss. The term usually means actual dehydration together with the ketoacidosis which often accompanies it. It occurs in severe vomiting in pregnancy and in prolonged labour. The skin is dry and inelastic, the tongue is dry and the eyes are sunken. The breath may smell of acetone, and the urine is scanty and contains ketone bodies. The electrolyte balance and the reaction of the blood are disturbed. Dehydration with ketoacidosis in the mother is dangerous to the fetus. It is treated by giving intravenous dextrose, with saline if the urinary chlorides are much diminished. In babies, dehydration fever may occur if insufficient fluid is taken. Severe dehydration is usually caused by diarrhoea; the fontanelle is depressed, skin turgor poor and weight loss occurs. This condition can be corrected orally if mild, or intravenously if severe.

delay in labour unusual prolongation of any one of the three stages of labour, especially of the first stage. In the first stage diagnosis of prolonged labour is usually made via the partogram. Average rates of cervical dilatation show two phases: latent and active. The latent phase lasts until the cervix is fully effaced and 2–3 cm dilated; in the active phase the rate in a primigravida is normally classified as 1 cm per hour, and in a multipara as 1.5 cm per hour. If the partogram is used, it can be seen at a glance if the rate of cervical dilatation is lagging behind the expected rate; if the lag is two hours or more, action to augment labour may be taken. *See* AUGMENTATION OF LABOUR.

In the second stage of labour, the usual duration is 30–120 minutes in a nullipara and 10–60 minutes in a multipara. However, time limits are not adhered to rigidly as long as the fetal and maternal conditions remain satisfactory and gradual progressive descent of the presenting part is being made.

The third stage of labour, when managed physiologically, may last anything up to 2 hours, although actively managed third stage may be as short as 5 minutes. Delay in separation and expulsion of the placenta may require a manual removal of the placenta and membranes to be carried out.

deletion in genetics, loss from a chromosome of genetic material.

delirium a mental disturbance of relatively short duration usually reflecting a toxic state, marked by illusions, hallucinations, delusions, excitement, restlessness and incoherence. Almost any acute illness accompanied by a very high fever can bring on delirium.

delivery natural expulsion or extraction of the child, placenta and fetal membranes at birth. *Abdominal d.* delivery of an infant through an incision made into the uterus through the abdominal wall (CAESAREAN SECTION). *Instrumental d.* delivery facilitated by the use of instruments, particularly forceps. *Spontaneous d.* delivery occurring without assistance of forceps or other mechanical aid. *Vaginal d.* complete expulsion of the baby, placenta and membranes via the birth canal. Normally the head comes first presenting by the vertex. Breech delivery is also possible.

demand feeding feeding when the baby appears hungry and not according to a fixed timetable. Sometimes called 'on demand' feeding or baby-led feeding.

demography the statistical science dealing with populations, including matters of health, disease, births, and mortality.

denaturation test Singer's test; a blood test to distinguish fetal from maternal blood.

denidation the degeneration and expulsion during menstruation, of certain epithelial elements, potentially the nidus of an embryo. The term used to describe the intended shedding of uterine lining when postcoital contraceptive pills are used.

Denis Browne splint a special boot designed for the correction of TALIPES.

denominator in obstetrics, a particular point on the presenting part of the fetus used to indicate its position in relation to a particular part of the mother's pelvis. In a vertex presentation the denominator is the occiput, in a breech presentation it is the sacrum, and in a face presentation the mentum or chin.

dental care See Appendix 12.

dental caries decay of teeth.

dentition teething. *Primary d.* cutting of the temporary or milk teeth, beginning at the age of 6 or 7 months and continuing until the end of the second year. A full set consists of 8 incisors, 4 canines and 8 premolars; 20 in all. *Secondary d.* appearance of the permanent teeth, beginning at 6 or 7 years and complete by 12 to 15 years, except for the posterior molars or 'wisdom teeth' which appear between the ages of 17 and 25.

There are 32 permanent teeth: 8 incisors, 4 canines, 8 premolars or bicuspids, and 12 molars.

deoxygenated deprived of oxygen. *D. blood* blood which has lost much of its oxygen in the tissues and is returning to the lungs for a fresh supply.

deoxyribonucleic acid (DNA) a nucleic acid of complex molecular structure occurring in cell nuclei as the basic structure of the GENES. DNA is present in all body cells of every species, including unicellular organisms and DNA viruses. DNA is the molecule that directs all the activities of living cells, including its own reproduction and perpetuation in generation after generation.

Department of Health (DH) the body responsible for administering the National Health Service.

Department of Social Security (DSS) central government department responsible for administering social security matters, including national insurance scheme, income support, child support, welfare benefits and social services.

Depo-Provera See MEDROXYPROGESTERONE ACETATE.

depression 1. a lowering of the spirits. A mood change experienced as sadness or melancholy. *Endogenous d.* occurs in the course of manic-depressive psychosis. The mood change is associated with slowing of thought and action and feelings of guilt. *Reactive d.* depression occurring as a result of some event which influences the person unfavourably. Either type may occur in the puerperium and usually starts in the first 2 weeks after delivery, but develops gradually. Early recognition and treatment with support, psychotherapy and often antidepressant drugs are required for those less severely disturbed. Mothers with severe depressive illness are treated in a psychiatric hospital, preferably a mother and baby unit where antidepressant drugs and sometimes ECT are necessary. About 60% of postnatal women experience the 'blues' on or around the fifth day after delivery. This normally lasts only a day or so, the mother quickly responding to emotional support and reassurance. 2. a dip, felt on palpation.

dermoid cyst a tumour consisting of a fibrous wall lined with stratified epithelium containing pulpy material in which epithelial elements such as hair are found.

descent a downward movement, e.g. of the fetus. During labour the fetus must descend through the brim, cavity and outlet of the pelvis in order to be born. The descent may be measured in fifths.

desquamation the shedding of the superficial cells from the epithelium of any part of the body.

destruction of controlled drugs should a midwife need to destroy controlled drugs which have been obtained through a supply order procedure, she should do this in the presence of an 'authorized' person: a supervisor of midwives in England, Wales and Northern Ireland, a Regional Pharmaceutical Officer in England, a Pharmaceutical Adviser for the Welsh Office, a Chief Administrative Pharmaceutical Officer of Health Boards in Scotland, a Northern Ireland Department of Health inspector appointed under the Misuse of Drugs Act 1971, Regional Medical Officers in England, Scotland and Wales, an inspector of the Pharmaceutical Society of Great Britain, a police officer or an inspector of the Home Office Drugs Branch.

detoxication the process of neutralizing toxic substances. A function of the liver.

detrusor a general term for a body part, e.g. a muscle, that pushes down.

development the process of growth and differentiation.

developmental pertaining to development. *D. anomaly* absence, deformity, or excess of body parts as a result of faulty development of the embryo. *D. milestones* significant behaviours which are used to mark the process of development, e.g. sitting, walking, talking, etc. *D. tests* a standard series of tests performed on children to assess their development.

dexamethasone a synthetic glucocorticoid used primarily as an anti-inflammatory agent in various conditions, including diseases and allergic states; it is also used in a screening test for the diagnosis of CUSHING'S SYNDROME. Dexamethasone is given to some women prior to preterm delivery because of the suggestion that it accelerates the maturation of the fetal lungs and therefore reduces the incidence of respiratory distress syndrome.

dextran a polysaccharide preparation used as a plasma substitute in the treatment of shock. Its advantages are: (*a*) that it restores the circulatory volume; (*b*) it does not leak out of the blood vessels in the same way as physiological saline; (*c*) it can be used when blood grouping is not possible; and (*d*) it carries no risk, as does genuine plasma, of viral infections.

dextropropoxyphene hydrochloride oral analgesic. Safety in pregnancy has not been established. May be addictive, especially if taken with alcohol.

Descent of the Fetal Head into the Pelvis

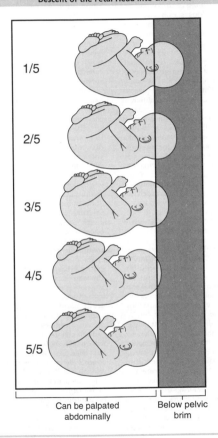

1/5

2/5

3/5

4/5

5/5

Can be palpated
abdominally

Below pelvic
brim

dextrose glucose. A monosaccharide. The simplest form of carbohydrate.

diabetes insipidus a rare disease of deficiency in secretion of the antidiuretic hormone of the posterior lobe of the pituitary gland. It is characterized by polyuria and consequent dehydration and thirst. Treated by the administration of vasopressin.

diabetes mellitus a familial disease of deficient secretion of insulin from the islet cells of the pancreas or increased resistance to the action of insulin, possibly caused by anterior pituitary growth hormone. Insulin resistance increases during pregnancy and gestational diabetes may develop. Pregnancy has a diabetogenic influence because of the increased metabolic workload and insulin resistance. However, this occurs only in women who have a genetic predisposition to the disease. The symptoms are polyuria, weight loss, thirst and lassitude. There is hyperglycaemia and later ketosis which may be severe enough to cause coma. Diabetes may be insulin dependent, in which the glucose tolerance test is abnormal and the woman exhibits the signs and symptoms of the disease; non-insulin dependent, when there is an abnormal glucose tolerance test but no signs and symptoms; gestational, with an abnormal glucose tolerance test due to the stress of pregnancy, which reverts to normal following delivery – these women often develop clinical diabetes in later life. Some women are also more at risk of developing diabetes, such as those who have had a previous baby weighing more than 4.5 kg; an unexplained stillbirth or neonatal death; and those with a close family history of diabetes.

Possible complications of diabetes during pregnancy include infections, pregnancy-induced hypertension, polyhydramnios, ketoacidosis; and fetal abnormalities, death or hypoxia, large fetus leading to cephalopelvic disproportion and birth trauma; neonatal hypoglycaemia or respiratory distress syndrome.

Care in pregnancy and labour is usually shared between the obstetrician and the physician to ensure close monitoring of mother and fetus. If problems arise the baby may be delivered early by caesarean section; otherwise hospital delivery with careful observation of the blood sugar levels is carried out. This should be continued postnatally when the mother's insulin requirements fall sharply. Extra carbohydrate is required if the mother is breastfeeding.

diabetic pertaining to diabetes. *D. coma* loss of consciousness occurring as a result of severe ketosis.

diabetogenic inducing diabetes. Pregnancy can, in susceptible women, induce a diabetic state which is usually temporary but which may recur in subsequent pregnancies and in later life.

diacetic acid acetoacetic acid, a colourless compound found in minute quantities in normal urine and in abnormal amounts in the urine of diabetic women and of those who have excessive vomiting.

diagnosis determination of the nature of a disease. *Clinical d.* is made by study of actual signs and symptoms. *Differential d.* the patient's symptoms are compared and contrasted with those of other diseases. *Tentative d.* a provisional one judged by apparent facts and observations. Denoted by the symbol $\triangle$.

diagonal conjugate an internal measurement of the pelvis, taken from the promontory of the sacrum to the lower border of the symphysis pubis; it should measure 12.5 cm in a normal pelvis. By subtracting 1.3 cm from the measurement, the true conjugate can be estimated. In practice, the examining finger cannot as a rule reach the sacral promontory unless the pelvis is unusually small, and in normal cases the true conjugate is inferred to be of average size because the promontory is not felt, i.e. is out of reach.

dialysis the passage of salts, water and metabolites through a semipermeable membrane. *Renal d.* the use of an artificial kidney. The patient's blood is separated from the dialysing fluid by the membrane, retaining blood cells and plasma proteins and losing the toxic substances normally excreted by the kidney.

diameter a straight line passing through the centre of a circle or sphere. The pelvic girdle is nearly circular at certain levels and the fetal skull is nearly spherical, hence a number of diameters are described in both. *See* FETAL SKULL *and* PELVIS.

diamorphine hydrochloride heroin. A powerful analgesic and drug of addiction.

diaphragm the muscular dome-shaped partition separating the thorax from the abdomen. It is an important muscle of respiration, and, as such, it is one of the secondary forces in labour. When relaxed, the diaphragm is convex but it flattens as it contracts during inhalation, thereby enlarging the chest cavity and allowing for expansion of the lungs. In the second stage of labour the contraction of the diaphragm and abdominal muscles aids the

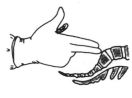

Measurement of the Diagonal Conjugate

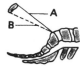

A, True conjugate; B, diagonal conjugate.

expulsive force of the uterine contractions. *Contraceptive d.* a device of moulded rubber or other soft plastic material, fitted over the cervix uteri to prevent entrance of spermatozoa.

diaphragmatic hernia protrusion of any or part of an abdominal organ through the diaphragm into the thoracic cavity.

diaphysis the shaft of a long bone.

diarrhoea the frequent passage of loose stools. It is usually caused by infection. In the neonate it is dangerous, as the baby may become rapidly dehydrated, with a disturbed electrolyte balance. If caused by infection it is very dangerous in a maternity unit, as it is rapidly transmitted. *See also* ESCHERICHIA COLI.

diastole the resting stage of the cardiac cycle. Following atrial and ventricular SYSTOLE the cardiac muscle is now in a state of relaxation.

diastolic murmur an abnormal sound produced during diastole, and occurring in valvular disease of the heart.

diastolic pressure the pressure of blood in the arteries during the resting stage of the heart. *See* BLOOD PRESSURE.

diathermy the use of high-frequency electrical currents as a form of physiotherapy and as a coagulative, cutting and haemostatic agent in surgical procedures. The term diathermy is derived from the Greek words *dia* and *therma*, and literally means 'heating through'. Surgically it is commonly used to treat neoplasms, warts, infected tissues and to cauterize blood vessels to prevent excessive bleeding. In obstetrics and gynaecology it is often used to treat cervical lesions. *See also* CRYOSURGERY.

diazepam a benzodiazepine tranquillizer used primarily as an anti-anxiety agent, and also used as a skeletal muscle relaxant, as an anticonvulsant for example, in eclampsia, as preoperative medication to relieve anxiety and tension, and in the management of alcohol withdrawal symptoms. May be given orally, intramuscularly or intravenously.

dicephalus a fetus or infant with two heads.

dichorial, dichorionic having two distinct chorions, said of dizygotic twins.

didactylism the presence of only two digits on a hand or foot.

didelphia the condition of having a double uterus.

didymitis inflammation of the testicle. Also called orchitis.

didymus a testis; also used as a word termination designating a fetus with a duplication of parts or one consisting of conjoined symmetrical twins.

diembryony the production of two embryos from a single egg.

dienestrol a synthetic oestrogen used in the treatment of atrophic vaginitis and kraurosis vulvae.

dietetics the branch of medical science concerned with diet, for both maintenance of health and cure of disease.

diethylstilbestrol a synthetic OESTROGEN.

dietician one who is concerned with the promotion of good health through proper diet and with the therapeutic use of diet in the treatment of disease.

differential making a difference. *D. blood count* comparison of the numbers of the different white cells present in the blood. *D. diagnosis See* DIAGNOSIS.

diffusion the passage of substances in solution into an area of weaker concentration through a semi-permeable membrane. Oxygen, carbon dioxide, some minerals and urea diffuse across the CHORIONIC VILLI of the placenta. More complex substances such as protein, lipids and carbohydrates are conveyed by active transport.

digestion the process by which food taken into the body is changed and rendered suitable for absorption into the blood.

digit a finger or toe.

digital pertaining to the finger or toe, usually the former, e.g. digital examination. An examination carried out with one or more fingers.

digitalis the active principle of the foxglove plant, *Digitalis purpurea*. It is used in congestive heart failure and atrial fibrillation to slow and strengthen the heart beat.

digoxin a drug obtained from the leaves of *Digitalis lanata*; used in the treatment of congestive heart failure.

dihydrocodeine tartrate oral and intramuscular analgesic. Side-effects include nausea, headaches vertigo. Should be avoided in asthmatics as it causes histamine release. Proprietary brand is DF 118.

dilatation stretching of either an orifice or, rarely, a hollow organ. It may be natural, as in the cervix during the first stage of labour, or artificial, as in that of the cervix preceding curettage of the uterine cavity.

dilator an instrument used to effect dilatation, e.g. HEGAR'S DILATORS.

dimenhydrinate an antiemetic preparation.

dimetria a condition characterized by a double uterus.

dimorphism the quality of existing in two distinct forms. *Sexual d.* 1. physical or behavioural differences associated with sex. 2. having some properties of both sexes, as in the early embryo and in some hermaphrodites.

diodone a contrast medium similar to iodoxyl, used in radiography.

diphtheria an acute, specific infectious disease caused by infection with *Corynebacterium diphtheriae* (Klebs–Loeffler bacillus). Highly dangerous prior to the introduction of diphtheria immunization. In the UK diphtheria toxoid is given in combination with tetanus toxoid and pertussis vaccine as 'triple-antigen' at 3 months, $4\frac{1}{2}$–5 months and $8\frac{1}{2}$–11 months of age. A booster dose of triple vaccine against diphtheria, tetanus and whooping cough is given just before the child starts school at the age of 5 years.

diphtheroids non-pathogenic corynebacteria resembling the bacilli of diphtheria, common COMMENSALS of the throat, nose, ear, conjunctiva and skin.

diplococci cocci found always in pairs. They may be encapsulated, e.g. pneumococci, or intracellular, e.g. gonococci. See GONOCOCCUS.

diploid the condition in which the cell contains two sets of CHROMOSOMES. In humans the diploid number is 46, i.e. 23 pairs.

diplosomatia a condition in which complete twins are joined at some of their body parts.

disability any restriction or lack (resulting from an impairment) of ability to perform an activity in the manner or within the range considered normal for a human being. *Developmental d.* a substantial handicap of indefinite duration, with onset before the age of 18 years, and attributable to mental handicap, autism, cerebral palsy, epilepsy, or other neuropathy.

disaccharide a carbohydrate formed of two simple sugar units. Examples are lactose in milk, sucrose and maltose. These may be broken down into MONOSACCHARIDES.

disc a circular or rounded flat plate. *Embryonic d.* a flattish area in a cleaved ovum in which the first traces of the embryo are seen. *Intervertebral d.* the layer of fibrocartilage between the bodies of adjoining vertebrae. *Prolapsed intervertebral d.* rupture of an intervertebral disc. Most commonly occurs in the lower back and occasionally in the neck.

discharge the flow of substances from the body. *Vaginal d.* in pregnancy is normal due to changes in hormone levels and vaginal pH. It should be white, mucoid and non-irritating. Profuse, offensive or irritating discharge should be investigated.

discoloration an alteration in the colour of the skin or mucous membranes. A bluish discoloration of the cervix and vagina is seen in early pregnancy and is known as Jacquemier's sign.

discus proligerus the compact mass of follicular cells surrounding the ovum before it is expelled from the Graafian follicle.

disease any abnormal condition which causes a local or general disturbance in the structure or function of the body.

disinfect to destroy micro-organisms but not usually bacterial spores, reducing the number of microorganisms to a level which is not harmful to health.

dislocation the displacement of a bone from its natural position. Some dislocations, especially of the hip, are congenital, usually resulting from a faulty construction of the joint.

displacement a movement to an unusual position. The non-gravid uterus normally lies in the centre of the pelvic cavity, anteverted and anteflexed. Retroversion and PRO-LAPSE are displacements.

disproportion lack of harmony or lack of a proper relationship between one object and another. *Cephalopelvic d.* disparity between the fetal head and the particular pelvis through which it is to pass. The fault lies either in the maternal pelvis, which is too small or abnormally shaped, or in the child's head, which is presenting by an unfavourable diameter, or is unusually large. It is recognized in the last 3 weeks of pregnancy by failure of the fetal head to engage, either spontaneously or on pressure. The degree of disproportion may be assessed accurately by means of X-rays or ultrasound. In minor degrees the action of the uterus in labour is sufficient to mould the fetal head through the pelvis, often with increased flexion, and labour may proceed without complication

to mother or child. This is anticipated in TRIAL LABOUR. In moderate and severe degrees, delivery is by caesarean section.

disseminated intravascular coagulation (DIC) widespread formation of thromboses in the microcirculation, mainly within the capillaries. It is a secondary complication of conditions which introduce coagulation-promoting factors into the circulation, such as abruptio placentae, retained dead fetus, amniotic fluid embolism and various types of infections and bacteraemias. Paradoxically, the intravascular clotting ultimately produces haemorrhage because of rapid consumption of fibrinogen, platelets, prothrombin and clotting factors, V, VIII and X. Treatment of DIC consists of replacement of the inadequate blood products and correction, when possible, of the underlying cause. When the primary condition cannot be treated, intravenous injections of heparin may inhibit the clotting process and raise the level of the depleted clotting factors.

distal situated away from the centre of the body or point of origin. Opposite of proximal.

Distalgesic *See* DEXTROPROPOXYPHENE HYDROCHLORIDE.

district general hospital a hospital equipped to provide a full range of specialist services to a natural catchment area.

diuresis increased secretion of urine.

diuretic a drug which increases the excretion of urine, e.g. furosemide (frusemide).

diurnal pertaining to or occurring during the daytime, or period of light.

dizygotic pertaining to or derived from two separate zygotes (fertilized ova). *D. twins* are more common than MONOZYGOTIC. Two ova are fertilized by two spermatozoa, and the fetuses may be the same or different sexes. There are two placentae, chorions and amnions. Sometimes termed binovular twins. *See also* MULTIPLE PREGNANCY.

Döderlein's bacillus a non-pathogenic lactobacillus occurring normally in vaginal secretions. Metabolism of glycogen within the squamous epithelium lining the vagina produces lactic acid. The resulting pH of 4.5 effectively counteracts the alkalinity of cervical mucus and proves hostile to pathogenic organisms.

dolichocephalic having a long head, where the anteroposterior diameter is increased.

domiciliary within or at home. *D. midwife* community-based midwife.

dominant inheritance the mode of inheritance by which one parent passes on a characteristic to the offspring. One of the pair of GENES carries the characteristic and is dominant over the other gene. There is a 1 in 2 chance of the offspring being affected, as in ACHONDROPLASIA. cf. RECESSIVE inheritance.

'domino' booking a plan of maternity care whereby a mother has her baby in a consultant unit, cared for by the community midwife. They return home any time after 6 hours following delivery. The name derives from *domi*ciliary midwife *in* and out.

donor one who gives. A blood donor is a person who gives blood for transfusion. A milk donor is one whose abundant lactation enables her to supply milk for a human milk bank.

dopamine an intermediate product in the synthesis of noradrenaline. It is a neurotransmitter in the central nervous system. Dopamine is administered intravenously to correct haemodynamic imbalance in shock syndrome.

Doppler ultrasound that in which measurement and a visual record are made of the shift in frequency of a continuous or pulsed ultrasonic wave proportional to the blood flow velocity in underlying vessels; used in diagnosis of occlusive vascular disease. It is also used in detection of the fetal heart beat and the velocity of blood across a stenotic heart valve.

dorsal concerning the back. *D. position* the woman lies on her back with her head and shoulders slightly elevated.

double-blind trial a test for the real effect of a new drug or treatment in clinical practice. Neither the patient nor the staff administering the treatment know which of two apparently identical treatments is the new one being tested.

double uterus abnormal development of the uterus resulting from failure of fusion of the Müllerian ducts. There are two uterine bodies with or without duplication of the cervix and/or the vagina. A cause of repeated miscarriages in some women; very occasionally two independent conceptions take place and implant into the two sections of the uterus; preterm labour is common.

douche 1. a stream or jet of water or other fluid applied to some part of the body. A vaginal douche of up to 5 litres of warm saline is occasionally used to provide hydrostatic pressure to distend the vagina and thus cause INVERSION OF THE UTERUS to revert to its normal position. 2. the apparatus used for a douche.

Douglas' pouch a pouch of peritoneum between the upper third of the vagina in front and the anterior wall of the rectum behind.

doula from the Greek word meaning 'woman who serves other women'; in maternity terms, one who provides emotional and practical support throughout pregnancy and labour. Doula birth companion training has been available in the UK since 1990, with a reduced training for qualified midwives, through the Birth and Bonding International organization.

Down's syndrome a chromosome abnormality, the commonest type having 47 instead of 46 chromosomes. The extra one is attached to the 21st pair, so that the condition is also called *trisomy 21*. This condition is associated with increasing maternal age. In the other form of Down's syndrome a translocation occurs, usually between chromosomes 14 and 21, as a *de novo* structural arrangement in the child, although the parents have normal chromosomes. Alternatively the translocations may occur as a result of a similar translocated chromosome in the parents, in which case there is a 10% chance of the condition recurring in a further pregnancy. The child exhibits certain characteristics and has learning difficulties. The child has slanting eyes, broad flat nose, brachycephaly, a short neck with loose skin, and HYPOTONIA. The hands are broad, with a single palmar crease. A third fontanelle is often present, as well as BRUSHFIELD'S SPOTS in the iris. Many of these individuals have other congenital abnormalities, i.e. congenital heart disease, and may not survive infancy. These children are often friendly and affectionate and benefit from special education.

drainage tube a tube inserted into a cavity, wound or infected area, to allow the exit of excess fluids or purulent material.

dramatherapy the therapeutic use of drama, in which clients are encouraged to act out their feelings in order to overcome problems. Has been used successfully in cases of infertility.

draught reflex *See* MILK FLOW MECHANISM.

drepanocyte sickle cell.

drepanocytosis occurrence of drepanocytes (sickle cells) in the blood.

dressing the covering applied to a wound surface.

Drew–Smythe cannula an S-shaped metal CATHETER designed for introduction into the birth canal to pass into the cervical os past the fetal head. The purpose is to puncture the hindwaters when the head is not engaged. It is rarely used now, as it can cause placental separation.

droplet infection the passage of pathogenic bacteria, conveyed during talking, coughing, sneezing, etc., in minute droplets, from the respiratory tract of an infected person.

drug 1. any medicinal substance. 2. a narcotic. 3. to administer a drug. *D. abuse* the use of one or more drugs for purposes other than those for which they are prescribed or recommended. *D. addiction* a state of periodic or chronic intoxication produced by the repeated consumption of a drug characterized by: (*a*) an overwhelming desire or need (compulsion) to continue use of the drug and to obtain it by any means; (*b*) a tendency to increase the dosage; (*c*) a psychological and usually a physical dependence on its effects; and (*d*) a detrimental effect on the individual and on society. *D. interaction* modification of the potency of one drug by another (or others) taken concurrently or sequentially. Some drug interactions are harmful and some may have therapeutic effects.

drugs in midwifery the need for drugs in midwifery can be divided into several categories: (*a*) Analgesia in labour. (*b*) Induction and acceleration of labour. (*c*) Management of haemorrhage. (*d*) Resuscitation. (*e*) Treatment of physiological and pathological disorders.

Dubowitz score a method used to assess gestational age in a low-birth-weight infant.

Duchenne's muscular dystrophy the childhood type of muscular dystrophy. 1. spinal muscular atrophy. 2. bulbar paralysis. 3. tabes dorsalis.

Ducrey's bacillus the organism which causes soft chancre (*Haemophilus ducreyi*).

duct (ductus) a tube or channel for conveying away the secretion of a gland.

ductus arteriosus a fetal blood vessel which bypasses the pulmonary circulation by connecting the pulmonary artery and the descending aorta, and which normally closes at birth. The umbilical vein travels in the cord to the fetus and divides into two branches, one of which is the *ductus venosus*, and this joins the inferior vena cava.

Duffy blood group a type of blood containing a rare antigen.

Dulco-lax *See* BISACODYL.

dunken *See* TRADITIONAL BIRTH ATTENDANT.

duodenum the first part of small intestine, from the pylorus to the jejunum. It is about 25–27 cm (10–11 in) in length. *Duodenal atresia* incomplete canalization of the duodenum. Projectile vomiting will occur as soon as the infant begins to be fed. Characteristically the vomitus contains bile.

dura mater the tough fibrous membrane lining the skull and forming the outermost covering of the brain and spinal cord. A double fold of the inner layer of dura mater, the falx cerebri, dips down between the cerebral hemispheres, and a horizontal fold, the tentorium cerebelli, separates the cerebellum from the cerebral hemispheres above. These two membranes carry the large venous sinuses which drain blood from the skull. They may be stretched and are sometimes torn during delivery, causing serious intracranial HAEMORRHAGE.

dural tap puncture of the dura mater, usually following regional anaesthesia, causing a leakage of cerebrospinal fluid. This causes a headache which may persist for about a week. Undue exertion and straining may cause further loss of cerebrospinal fluid so should be avoided.

duration of pregnancy duration averages 266 days from conception to delivery and 280 days (40 weeks or 9 months and 1 week) from the date of the last menstrual period to the date of delivery. If the woman knows the date of the first day of her last menstrual period, a useful calculation of the estimated date of delivery (EDD) can be obtained by adding 40 weeks. If the cycle is x days less than 28, the EDD will be x days earlier. Similarly, it will be 28 days plus x if the cycle is longer. About 67% of women may be expected to begin labour within a period of 7 days before or 7 days after the calculated date. Other symptoms of pregnancy, such as quickening, the size of the uterus and liquor studies, may be of value in determining the duration of a pregnancy. However, the most accurate method is by ultrasound. At 7–14 weeks the CROWN–RUMP LENGTH (CRL) is very accurate. A biparietal measurement between 13 and 20 weeks is as accurate as the CRL in the first trimester of pregnancy.

Dutch cap a contraceptive device. *See* DIAPHRAGM.

duty of care anyone who offers themselves as a skilled professional midwife, nurse or medical practitioner has an accepted duty to a patient or client irrespective of any contractual agreement existing between the parties. The law has developed a set of rules on the expected standard of care to assist in determining whether or not a professional has neglected their duty of care, based on the standards prevailing at the time of any case questioning the issue.

dydrogesterone an orally effective, synthetic progestin used mainly in the diagnosis and treatment of primary amenorrhoea and severe dysmenorrhoea, and in combination with oestrogen in dysfunctional menorrhagia.

dys- prefix meaning 'difficult', 'disordered' or 'painful'.

dysentery a notifiable intestinal infection characterized by severe diarrhoea, with the passage of blood or mucus and pus usually caused by a *Shigella* species or *Entamoeba histolytica*.

dyslexia impairment of ability to comprehend written language, due to a central lesion. adj. dyslexic.

dysmature a vague term commonly used to describe a baby who is small for gestational age.

dysmenorrhoea difficult or painful menstruation. It is characterized by cramp-like pains in the lower abdomen, and sometimes by headache, irritability, mental depression, malaise and fatigue.

dyspareunia difficult or painful coitus.

dyspepsia indigestion.

dyspnoea difficult or laboured breathing.

dystocia difficult or abnormal labour.

dystrophia literally, difficult or abnormal-growth. *Dystocia d.* **syndrome** a rare unfortunate obstetric sequence to which a certain type of woman is said to be prone. She is short, heavily built, subfertile, hirsute and often has pre-eclampsia. She has an android pelvis, an occipitoposterior position of the fetus with its many possible complications.

dysuria difficult or painful micturition.

E

early transfer the transfer home of mother and baby from a maternity unit within the early POSTNATAL PERIOD.

ecbolic oxytocic, i.e. makes uterine muscles contract.

ecchymosis effusion of blood beneath the skin, causing discoloration. Bruising.

echovirus a group of viruses (enteroviruses) isolated from humans which produce many different types of human disease, especially aseptic meningitis, diarrhoea and various respiratory diseases.

eclampsia a serious complication of pregnancy characterized by fits and accompanied by severe hypertension, oedema and proteinuria. adj. *eclamptic*. It is rare, with fits occurring occasionally towards the end of pregnancy, but more commonly during or shortly after labour. Fits are epileptiform, with a tonic phase of violent muscular spasm, rigidity, apnoea and cyanosis; a clonic phase with jerky, violent, uncontrollable movements; and a return to breathing with the risk of inhaling mucus or blood from the mouth or pharynx. A period of coma follows. Repeated fits are very dangerous for both mother and fetus. The mother may suffer cerebral haemorrhage, pulmonary oedema or renal or hepatic failure. Pneumonia may result from inhalation of debris. The fetus, already at risk of hypoxia, may die *in utero*, especially during the mother's apnoeic phase.

Prompt recognition and early treatment of pre-eclampsia should prevent all except the rare cases of sudden fulminating pre-eclampsia, with impending eclampsia.

If eclamptic fits occur, the doctor should be summoned urgently. The mother is laid on her side, an airway inserted if possible and oxygen administered until breathing resumes. Care should be taken to prevent the mother from harming herself during the violent phase.

Drugs such as intravenous magnesium sulphate or phenytoin to control the fits may be given. Hydralazine hydrochloride acts as a vasodilator, and diuretics may occasionally be given, although it is important to monitor fluid balance to avoid dehydrating the mother. Ergometrine is contraindicated. Once the fits are controlled, management consists of prevention of further fits until such time as delivery can be expedited. Often the mother goes into spontaneous labour, a factor which should be considered if she is strongly sedated, as signs of distress from contraction pain may be misinterpreted as the onset of more fits.

econazole an antifungal agent similar to clotrimazole or miconazole.

'ecstasy' methylenedioxymethamfetamine (MDMA) or 'E', One of the most widely used illicit drugs, a synthetic hallucinogenic amfetamine which comes in tablet and capsule form for oral or rectal use. As it is complex and expensive to produce the concentration of MDMA may vary from 2–200 mg and tablets and capsules may contain other substances such as caffeine, paracetamol or ketamine (an anaesthetic). MDMA inhibits reabsorption of serotonin so reduces brain reserves, affects moods and gives users boundless energy in the early stages. Prolonged use leads to loss of appetite, sweats, palpitations, insomnia, jaw stiffness, teeth grinding and a desire to urinate frequently. Eventually cardiac arrhythmias, hepatotoxicity, neurological and psychiatric damage occur. Hyperthermia is the most lethal effect, and disseminated intravascular coagulation, metabolic acidosis, hyperkalaemia and acute renal failure are associated with the thermoregulatory problems.

ecto- a prefix meaning 'outside'.

ectoblast the ectoderm.

ectocervix portio vaginalis.

ectoderm the outer germinal layer of the developing embryo from which the skin, external sense organs, mucous membrane of the mouth and anus and nervous system are derived.

-ectomy a suffix meaning 'cutting out', e.g. appendicectomy, hysterectomy.

ectopia abnormal position of any structure. *E. vesicae* an uncommon congenital defect of the abdominal wall in which the interior of the bladder is exposed.

ectopic gestation the embedding of a fertilized ovum, usually in the fallopian tube, but occasionally in the ovary, abdominal cavity, or rarely, in the cornu of the uterus, when it is termed an interstitial or angular pregnancy. The pregnancy usually terminates within 4–10 weeks due to tubal abortion, in which the gestation sac separates from the lining of

Ectopic Gestation

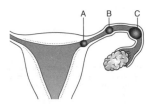

A, Interstitial (angular); B, isthmic; C, ampullar.

the tube and is carried to the peritoneal cavity by peristaltic action of the tube; slight vaginal bleeding occurs as the decidua is shed. Alternatively, tubal rupture occurs when the trophoblast has penetrated the fallopian tube more deeply. This causes severe pain, intraperitoneal or intraligamentary haemorrhage and profound shock. The woman needs an immediate blood transfusion and laparotomy to locate and ligate the bleeding vessels. The midwife's role involves management of the shock and haemorrhage until medical aid arrives, and follow-up support and care.

A few cases of abdominal pregnancy have been reported as having progressed almost to term and resulting in the birth of a live baby, delivered by laparotomy. The placenta, which is often adherent to a major abdominal organ such as the maternal liver, is left *in situ* to reabsorb slowly, over a period of months.

ectro- a prefix meaning miscarriage, congenital absence.

ectrodactyly congenital absence of all or part of a digit.

ectromelia gross hypoplasia or aplasia of one or more long bones of one or more limbs. adj. *ectromelic*.

ectrosyndactyly a condition in which some digits are absent and those that remain are webbed.

eczema a serious allergic skin condition. There are hereditary traits, and infantile eczema can be precipitated by giving cows' milk feeds. A mother with a family history of eczema, hay fever or asthma should be encouraged to breastfeed her baby totally, as even one complementary feed can induce these conditions.

Edwards' syndrome trisomy 18 syndrome. The baby is small for gestational age and has typical face, hands and feet and a shield-shaped chest. Most of these children have severe congenital heart disease and all are mentally retarded.

effacement 'taking up' of the cervix. The process by which the internal os dilates, so opening out the cervical canal and leaving only a circular orifice, the external os. This process precedes cervical dilatation, particularly in a nullipara whilst both occur simultaneously in a multigravida during labour.

efferent carrying outward, i.e. from the centre to the periphery. The *e. nerves*, also called motor nerves, obey impulses from the nerve centres of the brain.

effleurage a light, circular, stroking movement in massage. Abdominal effleurage in labour can act as a means of reducing the woman's perception of pain, as touch impulses reach the brain before pain impulses.

effusion the escape of blood or serum into surrounding tissues or cavities.

egg 1. an ovum; a female gamete. 2. an oocyte. 3. a female reproductive cell at any stage before fertilization and in derivatives after fertilization, and even after some development. *E. donation* the donor takes drugs to induce multiple ovulation; the ova are removed by laparoscopy, fertilized *in vitro* and then placed in the recipient's uterus.

Eisenmenger's syndrome large ventricular septal defect, overriding of the aorta and right ventricular hypertrophy. It is associated with a high maternal mortality.

ejaculation forcible, sudden expulsion; especially expulsion of semen from the male urethra, a reflex action that occurs as a result of sexual stimulation.

elective planned, as in elective caesarean section, when circumstances suggest that a surgical delivery is the only possibility for safe delivery of the baby, due to either the maternal or the fetal condition.

electrocardiogram (ECG) a tracing of the heart's action shown by electrical waves, used in the diagnosis of heart disease.

electrode a conductor through which electricity leaves its source to enter another medium. *Fetal scalp e.* an electrode applied to the fetal scalp to record the fetal condition.

electroencephalogram (EEG) a tracing of electrical waves from the brain. Epileptic patients show a characteristic abnormal pattern which has also been noted in some women with eclampsia.

electrolyte a substance which in solution dissociates into electrically charged particles (IONS), e.g. sodium bicarbonate, potassium chloride. Imbalance, e.g. from severe vomiting or renal failure, is diagnosed by examination of the serum.

electrophoresis the movement of charged particles suspended in a liquid or various media under the influence of an applied electric field.

The various charged particles of a particular substance migrate in a definite and characteristic direction – toward either the anode or the cathode – and at a characteristic speed. This principle has been widely used in the separation of proteins and is therefore valuable in the study of diseases in which the serum and plasma proteins are altered. The principle has also been applied in the separation and identification of various types of human haemoglobin.

eliminate to expel waste substances of the body; e.g. the kidney eliminates urea, the bowel eliminates the unabsorbed food products, the lungs eliminate carbon dioxide.

embolism the blocking of a blood vessel by a solid or foreign substance introduced into the circulation. *Air e.* air bubbles entering the circulation, possibly in vaginal or intrauterine douching in pregnancy. *Amniotic fluid e.* amniotic fluid with the substances it may contain entering the circulation; an occasional complication of labour. *Pulmonary e.* following labour in the event of pelvic or leg vein thrombosis, part of the clot is detached and travels in the blood stream until it is arrested in a branch of the pulmonary artery. Any large embolus will cause immediate death. A smaller embolus will cause the patient to collapse with pain in the chest, dyspnoea and cyanosis. Oestrogens appear to increase the risk of venous thrombosis, so that most authorities have abandoned their use to suppress lactation.

embolus a foreign particle or substance circulating in the blood, e.g. a detached portion of thrombus, a mass of bacteria, an air bubble or amniotic fluid.

embryo the developing offspring of viviparous animals before birth. The human embryo is usually so called for the first 8 weeks after conception, the term fetus being employed subsequently.

embryology the science of the development of the embryo.

embryonic plate that portion of the inner cell mass of the blastocyst from which the embryo itself is formed.

embryotomy cutting up the fetus to make delivery possible, occasionally necessary in neglected obstructed labour where there are no facilities for operative procedures. Extremely rare in modern obstetrics.

emergency a condition requiring immediate attention. The NMC Midwives' Rules state that 'A practising midwife shall not, except in an emergency, undertake any treatment which she has not been trained to give, either before or after registration as a midwife, and which is outside her sphere of practice'. *E. obstetric unit* an emergency team from a consultant obstetric unit which goes out to obstetric emergencies in the community or, in general practitioner units, taking the appropriate equipment, including O-negative blood for transfusion. *E. protection order* a court order whereby a child is arbitrarily removed from the care of its parents in the interests of his/her safety.

emetic a substance which induces vomiting. Examples are common salt in water, and apomorphine.

emmenagogue any substance which may induce menstrual bleeding.

empowerment the capacity to empower, to give power or authority. A recommendation of the 'CHANGING CHILDBIRTH' REPORT 1993 is that women should be empowered during pregnancy, labour and the puerperium to take control over their own care and to work in partnership with maternity care providers.

emulsion a mixture of minute particles of a fatty or oily substance suspended in fluid.

encephalins *See* ENKEPHALINS.

encephalitis inflammation of the brain. Viral encephalitis may be caused by such conditions as herpes simplex; it may also be caused by bacterial infections such as tuberculosis or syphilis, by fungal infections such as histoplasmosis and protozoal infections such as toxoplasmosis.

encephalocele hernia of the brain through a congenital or traumatic opening of the skull.

encephalopathy a non-specific term meaning diffuse disease or damage of the brain. *Wernicke's e.* an inflammatory haemorrhagic encephalopathy due to thiamine deficiency. It may be a complication of hyperemesis gravidarum.

encopresis incontinence of faeces, not due to organic defect or illness.

endemic pertaining to an infectious disease which, to a greater or lesser degree, is always present in the locality.

endo- a prefix meaning 'inside' or 'within'.

endocarditis inflammation of the endocardium or lining of the heart.

endocervicitis inflammation of the lining membrane of the cervix uteri, more commonly termed CERVICITIS.

endocervix the mucous membrane lining the cervical canal.

endocrine secreting within. Applied to those glands whose secretions (hormones) pass directly into the blood stream.

endoderm entoderm.

endogenous originating inside the body. In puerperal sepsis, inside the birth canal.

endometriosis tissue resembling endometrium, and functioning similarly, developing outside the uterus. Chocolate cyst of the ovary contains some endometrial material.

endometritis inflammation of the endometrium, or lining of the uterus.

endometrium the mucous membrane lining the body of the uterus.

endorphins a group of opiate-like peptides produced naturally by the body at neural synapses at various points in the central nervous system pathways where they modulate the transmission of pain perceptions. Endorphins raise the pain threshold and produce sedation and euphoria; the effects are blocked by naloxone, a narcotic antagonist.

endoscope an instrument, fitted with a light, used to inspect hollow organs and structures. CYSTOSCOPES and LAPAROSCOPES are examples.

endotoxic shock a rare condition associated with septicaemia caused by Gram-negative organisms, especially *Escherichia coli* and *Clostridium welchii* and, more recently, betahaemolytic streptococcus. The endotoxins released from the bacteria are thought to cause widespread dilatation of arterioles in liver, lungs and other organs, so that diminished venous return causes profound shock. The signs are similar to hypovolaemic shock but sometimes rigors occur also. Urgent administration of appropriate antibiotics is required.

endotracheal within the trachea. *E. tube* an airway catheter inserted in the trachea during endotracheal intubation to assure patency of the upper airway and enable removal of secretions. Endotracheal intubation is carried out for resuscitation purposes, when it may be accompanied by cardiac massage, and also during general anaesthesia. In the latter case a 'cuffed' tube is used which protects the lungs because, when inflated, it prevents any regurgitated gastric fluid from passing the 'cuffed' area and entering the lungs.

enema an injection of fluid into the rectum.

energy (calorie) requirement every bodily process – the building up of cells, motion of the muscles, the maintenance of body temperature – requires energy, and the body derives this energy from the food it consumes. Digestive processes reduce food to usable 'fuel' which the body 'burns' in the complex chemical reactions that sustain life. The amount of energy required for these chemical processes varies. A woman during pregnancy requires about 2500 Cal (625 kJ) per day. Excess energy foods are stored as fat. This fat provides a supplementary source of energy if the diet is inadequate.

engagement the entry of the presenting part of the fetus, generally the head, into the true pelvis. A head is said to be engaged when its greatest presenting transverse diameter, the BIPARIETAL DIAMETER, has passed the plane of the pelvic brim. In a primigravida the fetal head usually becomes engaged after the 36th week of pregnancy; in a multigravida it is usually later and may not occur until after the onset of labour.

engorgement of the breasts painful accumulation of secretion in the breasts, often accompanied by lymphatic and venous stasis and oedema at the onset of lactation. Early on-demand breastfeeding with the baby correctly positioned at the breast should be encouraged to prevent engorgement. A natural means of relieving breast engorgement is the application of cabbage leaves. Dark green cabbage leaves are wiped (not washed) and cooled in the refrigerator. Leaves are applied over the breasts; when they become wet, often within seconds, they are replaced with dry leaves. This process is repeated until relief is obtained. A firm supporting brassiere or breast binder may be helpful but care should be taken not to create pressure on the oedematous tissue.

enkephalin either of two naturally occurring pentapeptides isolated from the brain, which have potent opiate-like effects and probably serve as neurotransmitters. They are classified as ENDORPHINS.

ensiform cartilage the lowest part of the sternum, the xiphisternum, used as a marker when undertaking antenatal abdominal examination, to estimate the gestation.

enteritis intestinal infection. *See* DYSENTERY.

entoderm those cells in the inner cell mass which line the yolk sac and which later develop into the epithelium of the alimentary tract, trachea, bronchi, bladder and urethra.

Entonox nitrous oxide and oxygen, 50% of each, premixed in one cylinder and used as an analgesic. The Entonox apparatus, which is approved by the Nursing and Midwifery Council for use by midwives as a means of administering analgesia in labour, is attached to a cylinder of oxygen and nitrous oxide; the cylinder is blue with a white collar. The mother controls the amount of gas received by inhaling as required, either through a face mask or a mouth piece.

enuresis involuntary micturition; bedwetting. Causes may be psychological, neurological or pathological.

environmental health the concept that the health of any individual can be affected by his or her environment. Levels of pollution and poor housing are two instances of factors which can affect health.

environmental health officer the person employed by the local authority to improve and regulate environment and to enforce statutory regulations. Responsibilities include housing, food hygiene and refuse collection, and also infestation, air pollutants and noise. Some authorities employ several officers, each specializing and responsible to a chief officer.

enzyme a biological catalyst, i.e. a substance present in small amounts that brings about a chemical reaction; e.g. milk sugar (lactose) is broken down by the enzyme lactase in the small intestine to form GLUCOSE and GALACTOSE.

eosin a red stain used in identifying cells and bacteria.

eosinophil a white blood cell in which the granules can be stained red with eosin.

Epanutin *See* PHENYTOIN SODIUM.

ephedrine an adrenergic alkaloid; used as a bronchodilator, antiallergic, central nervous system stimulant in narcolepsy, mydriatic and pressor agent.

epicanthus a vertical fold of skin on either side of the nose, sometimes covering the inner canthus (junction of eyelids). Prominent in certain races and in infants with Down's syndrome.

epidemic a situation in which any disease has attacked a large number of people at one time.

epidemiology the study of the distribution of factors determining health and disease in human populations, and the application of this study to the prevention and control of disease.

epidermis the non-vascular outer layer or cuticle of the skin.

epidermolysis bullosa a severe, usually fatal, skin disorder characterized by a profusion of fluid-filled blisters resembling PEMPHIGUS NEONATORUM. It is inherited as an autosomal RECESSIVE trait.

epididymis an elongated, cord-like structure along the posterior border of the testis, whose coiled duct provides for the storage, transport and maturation of spermatozoa.

epidural analgesia also known as extradural or peridural anaesthesia. A form of pain relief for both first and second stages of labour, obtained by the injection of a local analgesic, e.g. BUPIVACAINE, into the epidural space in order to block the spinal nerves. It may be approached by two routes: (*a*) caudal, through the sacrococcygeal membrane covering the sacral hiatus, or (*b*) lumbar, through the intervertebral space and ligamentum flavum. Indications for epidural analgesia include prolonged labour, particularly when the occiput is posterior, breech labour and delivery; certain forceps deliveries; to reduce hypertension in cases of pre-eclampsia or eclampsia; multiple or preterm delivery; caesarean section; maternal cardiac or respiratory disease; client preference.

Dangers of epidural analgesia include sudden hypotension leading to fetal hypoxia; spinal or dural tap; toxic reactions to the drug; neurological sequelae from injury or haematoma; higher risk of instrumental delivery due to poor head flexion as a result of the relaxed pelvic floor; infection. The mother should have an intravenous infusion commenced as a means of immediate treatment in the event of a problem. She should be cared for in a position which will not lead to postural hypotension. The midwife should monitor the maternal blood pressure and fetal heart rate frequently, especially after the first dose of bupivacaine – given by the anaesthetist who inserts the epidural cannula – and after each 'top up', which midwives may be trained to administer. *See also* MOBILE EPIDURAL *and* SPINAL ANAESTHESIA.

epigastrium the upper and middle region of the abdomen, located within the sternal angle. adj. *epigastric*. In women with severe pre-eclampsia, pain in the epigastric region may herald the onset of ECLAMPSIA and is due to hepatic oedema and/or haemorrhage.

epiglottis the lid-like cartilaginous structure overhanging the entrance to the larynx.

epilepsy paroxysmal transient disturbances of nervous system function resulting from abnormal electrical activity of the brain. Anticonvulsive drugs are required to prevent convulsive seizures. These drugs may have a teratogenic effect on the fetus, most commonly affecting the lip, palate and heart. Maternal fits cause intrauterine hypoxia so must be controlled.

epileptiform resembling an epileptic fit, as in eclampsia.

epiphysis the end of a long bone from which in childhood the shaft is separated by a piece of cartilage. The appearance of ossification in the fetal epiphyses may give a rough guide to its maturity. pl. *epiphyses*.

episiorrhaphy repair of an EPISIOTOMY.

episiotomy an incision made into the thinned-out perineal body to enlarge the vaginal orifice during delivery. Prior to the incision the perineum should be infiltrated with local anaesthetic, usually lidocaine (lignocaine) 0.5% 10 ml or 1% 5 ml. The incision may be mediolateral or median (midline). There is evidence

Episiotomy

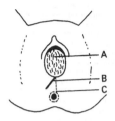

A, Fetal head; B, mediolateral incision; C, midline incision.

that the only justifiable indications for episiotomy are: 1. to expedite delivery in cases of fetal distress; 2. prior to an operative delivery such as forceps or ventouse extraction; 3. to minimize the risk of intracranial damage during preterm and breech delivery. The Nursing and Midwifery Council sanctions midwives to infiltrate the perineum, perform an episiotomy and repair perineal trauma, provided they have been instructed and have attained competence in these procedures.

epispadias a condition in which there is an abnormal urethral opening on the dorsal surface of the penis.

epistaxis nose bleeding.

epithelial tissue *See* EPITHELIUM.

epithelium a layer of cells covering all outer and lining all inner surfaces, including cavities, glands and vessels.

epsilon-aminocaproic acid an antifibrinolytic drug used to prevent the breakdown of FIBRIN by PLASMIN. It may be used in cases of severe abruptio placentae.

Epstein's pearls small white epithelial spots seen at the junction of the hard and soft palate.

Equal Opportunities Commission an *ad hoc* body set up in 1975 to help enforce the Sex Discrimination Act and the EQUAL PAY ACT 1970.

Equal Pay Act 1970 an Act which came into force in 1975 to eliminate discrimination between men and women with regard to their pay and conditions of employment.

Erb's paralysis paralysis of the upper arm due to injury, during birth, of the upper trunk of the brachial plexus nerves as they leave the spinal cord in the cervical region. A number of muscles are paralysed, so that the arm hangs medially rotated with the elbow extended and the wrist and fingers flexed. It results from traction on the child's neck, as in a breech delivery during the birth of the head or where there has been SHOULDER PRESENTATION prior to vertex delivery.

erectile having the power of becoming erect. *E. tissue* vascular tissue which, under stimulus, becomes congested and swollen, causing erection of the part, e.g. the nipple of the female breast.

ergometrine an alkaloid which is the active principle of ergot. A valuable oxytocic drug which is effective in preventing or controlling postpartum haemorrhage. It is very commonly used in conjunction with oxytocin as Syntometrine. If given intravenously, ergometrine acts in 45 seconds; intramuscular administration is effective in 7 minutes and gives a sustained uterine contraction. Secondary postpartum haemorrhage due to retained products of conception may be treated with oral ergometrine.

ergonomics scientific study of human beings in relation to their work and the effective use of human energy.

ergot a drug obtained from a fungus which grows on rye. It causes strong sustained contraction of muscle, especially of the uterus.

erosion of the cervix during pregnancy hormonal changes cause softening and an increase in HYGROSCOPIC qualities of the collagen connective tissue. This results in the columnar epithelium near the external os being drawn out to form a red zone around it known as an erosion. Many cervical erosions disappear after delivery.

erythema redness of the skin.

erythroblast an immature, nucleated red blood cell.

erythroblastosis fetalis a condition in which ERYTHROBLASTS are found in the neonatal circulation. More commonly called haemolytic disease of the newborn (HDN).

erythrocyte a red blood cell. A minute biconcave disc containing haemoglobin which acts as a carrier of oxygen. *E. sedimentation rate* the rate at which red blood cells settle at the bottom of a tube of blood. The normal rate is no more than 10 mm/hour; this is increased in infection and normal pregnancy to an average of 78 mm/hour.

erythromycin an antibiotic with an action similar to that of penicillin.

erythropoiesis the formation of red blood cells.

Esbach's albuminometer a graduated glass tube for estimating the approximate amount of albumin in urine.

Escherichia coli a Gram-negative bacillus (*see* GRAM STAIN) normally inhabiting the intestine. Pathogenic strains are the cause of many cases of urinary tract infections and of epidemic diarrhoeal diseases, especially in infants and children. If it enters the blood stream it may cause endotoxic shock.

essential hypertension persistently high blood pressure; cause unknown, but heredity a major predisposing factor. Diagnosis is made if the first trimester blood pressure is above 140/90 mmHg. During pregnancy the condition may worsen, remain static or improve. Antihypertensive drugs are used only with caution as they decrease renal and placental blood flow. Dangers are superimposed pre-eclampsia, ECLAMPSIA, ABRUPTIO placentae, subarachnoid haemorrhage, cardiac or renal failure. The fetus is at risk of placental insufficiency, producing a baby small for gestational age, or resulting in stillbirth.

essential oils highly concentrated substances extracted from plants and used in aromatherapy for their therapeutic properties resulting from the chemical constituents. They should always be diluted in carrier oil and rarely taken by mouth. Many essential oils are contra-indicated in pregnancy, labour and during breast feeding.

estimated date of delivery *See* EXPECTED DATE OF DELIVERY.

ethambutol a tuberculostatic agent.

ethics rules or principles which govern correct conduct, and personal and social values. Each practitioner, upon entering a profession, is also invested with the responsibility to adhere to the standards of ethical practice and conduct set by that profession. The Code of Professional Conduct for the Nurse, Midwife and Health Visitor, adopted by the NMC in 2000 provides guidance and advice for standards of practice and conduct that are essential for the ethical discharge of the practitioner's responsibility. Similarly, the Midwives' Code of Practice, provides guidance specifically related to the role of the midwife.

ethinylestradiol contraceptive pills containing oestrogen and progesterone. Usual dose is 30 μg. They can be commenced 3–4 weeks postpartum, but are contraindicated during the breastfeeding period.

ethnic pertaining to a social group which shares cultural bonds or physical (racial) characteristics. *E. minority* a social grouping of people who share cultural or racial factors but who constitute a minority within the greater culture or society.

ethnography study of the culture of a single race. Data are collected through observation, usually during a period of residence with the group being studied.

ethnomethodology a sociological theory which concentrates on the case study using participant or non-participant observation.

ethyl chloride a local anaesthetic applied topically to intact skin.

etiology *See* AETIOLOGY.

eugenics the study of measures which may be taken to improve future generations.

Eugynon 30, Eugynon 50 contraceptive tablets containing oestrogen and progesterone.

euphoria a feeling of well-being, not always justified by the circumstances.

eustachian tube the narrow tube which connects the tympanum (middle ear) with the nasopharynx.

eutocia normal labour, or childbirth.

evacuation an emptying; *e. retained products of conception* (ERPC) surgical emptying of the uterus to remove blood clots and placental tissue, in order to prevent or control severe uterine postpartum haemorrhage.

evaluation the fourth stage in a process approach to care, in which the effectiveness of care is judged.

eversion a turning inside out; to turn outward.

evidence-based practice systematic appraisal of clinical situations and use of contemporary research findings as a justification for clinical decision-making.

evisceration a destructive operation, rarely necessary nowadays, involving removal of the organs of the abdomen and thorax of a dead fetus where a tumour or gross ascites has delayed vaginal delivery.

evolution natural development; the process of unfolding or opening out. *Spontaneous e.* a rare delivery without obstetrical aid of a fetus in the transverse lie by shoulder presentation. The shoulder escapes first, the thorax, pelvis and limbs next, and finally the head. cf. Spontaneous EXPULSION.

ex- prefix meaning 'out of', 'outside', 'away from'.

exacerbation increase in the gravity or seriousness of disease symptoms.

exchange transfusion a method of TRANSFUSION in which a sample of blood is withdrawn from the patient and replaced by the same volume of donor blood. It is used in the newborn to treat severe hyperbilirubinaemia and anaemia, usually resulting from Rhesus incompatibility. It is sometimes called a replacement transfusion.

excreta any waste matter excreted from the body. Used chiefly of faeces, but applies also to urine, sweat, sputum, etc.

exercise in pregnancy women should be encouraged to continue gentle exercise to which they are accustomed, for as long as they feel comfortable. Many antenatal classes now include yoga, aerobics or aquanatal exercises. *See also* POSTNATAL EXERCISES.

exfoliation a falling off in scales or layers. adj. *exfoliative. Lamellar e. of newborn* a congenital hereditary disorder in which the infant is born completely covered with a parchment-like membrane that peels off within 24 hours, after which there may be complete healing, or the scales may reform and the process repeated. In the more severe form, the baby (harlequin fetus) is completely covered with thick, horny, armour-like scales, and is usually stillborn or dies shortly after birth. Called also ichthyosis congenita, ichthyosis fetalis, and lamellar ichthyosis of newborn.

exocrine 1. secreting externally via a duct. 2. denoting such a gland or its secretion.

exogenous of external origin.

exomphalos a herniation of the umbilicus of abdominal contents covered with peritoneum. A midwife must endeavour to avoid damage leading to sepsis by covering it with a sterile non-adhesive dressing and then a pad of cotton wool if medical aid is not immediately available.

exotoxin a potent toxin formed and excreted by the bacterial cell, and found free in the surrounding medium. Bacteria of the genus *Clostridium* are the most frequent producers of exotoxins; diphtheria, botulism, and tetanus are all caused by bacterial toxins.

expected date of delivery (EDD) it is calculated by counting forwards 9 months and adding 7 days from the first day of the last normal menstrual period or counting back 3 months and adding 7 days. Adjustments have to be made for a regular long cycle by adding days in excess of 28 days and in a regular short cycle by subtracting days less than 28.

expression pressing out. 1. pressure on the uterus to facilitate the expulsion of the placenta. *See* CREDÉ'S EXPRESSION. 2. mechanical or digital pressure on the areola to compress the lacteal sinuses so that milk is removed from the breast.

expulsion forcible driving out, e.g. of the fetus from the uterus. *Spontaneous e.* the manner in which a very small macerated fetus can be forced through the pelvis with the shoulder presenting so that the head and trunk are born together.

exsanguinate to deprive of blood, as after a severe haemorrhage.

extension drawing out, lengthening. The opposite of flexion. Used to describe certain movements in the mechanism of labour, e.g. that by which the head is normally born. The occiput of the head escapes under the pubic arch, and, forced downwards by the uterine contractions and forwards by the pelvic floor muscles, the head extends, pivoting under the symphysis pubis.

external os the opening from the cervical canal into the vagina.

external version a manoeuvre designed to convert a malpresentation to one which is more likely to result in a vaginal delivery. This may be turning a breech presentation to cephalic, or a transverse or oblique lie to a longitudinal lie, either a cephalic or breech presentation. Complications include true cord knots, placental abruption, fetal distress; in many cases the procedure is unsuccessful.

extra- prefix meaning 'outside'.

extracellular fluid fluid outside the cells.

extrauterine pregnancy embedding of the fertilized ovum outside the uterine cavity. Theoretically this could be in the abdominal cavity, ovary or fallopian tube. In fact, almost all cases of extrauterine pregnancy are of the tubal variety. Also termed ECTOPIC GESTATION.

extravasation the discharge or leaking of fluid from its normal channel into surrounding tissue, e.g. the escape of blood or lymph from a vessel.

extrinsic of external origin. *e. factor* a haematopoietic vitamin that combines with intrinsic factor for absorption and is needed for erythrocyte maturation; called also VITAMIN B_{12} and CYANOCOBALAMIN.

extubation removal of a tube used in intubation.

exudation the outward flow of a liquid or semi-liquid substance, e.g. of sebum from the sebaceous glands.

F

face in the fetus, that area extending from the mentum or chin to the supraorbital ridges, composed of 14 bones, fused together.

face presentation a cephalic presentation in which the spine and head of the child are extended and the face lies lowest in the pelvis. In a mentoanterior position labour may be uncomplicated and delivery spontaneous, especially in a multigravida with a small baby. In a mentoposterior position there is little possibility of spontaneous delivery, unless the chin rotates anteriorly, but a considerable risk of persistent mentoposterior position and obstructed labour. The incidence is 1 in about 500–600 deliveries. Face presentation may result from an occipitoposterior position when insufficient flexion causes the biparietal diameter to be caught in the sacrocotyloid diameter until the head is extended. This may be due to an android pelvis. Anencephaly may also result in face presentation.

Caesarean section is usually performed if the diagnosis is confirmed, particularly in a nullipara. The baby's face will be very bruised and oedematous at delivery.

face-to-pubes persistent occipitoposterior position. An occipitoposterior position of the vertex in which the attitude of the head is military, neither flexed nor extended, and the sinciput, meeting the pelvic floor first, has rotated forwards bringing

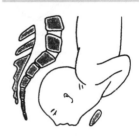

the occiput to the hollow of the sacrum. Note that face to pubes is a *position* of the vertex presentation, totally different from FACE PRESENTATION. *See* PERSISTENT OCCIPITOPOSTERIOR. Delay in the first and second stages is common. An upright maternal position such as squatting may enlarge the outlet sufficiently to facilitate vaginal delivery but severe stretching and laceration of the pelvic floor often occurs. Forceps delivery is sometimes necessary.

facial paralysis paralysis of the muscles of the face, usually one side only, resulting from injury to the seventh cranial (facial) nerve, for example, following forceps delivery. It usually resolves spontaneously within a few days.

factor an agent or element that contributes to the production of a result.

Face-to-Pubes Delivery

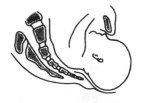

Anti-haemophilic f. (AHF) factor VIII, one of the CLOTTING factors. *Anti-haemorrhagic f.* vitamin K. *Clotting f's, coagulation f's* factors essential to normal blood clotting, whose absence, diminution or excess may lead to abnormality of the clotting mechanism; at least 12 factors have been described. *Extrinsic f. see* EXTRINSIC. *Intrinsic f.* glycoprotein secreted by the parietal cells of the gastric glands, necessary for the absorption of VITAMIN B_{12}. Its absence results in pernicious anaemia. *Releasing f's* factors elaborated in one structure that effect the release of hormones from another structure. *Rhesus f.* genetically determined antigens present on the surface of erythrocytes. *See* RHESUS FACTOR.

faeces food residue and other waste products excreted from the bowels.

Fahrenheit a scale of temperature measurement. It registers the freezing point of water at 32°, the normal temperature of the human body at 98.4°, and the boiling point of water at 212°. For comparison with Celsius, *see* Appendix 8.

faint temporary loss of consciousness due to generalized cerebral ischaemia; syncope.

falciform sickle-shaped.

fallopian tubes the uterine tubes or oviducts. Two narrow canals, each 10 cm long, leading from the uterine cornua to the ovaries.

Fallot's tetralogy a combination of 4 congenital cardiac defects, namely, pulmonary stenosis, ventricular septal defects, dextroposition of the aorta, so that it overrides the interventricular septum and receives venous as well as arterial blood, and right ventricular hypertrophy.

false labour uterine contractions giving rise to discomfort and simulating labour, but not causing dilatation of the cervix. They are thought to be due to increasing muscle contractility but without the normal FUNDAL DOMINANCE of the uterus.

false pelvis the region between the brim of the true pelvis and the crests of the ilia.

falx a sickle, or a sickle-shaped structure.

falx cerebri the sickle-shaped fold of dura mater which separates the two cerebral hemispheres of the brain.

familial occurring in families. The term is applied to such inherited conditions as haemophilia and acholuric jaundice.

family a group of people who reside together, or who may be related by blood or marriage. *Extended f.* a nuclear family and their close relatives such as the children's grandparents, aunts and uncles. *Nuclear f.* a couple and their children by birth or adoption who are living together and are more or less isolated from their extended family. *Single-parent f.* a lone parent and offspring living together as a family unit.

family planning the arrangement spacing and limitation of the children in a family, depending upon the wishes and social circumstances of the parents. *See* CONTRACEPTION.

fascia a sheet or band of fibrous connective tissue. The fibres may be arranged loosely as around organs and blood vessels, or in dense strong sheets often between muscles forming their attachments. *Pelvic f.* the fascia of the pelvic cavity is in two layers: a parietal layer, lining the walls and covering the pelvic floor; and a visceral layer, surrounding and supporting the pelvic organs, the part around the uterus being termed the parametrium.

fat 1. adipose or fatty tissue of the body. 2. neutral fat; a triglyceride (or triacylglycerol) which is a compound of fatty acids and glycerol.

fat soluble capable of being dissolved in fats, e.g. vitamins.

favism an acute haemolytic anaemia caused by ingestion of fava beans. *See* GLUCOSE-6-PHOSPHATE DEHYDROGENASE.

febrile feverish; pyrexial.

fecundation fertilization.

fecundity the ability to produce offspring.

female genital mutilation female circumcision involving excision of the labia majora, labia minora and clitoris and in some cases, partial closure of the introitus. It is prevalent in certain areas such as the Sudan. Prior to pregnancy it may cause problems with micturition and intercourse; special care will be required during labour and delivery and excision and separation of the tissues may be carried out, or caesarean section may be necessary.

feminization 1. normal development of female sexual characteristics. 2. development of female sexual characteristics in the male. *Testicular f.* condition in which subject is phenotypically female but lacks nuclear sex chromatin and is of XY chromosomal sex.

femoral pertaining to the femur. *F. artery* the principal artery of the thigh, a continuation of the external iliac artery. *F. vein* the main vein of the thigh, a continuation of the popliteal vein. It passes up the leg through the groin, whence it continues as the external iliac vein.

femur the thigh bone, which extends from the hip to the knee, articulating with the innominate bone at the acetabulum.

fenestrated possessing a window-like opening or *fenestra*. The blade of the midwifery forceps is fenestrated. *F. placenta* or *placenta fenestrata*. *See* PLACENTA.

fentanyl intravenous or intramuscular analgesic for intra- and post-operative pain.

Fentazin *See* PERPHENAZINE.

ferment an enzyme, having a specific action.

Fern test cervical cytology undertaken to determine the amount of oestrogen in cervical mucus. When oestrogen is adequate the dried cervical mucus has a fern-like appearance on low power microscopy.

ferritin the iron–apoferritin complex; one of the forms in which iron is stored in the body.

ferrous containing iron in its plus-two oxidation state. *F. fumarate* the anhydrous salt of a combination of ferrous iron and fumaric acid; used as a haematinic. *F. gluconate* a haematinic that is less irritating to the gastrointestinal tract than other haematinics, and generally used as a substitute when ferrous sulphate cannot be tolerated. *F. sulphate* the most widely used haematinic for the treatment of iron deficiency anaemia. It is believed to be less irritating than equivalent amounts of ferric salts and is more effective.

fertile capable of producing offspring. *F. period* 1. the 9 days surrounding ovulation when fertilization of the ovum is theoretically possible. It is usually taken to be the 5 days before, the day of, and the 3 days following ovulation, which is assessed over a period of months by recording the basal temperature. 2. that period of a woman's life during which she has potential for childbearing. Usually taken to be between the ages of 15 and 45.

fertility the ability to produce young. *See also* SUBFERTILITY *and* INFERTILITY.

fertilization impregnation. The union of the spermatozoon and the ovum. By this event, also called conception, a new life is created and the sex and other biological traits of the new individual are determined. These traits are determined by the combined genes and chromosomes that exist. *In vitro f.* artificial fertilization of the ovum in laboratory conditions. *In vivo f.* that which takes place by artificial means in the living situation, i.e. within the mother's reproductive tract.

fetal pertaining to the fetus. *F. abnormalities see* MALFORMATION. *F. alcohol syndrome* a syndrome resulting from heavy consumption of alcohol in pregnancy. Clinical signs seen are abnormalities of facial features, some degree of mental retardation, and these babies are often small for dates. *F. death see* INTRAUTERINE DEATH. *F. haemoglobin* haemoglobin F. It differs from adult haemoglobin in having a greater affinity for and higher capacity for oxygen. It forms 85% of the haemoglobin of a baby born at full term. *F. heart sounds*, the heart beat of the fetus, auscultated and counted through the abdominal wall, uterus and liquor amnii. It may be continuously recorded by a fetal heart monitor. *F. maturity* the most satisfactory method of estimating this is by ultrasound CEPHALOMETRY.

fetal blood sampling a technique for obtaining a minute quantity of fetal scalp blood to estimate its pH and sometimes the blood gases, to exclude fetal hypoxia, which is indicated by acidosis. Normal values are a pH of 7.25–7.4. When the fetus is hypoxic it becomes acidotic; values of 7.20–7.24 indicate moderate hypoxia, whereas a pH of below 7.20 indicates severe hypoxia and urgent delivery is required. A sample of fetal blood is obtained by visualizing the presenting part through an amnioscope via the dilating cervix. The area is cleaned, dried and sprayed with ethyl chloride to cause hyperaemia. Blood is collected into a capillary tube and the fetal pH levels obtained from analysis of the blood sample in a computerized machine.

fetal distress the clinical manifestation of fetal hypoxia. This may be caused by interference with the maternal respiration as in eclamptic fits or epilepsy; inadequate circulation in cases of cardiac failure, profound anaemia, hyper- or hypotension; diabetes mellitus or maternal infection. Fetal causes include intracranial birth trauma, severe Rhesus incompatibility leading to gross anaemia, some congenital abnormalities, intrauterine infections, multiple pregnancy, malpresentations and malpositions. Uterine causes include hypertonicity, or excessive retraction in obstructed labour, partial separation of the placenta or placental insufficiency. Umbilical cord factors include prolapse of the cord, true knots, traction or coiling.

Fetal distress can be detected on auscultation of the fetal heart either with a Pinard's stethoscope or via

Vault of the Fetal Skull

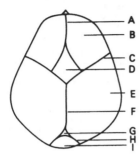

A, Frontal suture; B, frontal bone;
C, coronal suture; D, anterior
fontanelle or bregma; E, parietal
bone; F, sagittal suture;
G, posterior fontanelle;
H, lambdoid suture; I, occipital
bone.

cardiotocography, meconium-stained amniotic fluid, tumultuous movement of the fetus. Immediate delivery is required once the diagnosis is confirmed. *See also* CARDIOTOCOGRAPHY.

fetal skull the bony structure of the head of the fetus. The *vault* is the most significant area in obstetrics, and contains the brain; it is composed of 2 frontal bones divided by a frontal suture, 2 parietal bones divided by the sagittal suture and separated from the frontal bones by the coronal suture, and 1 occipital bone separated from the parietal bones by the lambdoidal suture. Where three or more sutures meet, the anterior fontanelle or BREGMA and the posterior fontanelle or LAMBDA

are formed of membrane. Sutures and fontanelles are felt on vaginal examination in labour and enable the midwife to determine the position of the head in a cephalic presentation. *See* Figure and Appendix 4.

The *base* of the skull is composed of 2 temporal, 1 ethmoid, 1 sphenoid and part of the occipital bone, and contains an opening called the foramen magnum through which passes the spinal cord. The *face* is composed of 14 fused bones. *Diameters of* the skull are assessed to estimate progress in labour, and are taken longitudinally or transversely. Circumferences may also be assessed.

Within the skull are the brain and intracranial membranes, the FALX CEREBRI and the TENTORIUM CEREBELLI which carry the venous sinuses by which blood is drained from the head: the SUPERIOR and INFERIOR LONGITUDINAL SINUSES, the STRAIGHT SINUS, the TRANSVERSE SINUS and the GREAT VEIN OF GALEN. If delivery or MOULDING are excessive the membranes and sinuses may be torn, causing intracranial haemorrhage.

fetoscopy the inspection of a fetus through the uterine wall by means of a fetoscope.

fetus the unborn offspring of a mammal. The human embryo from the 8th week of pregnancy to the time of birth. *F. papyraceus* one of twins which, dying in utero at an early stage of pregnancy, becomes flattened against the uterine wall. It is usually expelled with the placenta and resembles a piece of parchment.

fever pyrexia. A high body temperature. An illness characterized by pyrexia.

fibre a thread-like structure. A muscle cell. *Dietary f.* that portion of ingested foodstuffs that cannot be broken down by intestinal enzymes

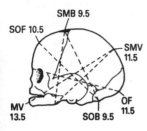

Longitudinal Diameters
(with diameters (cm))

SOF, Suboccipitofrontal;
SMB, submentobregmatic;
MV, mentovertical;
SOB, suboccipitobregmatic;
OF, occipitofrontal;
SMV, submentovertical.

and juices and, therefore, passes through the small intestine and colon undigested. Vegetables, cereals and fruits are the main sources of dietary fibre. Helps to prevent constipation.

fibrin an insoluble protein formed by the action of thrombin upon fibrinogen. Necessary in the process of blood clotting, where it forms a network of minute long strands in which blood cells get caught.

fibrinogen a protein formed in the liver and circulating in the blood plasma. In tissue injury it is activated by THROMBIN, to form FIBRIN and thus to arrest haemorrhage by clotting. Preparations containing human fibrinogen used to restore blood fibrinogen levels after extensive surgery, or to treat diseases or haemorrhagic conditions that are complicated by AFIBRINOGENAEMIA include fresh frozen plasma and cryoprecipitate. Pure

fibrinogen is rarely used because of the risk of transmitting hepatitis.

fibrinolysin 1. PLASMIN. 2. a preparation of proteolytic enzyme formed from profibrinolysin (plasminogen) by action of physical agents or by specific bacterial kinases; used to promote dissolution of thrombi.

fibrinolysis the dissolution of fibrin by enzymatic action. adj. *fibrinolytic.*

fibrocystic disease *See* CYSTIC FIBROSIS.

fibroid 1. composed of fibrous tissue. 2. a benign tumour. Uterine fibroids may be submucous, interstitial or subserous. Occasionally a cervical fibroid occurs. In midwifery they are most commonly seen in primigravid women over 30 years of age. In pregnancy they rarely create trouble, but may occasionally be the cause of abortion or undergo red degeneration. In labour, fibroids, unless of the cervix, are usually drawn out of the pelvis as the cervix dilates, and do not cause obstruction. Fibroids in the region of the placental site could interfere with the contraction of the uterus and cause postpartum haemorrhage. In the puerperium and subsequently fibroids may decrease in size so much that operative removal is unlikely to be necessary.

fibromyoma a fibroid.

fibroplasia the formation of fibrous tissue, as in the healing of a wound. *Retrolental f.* a condition characterized by retinal vascular proliferation and tortuosity and by the presence of fibrous tissue behind the lens, leading to detachment of the retina and arrest of growth of the eye, generally attributed to use of excessively high concentrations of oxygen in the care of preterm infants.

fibrosis formation of fibrous tissue; fibroid degeneration. adj. *fibrotic. Cystic f.* a generalized hereditary disorder with widespread dysfunction of exocrine glands, chronic pulmonary disease, pancreatic deficiency, high levels of electrolytes in sweat, and sometimes biliary cirrhosis. *See also* CYSTIC FIBROSIS.

fibula the lateral and smaller of the two bones of the leg.

filter a porous substance which permits fluids and materials in solution to pass through, but which holds back solids in solution. A filter of cellulose acetate which removes bacteria and therefore sterilizes a solution, as in EPIDURAL ANALGESIA.

filtrate fluid which has passed through a filter.

fimbria a finger-like fringe. The fringe-like extremity of the fallopian tube is described as fimbriated.

first degree perineal lacerations *See* PERINEAL LACERATIONS.

first stage of labour the period from the onset of labour until complete or full dilatation of the cervix.

fission cleavage or splitting. Reproduction by division of a cell into two equal parts. *Nuclear f.* the splitting of the nucleus of an atom.

fissure a cleft. This may be normal, e.g. cerebral fissure, or due to disease, e.g. anal fissure.

fistula an abnormal passage between two cavities or between a cavity and the surface of the body. *Rectovaginal f.* an opening between the vagina and the rectum, usually resulting from severe and/or neglected laceration of the perineal body. *Vesicovaginal f.* an opening between the bladder and the vagina, which might result from prolonged pressure in neglected obstructed labour.

fit a seizure. Convulsion, as in eclampsia or epilepsy.

flaccid limp; without tone. The condition of the muscles in a baby suffering from severe asphyxia.

flagellum the whip-like protoplasmic filament by which some bacteria move. *Trichomonas vaginalis*, a protozoon, is also flagellated. pl. *flagella*.

Flagyl *See* METRONIDAZOLE.

flank the side of the abdomen, between the ribs and the iliac crest.

flat pelvis a pelvis in which the anteroposterior diameter of the brim is much shorter than the transverse diameter. There are two described: the platypelloid and the rachitic. *See* PELVIS.

flatulence the presence of gas or air in the stomach or intestine; sometimes causing severe pain, but as a rule merely discomfort.

flatus gas in the bowel.

fleshy mole CARNEOUS MOLE, a mass of clotted blood surrounding a dead embryo and retained in the uterus.

flexion bending. A movement of a limb or organ out of alignment. *See* ANTEFLEXION *and* RETROFLEXION. Flexion is the normal attitude of the fetus *in utero*.

'flooding' severe bleeding from the uterus. A lay term used to describe MENORRHAGIA, METRORRHAGIA and severe bleeding in miscarriage.

flora *Intestinal f.* the bacteria normally residing within the lumen of the intestine.

flucloxacillin antibiotic which is active against most staphylococci and streptococci, including the majority of penicillinase-producing staphylococci. May be given orally, intramuscularly or intravenously.

fluid a liquid or gas; any liquid of the body. *Amniotic f.* the fluid within the amnion which bathes the developing fetus and protects it from mechanical injury. *Body f's* the fluids within the body, composed of water, electrolytes and non-electrolytes which are continuously in motion. *Intracellular f.* fluid within the cell membranes comprises about two-thirds of the total body fluids. The remaining one-third is outside the cell and is called *extracellular f. Cerebrospinal f.* fluid contained within the ventricles of the brain, the subarachnoid space, and the central canal of the spinal cord. *F. balance* a state in which the volume of body water and its solutes (electrolytes and non-electrolytes) is within normal limits and there is normal distribution of fluids within the intracellular and extracellular compartments. The total volume of body fluids should be 60% of the body weight. A fluid balance record is kept on each woman who is susceptible to or already suffering from a disturbance in the balance of body fluids, e.g. severe pre-eclampsia. All intake and output is accurately recorded on a *fluid balance chart.*

fluorescent treponemal antibody test a serological test for syphilis; the first to become positive after infection.

'flying squad' See EMERGENCY OBSTETRIC UNIT.

folate a general term used to describe a large group of compounds, i.e. the folates which are derived from the parent compound, FOLIC ACID. Folates are necessary for a variety of biochemical reactions in the body, the most important of which is required for DNA synthesis. Folate levels in the serum and red blood cells are measurable and are used to assess the body stores; low levels of both are found in megaloblastic anaemia secondary to folate deficiency.

folic acid a constituent of the vitamin B complex, necessary for the development of normal red blood cells. Deficiency in pregnancy causes megaloblastic anaemia as the rapidly dividing fetal cells compete for folic acid to form cell nuclei. Green

vegetables, liver and yeast are major sources of folic acid in the diet. It is also produced synthetically. Folic acid deficiency may result from the inability of the body to utilize the vitamin. Women planning to conceive are encouraged to take folic acid supplements preconceptionally to reduce the risk of fetal neural tube defects.

follicle a very small sac or gland. *Graafian f.* small vesicles formed in the ovary, each containing an ovum. One follicle matures during each menstrual cycle, which is controlled by pituitary hormones. See GONADO-TROPHIC.

follicle-stimulating hormone (FSH) a hormone released from the anterior pituitary gland, stimulating one or more GRAAFIAN FOLLICLES to mature, during each menstrual cycle.

fomites substances or objects which transmit infectious organisms by contamination.

fontanelle a membranous space where two or more sutures meet between the cranial bones of the fetus or newborn child. *Anterior f.* the bregma. *Posterior f.* the lambda. See FETAL SKULL.

footling presentation a type of breech presentation in which one or both feet lie in advance of the buttocks. See also BREECH PRESENTATION.

foramen an opening or hole, especially in a bone. *F. magnum* the opening in the occipital bone through which the medulla oblongata becomes continuous with the spinal cord. *Obturator f.* the large hole in the os innominatum of the pelvis. *F. ovale* the opening between the two atria of the fetal heart.

forceps surgical instruments with two blades used for lifting or compressing an object: e.g. *dressing f., dissecting f. Artery f.* compress bleeding points during an operation. *Mid-wifery f.* are used in the second stage of labour to extract the child's head, in cases where this mode of delivery is safer for the mother or child. These include KJELLAND'S, NEVILLE BARNES and WRIGLEY'S FORCEPS. *Vulsellum f.* have claw-like ends. *See* Appendix 3.

foreskin the prepuce. The skin covering the glans penis.

forewaters the liquor amnii contained in the membranes lying below the presenting part of the fetus. That part of the bag of membranes behind the presenting part is the HINDWATERS.

formaldehyde a powerful disinfectant gas whose solution is formalin.

formalin *See* FORMALDEHYDE.

formula 1. a prescription or recipe, especially for an infant's feed. 2. a group of symbols making a certain statement.

fornix an arch. The vaginal fornices are the recesses at the vault of the vagina in front of (*anterior f.*), behind (*posterior f.*) and at the sides (*lateral f.*) of the cervix. pl. *fornices*.

Fortral *See* PENTAZOCINE HYDROCHLORIDE.

fossa a pit or hollow, e.g. the iliac fossa, which is a depression on the inner surface of the iliac bone.

foster children children under the care of FOSTER PARENTS.

foster parents persons who undertake for reward the care of children who are not related to them within the meaning of the Children Act.

Fothergill's operation the Manchester operation for uterovaginal prolapse.

Foundation for the Study of Infant Deaths (SID) a registered charity, founded in 1971, giving support to parents whose child's demise apparently has been a 'cot death'. It also sponsors research into this mysterious syndrome.

fourchette a fold of skin between the posterior extremities of the labia minora.

fracture a break, usually of bone; a possible, though uncommon birth injury. Occasionally in a breech delivery the clavicle, humerus or femur may be fractured, and sometimes after any difficult delivery a depressed fracture of the skull can be found. This normally heals well.

fraenum, frenum, frenulum a small ligament that checks the movement of an organ, e.g. the *f. linguae*, the membranous connection between the floor of the mouth and the lower surface of the tongue. *See* TONGUE TIE.

fragilitas ossium OSTEOGENESIS IMPERFECTA. Fragile brittle bones.

Frankenhauser's plexus a ganglion near the uterine cervix from which sympathetic and parasympathetic nerves supply the vagina, uterus and other pelvic viscera.

friable easily torn, broken or crumbled. The chorion attached to the placenta is friable, and is often torn, portions being retained in the uterus.

Friars' balsam compound tincture of benzoin. This acts as a decongestant when inhaled as a vapour.

Friedman test one of the biological pregnancy tests. The urine of a pregnant woman contains an excess of GONADOTROPHIC HORMONE. If the urine is injected intravenously into female rabbits, on post-mortem examination 48 hours later the ovaries will show evidence of ruptured follicles. This test is about 98% accurate, but has largely been superseded by immunological tests.

frigidity coldness; especially sexual unresponsiveness of the female to physical stimulation, due to psychological causes.

frontal pertaining to the forehead. In the fetus the two *frontal bones* form the forehead. The *frontal suture* is the membranous channel between these two bones. *Frontal headache* in pregnancy may be a serious symptom of severe PRE-ECLAMPSIA or impending ECLAMPSIA caused by cerebral oedema.

fulminating bursting forth, violently explosive. The term is applied to conditions and diseases that appear with great suddenness and severity. In obstetrics, such conditions include severe pre-eclampsia and eclampsia, when they arise very suddenly.

fundal pertaining to the fundus, usually, in obstetrics, of the uterus. *F. dominance* normal uterine action is such that the contractions originate from a pacemaker in the fundus, the wave of contraction gradually weakening as it passes over the upper and lower segments of the uterus. *F. pressure* a rarely used method of using the contracted FUNDUS UTERI, following descent of the placenta and membranes into the vagina, as a piston to expel the placenta and complete the third stage of labour.

fundus the base of an organ, or the part farthest removed from the opening. *F. uteri* the top of the uterus – the part farthest from the cervix.

fungus a general term for a group of eukaryotic organisms (mushrooms, yeasts, moulds, etc.). Thrush is a fungal condition.

funic pertaining to the funis, i.e. the umbilical cord. *F. souffle* a soft whispering sound synchronizing with the fetal heart sounds and coming from the umbilical cord.

funis the umbilical cord.

funnel pelvis a pelvis the shape of a funnel, i.e. narrowing from above downwards. This is a characteristic of the ANDROID (or male type of) PELVIS, in which the outlet is considerably smaller than the brim.

Furadantin *See* NITROFURANTION.

furosemide (frusemide) a diuretic that acts by blocking reabsorption of sodium and chloride in the ascending loop of Henle; used for treatment of oedema and acute renal failure. May be administered intravenously or intramuscularly in doses of 20–40 mg. Normally reserved for women with pulmonary oedema and, occasionally, oliguria. May inhibit lactation.

Fybogel *See* ISPAGHULA.

G

gag 1. an instrument for holding open the jaws. 2. to retch, or strive to vomit. *G. reflex* elevation of the soft palate and retching elicited by touching the back of the tongue or the wall of the pharynx; called also pharyngeal reflex.

Gairdner headbox a Perspex box which is placed over the baby's head into which additional oxygen is provided in order to increase the oxygen concentration of inspired air.

gait walk or carriage. This should be observed in the pregnant woman. It may give rise to the suspicion of a pelvic deformity.

galact-, galacto- word element meaning 'milk'.

galactischia suppression of milk secretion.

galactogogue an agent which is said to increase the secretion of milk.

galactorrhoea an excessive flow of breast milk.

galactosaemia a genetically determined biochemical disorder in which there is a lack of an enzyme necessary for proper metabolism of galactose leading to high levels of galactose in the blood and tissues. This leads to failure to thrive, hepatomegaly and jaundice, and ultimately, mental retardation and death if the condition remains untreated. Treatment involves the exclusion of all galactose or lactose-containing foods from the diet.

galactose a MONOSACCHARIDE resulting from the digestion of LACTOSE. The liver converts it to glucose.

galactose-1-phosphate uridyl transferase an enzyme which converts galactose to glucose. Deficiency of the enzyme results in classic galactosaemia.

galea aponeurotica the tendon of the occipitofrontalis muscle, which forms a layer of the scalp.

Galen, vein of See GREAT VEIN OF GALEN

gallbladder a sac situated on the under part of the liver, holding and concentrating the bile secreted by that organ.

gamete a male or female reproductive cell.

gamete intrafallopian transfer (GIFT) infertility treatment involving the retrieval of oocytes from the ovary at laparoscopy and placing of the oocytes sequentially with sperm into the fallopian tubes. It is suitable for women with unexplained infertility and those with at least one patent, healthy fallopian tube when the male sperm parameters are near normal. *See also* ZYGOTE INTRAFALLOPIAN TRANSFER.

gamgee tissue absorbent wool covered with gauze and used for dressing wounds, etc.

gamma globulin γ globulin, a class of plasma proteins composed almost entirely of IgG, an IMMUNOGLOBULIN protein that contains most antibody activity. Commerical preparations of gamma globulin are derived from blood serum and are used for prevention, modification, and treatment of various infectious diseases. This type of gamma globulin contains almost all the known antibodies circulating in the blood. It can provide passive immunity, usually for about 6 weeks against infections to which most of the population has antibodies. Certain specific types of gamma globulin may be used to raise the body's resistance to measles, mumps and poliomyelitis. Gamma globulin containing a high concentration of anti-Rhesus antibody can be given to a Rhesus-negative mother within 72 hours of delivery to prevent her forming her own antibody.

ganglion a nerve centre from which nerve fibres proceed.

gangrene death of tissue, usually applied to a large area or definite organ. *Dry g.* is due to failure of arterial blood supply, e.g. the process by which the umbilical cord dries and separates from the umbilicus about 5–7 days after birth. *Moist g.* is caused by putrefactive changes, e.g. infection of the umbilical cord, when it remains moist, becomes offensive and separation is delayed. *See also* GAS GANGRENE.

Gardnerella a genus of Gram-negative rod-shaped bacteria having one species, *G. vaginalis* (formerly called *Haemophilus vaginalis*). It is found in the normal female genital tract and is the causative organism for non-specific vaginitis. *Gardnerella* infection is one of the most common and most infectious of the sexually transmitted diseases. The major symptom is increased vaginal discharge that is thin and grey and has a fishy odour, especially after sexual intercourse. Treatment is with metronidazole for both the woman and her sexual partner.

gargoylism a type of MUCOPOLY-SACCHARIDOSIS.

gas matter in its least dense form, neither solid nor liquid, where the molecules are in constant movement. A vapour. Air is a mixture of several gases: oxygen, nitrogen, traces of carbon dioxide, argon and helium.

'gas and oxygen' analgesia *See* INHALATION ANALGESIA *and* ENTONOX.

gas gangrene infection of damaged tissues by the anaerobic organism *Clostridium welchii*. The uterus may be thus infected following criminal abortion, and, very rarely, following labour.

gastric pertaining to the stomach.

gastritis inflammation of the lining of the stomach.

gastro- a prefix meaning 'relating to the stomach'.

gastroenteritis inflammation of the lining of stomach and intestine. An acute condition of diarrhoea and vomiting particularly dangerous in infants, producing rapid and severe dehydration. Any infant in whom this condition is suspected should be immediately isolated from other babies. The treatment is to administer fluids orally or intravenously, to combat the dehydration, correct the electrolyte balance and treat the infection.

gastrointestinal pertaining to the stomach and intestines. *G. tract* the alimentary tract.

gastrojejunostomy surgical anastomosis of the stomach to the jejunum. It may be performed to bypass the obstruction in cases of duodenal atresia in the newborn.

gastroschisis a congenital fissure of the abdominal wall.

gastrostomy the creation of an opening into the stomach. The procedure is done to provide for the administration of food and liquids when stricture of the oesophagus or other conditions make swallowing impossible.

gate control theory of pain this theory proposes that a neural mechanism in the dorsal horns of the spinal cord acts like a gate which can increase or decrease the flow of nerve impulses from peripheral fibres to the central nervous system. It is the position of the gate which determines how much information is transmitted to the brain and therefore on the amount of pain generated. Influences such as anxiety and anticipation cause the gate to open and therefore increase the level of pain experienced, whereas other factors may cause the gate to close, thereby reducing the pain. The theory was initially postulated by Melzack and Wall in 1965 but considerable research into the physiology and psychology of pain has been undertaken since then. Electrical stimulation applied to nerve fibres in the skin was found to impair the transmission of painful stimuli from the peripheral to the central nervous system, thereby closing the 'gate'. This, coupled with the release of endorphins from the brain, is the reason that TRANSCUTANEOUS ELECTRICAL NERVE STIMULATION (TENS) is effective as a method of pain relief.

gauze a large-mesh, thin cotton material, used for dressings.

Geiger counter an instrument used to detect radioactive substances.

gemellology the scientific study of twins and twinning.

gemeprost pessaries used to soften and dilate the cervix to facilitate transcervical procedures in the first trimester. 1 mg is administered 3 hours prior to surgery. Used also for second trimester termination of pregnancy; 1 mg is given every 3 hours up to a maximum of 5 doses; if necessary, a second course is commenced 24 hours later.

gender sex; the category to which an individual is assigned on the basis of sex.

gene a single unit of the hereditary factors located in a definite position on a CHROMOSOME. Genes are composed of DEOXYRIBONUCLEIC ACID (DNA), consisting of a complex double chain of molecules which carry the genetic code of an individual, so governing each characteristic. Through the genetic code of DNA they also control the day-to-day functions and reproduction of all cells in the body. For example, the genes control the synthesis of structural proteins and also the enzymes that regulate various chemical reactions that take place in a cell. The gene is capable of replication. When a cell multiplies by mitosis each daughter cell carries a set of genes that is an exact replica of that of the parent cell. This characteristic of replication explains how genes can carry hereditary traits through successive generations without change. Rarely there may be an abnormal or mutant gene. An example of a condition resulting from two abnormal RECESSIVE genes is PHENYLKETONURIA.

General Medical Council (GMC) the regulating body of all medical practitioners within the United Kingdom; the medical equivalent of the Nursing and Midwifery Council.

general practitioner obstetrician (GPO) a general practitioner qualified or having experience in obstetrics, who has agreed to provide maternity services on application. This is indicated by the prefix 'M' before the appropriate entry in the Family Practitioner List.

generic 1. pertaining to a genus. 2. non-proprietary; denoting a drug name not protected by a trademark, usually descriptive of the drug's chemical structure.

genetic counselling this is carried out in certain clinics, where the geneticist explains the chances of recurrence of hereditary diseases, and can advise a couple whether there is a risk to future children.

genetics the study of heredity.

genital relating to the organs of reproduction.

genitalia the organs of reproduction.

genitourinary pertaining to the genital and urinary organs.

genotype classification of the genetic make-up of an individual. *See* GENE.

gentamicin an antibiotic complex, effective against many Gram-negative bacteria, especially *Pseudomonas* species, as well as certain Gram-positive bacteria, especially *Staphylococcus aureus*. Should be avoided in pregnancy due to the risk of fetal VIIIth nerve damage. It is used for septicaemia, neonatal sepsis, particularly infections of the central nervous system.

gentian violet an antibacterial, antifungal, and antihelmintic dye, applied topically in the treatment of infections of the skin and mucous membranes associated with Gram-positive bacteria and moulds and administered orally in pin worm and liver fluke infections.

genu the knee.

genupectoral position knee–chest position, i.e. face downwards and resting on the knees and the chest. *See* POSITION.

genus a classificatory group of animals or plants comprising one or more species.

German measles *See* RUBELLA.

germicide an agent capable of destroying micro-organisms.

gestagen any hormone with progestational activity.

gestalt a whole perceptual configuration. *G. therapy* a psychotherapeutic approach which encourages the individual to cease intellectualizing his or her difficulties and instead to focus on feelings and emotions, and thereby to gain emotional insight and balance.

gestation pregnancy. *G. period* in the human species approximately 40 weeks from the first day of the last normal menstrual period or 38 weeks from the date of conception. *Ectopic g.* pregnancy outside the uterus. *G. sac* the placenta and membranes containing the liquor amnii and the fetus during pregnancy.

gestational pertaining to gestation. *G. hypertension* raised blood pressure during pregnancy, which may progress to pre-eclampsia or eclampsia. *G. diabetes* the former term for a situation in which a woman has impaired glucose tolerance during pregnancy. The glucose tolerance test reverts to normal following delivery but these women may develop overt clinical diabetes mellitus in later life.

gigantism abnormal overgrowth of the whole or part of the body, due to overactivity of the anterior pituitary growth hormone.

Gigli's operation pubiotomy. *See* SYMPHYSIOTOMY.

Gigli's saw a fine wire instrument for sawing through bone.

gingivitis inflammation and bleeding of the gums.

girdle a belt. *Pelvic g.* the bony ring of the pelvis formed by the two innominate bones and the sacrum.

glabella the area on the frontal bone above the nose and between the eyebrows.

gland a collection of cells specialized to secrete or excrete materials not related to their own metabolic needs. Endocrine glands secrete hormones into the blood stream, e.g. the thyroid gland secretes thyroxine. Exocrine glands discharge their secretion through one or more ducts, e.g. breast or liver.

glans an acorn-shaped body, such as the rounded end of the penis and the clitoris.

globin the protein constituent of haemoglobin; also, any member of a group of proteins similar to the typical globin.

globulin a subdivision of plasma proteins. Globulin is further subdivided into alpha (α), beta (β) and gamma (γ) globulins. *See also* GAMMA GLOBULIN *and* IMMUNOGLOBULIN.

glomerulus the tuft of capillaries which is invaginated in the kidney tubule at its commencement in the renal cortex.

glossal pertaining to the tongue.

glottis the vocal apparatus of the larynx, consisting of the true vocal cords and the opening between them.

glucagon a polypeptide hormone secreted by the alpha cells of the islets of Langerhans in response to hypoglycaemia or to stimulation by growth hormone. It increases blood glucose concentration by stimulating glycogenolysis in the liver and is administered to relieve hypoglycaemic coma from any cause, especially hyperinsulinism.

glucocorticoid any corticoid substance that increases gluconeogenesis, raising the concentration of liver glycogen and blood sugar, i.e. cortisol (hydrocortisone), cortisone and corticosterone.

glucose dextrose, a monosaccharide found in many fruits and honey. It is the monosaccharide to which carbohydrates are reduced by digestion, and therefore found in the blood. The metabolism of glucose produces energy for the body cells; the rate of metabolism is controlled by insulin. Glucose that is not needed for energy is stored in the form of glycogen as a source of potential energy, readily available when needed. Most of the glycogen is stored in the liver and muscle cells. The normal fasting level for glucose in the blood is between 70 and 90 mg per 100 ml (3.9–5.6 mmol/l). Unusually high levels of glucose in the blood (hyperglycaemia) may indicate such diseases as DIABETES MELLITUS, HYPERTHYROIDISM and hyperpituitarism. A GLUCOSE TOLERANCE TEST is done to assess the ability of the body to metabolize glucose. Glucose is present in the urine of women with untreated diabetes mellitus. In medicine glucose is used extensively, as it is an excellent source of energy and can be given by mouth or intravenously.

glucose-6-phosphate dehydrogenase (G6PD) an important enzyme, especially in red cells. The absence of this enzyme leads to attacks of HAEMOLYSIS and severe or fatal anaemia. The eating of fava beans can cause such an attack (favism), and the disease is common in coloured races, and in Mediterranean countries. It is inherited as an X-linked RECESSIVE trait.

glucose tolerance test (GTT) a test of the body's ability to utilize carbohydrates. It is used to detect abnormalities of carbohydrate metabolism such as occurs in diabetes mellitus. The client must be in a fasting state when the test is started and a blood sample is taken for measurement of the fasting blood glucose. A dose of 75 g of glucose is given orally. Blood samples are then obtained at intervals for glucose estimation. Abnormal findings would be as follows:

fasting blood glucose over 7.0 mmol/litre

two-hour blood glucose over 10.0 mmol/litre

glucuronyl transferase the liver enzyme which converts fat-soluble or toxic bilirubin to the water-soluble type which is not toxic.

glutaraldehyde an antiseptic used in the treatment of viral warts.

gluteal pertaining to the buttocks.

glycerol suppositories used as a rectal stimulant.

glycogen a polysaccharide. The form in which carbohydrate is stored in the liver and in the muscles.

glycosuria glucose in the urine. Glycosuria in pregnancy may be: (a) *alimentary*, related to the ingestion of a large quantity of carbohydrate and inability to store it; (b) *renal*, resulting from a lowering of the renal threshold for sugar – neither is of serious import; (c) due to DIABETES MELLITUS, which causes numerous hazards to both mother and child. In order that a differential diagnosis may be made, a midwife should always report the occurrence of glycosuria.

gnathic pertaining to the jaw or cheeks.

goblet cell a goblet-shaped cell, found in the cubical epithelium of the fallopian tubes. These cells produce a secretion containing glycogen to nourish the ovum.

goitre enlargement of the thyroid gland, causing a marked swelling in front of the neck, which sometimes results in pressure on the trachea.

gonad the organ which produces ova or spermatozoa; in the female the ovary and in the male the testis.

gonadotrophic stimulating the gonads. *G. hormones* those of the anterior pituitary lobe or placenta.

gonadotrophin any hormone having a stimulating effect on the gonads. Two such hormones are secreted by the anterior pituitary: follicule-stimulating hormone and luteinizing hormone. *Chorionic g.* a gonad-stimulating hormone produced by the cells of the cytotrophoblast of the chorionic tissue which later forms the placenta. Biological and immunological pregnancy tests depend on the detection of human chorionic gonadotrophin (HCG) in the urine.

gonococcal pertaining to or caused by the gonococcus. *G. ophthalmia* acute conjunctivitis resulting from gonococcal infection. This, occurring in newborn babies, can lead to ulceration of the cornea, and was at one time the commonest cause of blindness in babies and young children. *See* OPHTHALMIA NEONATORUM.

gonococcus *Neisseria gonorrhoeae*. The Gram-negative intracellular diplococcus which causes gonorrhoea.

gonorrhoea a sexually transmitted disease due to infection by the gonococcus, usually acquired by sexual intercourse, which infects the mucous membrane of the cervix, urethra and Bartholin's glands. Occasionally, the infection may spread causing salpingitis or septicaemia. The incubation period is 1–16 days. It may cause a purulent discharge from the vagina or urethra and burning pain on micturition, but is more often symptomless. Penicillin will effect a rapid cure. Any vaginal discharge during pregnancy which causes soreness or irritation, or is associated with pain, should be investigated without delay. Both smears and cultures may be used in diagnosis.

Goodell's sign softening of the cervix uteri and vagina; a sign of pregnancy.

Graafian follicle a cystic structure developing in the ovarian cortex

Graafian Follicle

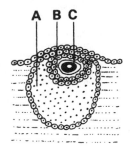

A, Follicular fluid; B, granulosa cells;
C, ovum.

during the menstrual cycle. It has outer covering or theca folliculi, and a lining of granulosa cells which also surround the ovum, which lies within the follicle. When it is ripe, the follicle ruptures, discharging the ovum (ovulation) and develops into a CORPUS LUTEUM. The Graafian follicle secretes several oestrogenic hormones.

gram the unit of weight of the metric system. Abbreviated 'g'.

Gram stain a special stain used in bacteriology. Micro-organisms which retain it are said to be Gram-positive (+), and those which lose it Gram-negative (−).

grand mal a major epileptic seizure attended by loss of consciousness and convulsive movements, as distinguished from PETIT MAL, a minor seizure.

grande multigravida a woman in her fourth or subsequent pregnancy, but who has not necessarily borne live children in previous pregnancies.

grande multipara a woman of high parity. Usually one who has borne 4 or more children. Increasing parity can lead to an increased risk of problems in pregnancy, labour and the puerperium.

granulation a process by which healing of a wound may take place. Granulations appear as small red projections on the surface of the wound, bringing a rich blood supply to the healing surface.

granulosa cells the lining cells in the Graafian follicle, which secrete oestradiol.

granulosa lutein cells granulosa cells after ovulation. They secrete oestradiol and progesterone.

gravid pregnant.

gravida a pregnant woman See PRIMIGRAVIDA and MULTIGRAVIDA.

Gravigard an intrauterine contraceptive device.

Gravindex an immunological pregnancy test.

gravity weight. The specific gravity of a substance is its weight compared with that of an equal volume of water. The specific gravity of water is 1000, and that of normal urine about 1010–1020. This is increased if more solids are dissolved in the urine, e.g. sugar, and decreased when the normal amount of urea is not being excreted, e.g. chronic nephritis.

great vein of Galen large cerebral vein which passes from the midbrain and enters the junction of the inferior longitudinal and straight sinuses. Extreme, abnormal or rapid moulding of the fetal skull during delivery may cause the cerebral membranes and the cerebral veins to be torn causing intracranial haemorrhage.

grey-scale display a method to show the texture of tissue on ULTRASOUND display. The amplitude of each echo is represented by varying shades of grey. A bright white outline is seen from SPECULAR REFLECTIVE surfaces, a mottled grey from various tissue areas, and black from collections of fluid such as the bladder and amniotic sac.

grey syndrome a potentially fatal condition seen in neonates, particularly preterm babies, due to a reaction to chloramphenicol, characterized by an ashen grey cyanosis, vomiting, abdominal distension, hypothermia and shock.

grief loss, usually caused by death. The normal grieving process may take 2 or 3 years and usually follows a pattern of numbness and denial, anger, guilt, bargaining and depression, and finally acceptance and readjustment.

groin the junction of the front of the thigh with the trunk.

group practice medical or midwifery practice carried out by a team of general practitioners or midwives (often independent midwives) working together.

growth hormone a substance that stimulates growth, especially a secretion of the anterior PITUITARY GLAND that directly influences protein, carbohydrate and lipid metabolism, and controls the rate of skeletal and visceral growth. Increased production of growth hormone occurs in the baby of the poorly controlled diabetic mother.

guardian *ad litem* a person, usually from the local authority social services department, who is appointed by a court to look after the interests of a child before its full Adoption Order is granted. Meanwhile the prospective adoptive parents have continuous possession of the child,

and are visited and interviewed by the guardian *ad litem* to ensure that the home will be satisfactory, and who makes a detailed report to the court.

guardian Caldicott named member of an NHS Trust responsible for agreeing and reviewing internal protocols governing the protection and use of patient identified information by staff within the healthcare system. Protocols must meet national requirements and be monitored regularly.

gum gingiva in pregnancy oestrogen causes the gums to retain fluid and they become enlarged and spongy.

gumma a syphilitic lesion found in the third or tertiary stage of syphilis in any part of the body.

Guthrie test a blood test carried out on a neonate between the 6th and 14th days of life to diagnose PHENYL-KETONURIA. The baby must be well established on milk feeds before the test is carried out. If the baby is receiving antibiotics the test is deferred.

gynae- prefix meaning 'woman'.

gynaecoid woman-like. Having feminine characteristics. *G. pelvis* a pelvis of typical female conformation.

gynaecologist doctor specializing in women's health, particularly conditions of the reproductive tract.

gynaecology the branch of medicine which treats diseases of the female genital tract.

gynandroid a hermaphrodite or a female pseudohermaphrodite.

gynandromorphism the presence of chromosomes of both sexes in different tissues of the body, which produces a mosaic of male and female sexual characteristics. adj. *gynandromorphous*.

H

habitual abortion sequence of 3 or more spontaneous abortions. Treatment may be hormone therapy, cervical CERCLAGE or antibiotics, depending on the cause. *See also* ABORTION.

haem the non-protein, insoluble, iron protoporphyrin constituent of haemoglobin, other respiratory pigments and of many cells. It is an iron compound of protoporphyrin and is responsible for the oxygen-carrying properties of the haemoglobin molecule.

haema-, haemo-, haemato- prefixes denoting or relating to blood.

haemagglutination agglutination of erythrocytes.

haemagglutinin an antibody that causes agglutination of erythrocytes.

haemangioma a tumour made up of blood vessels, clustered together. Haemangiomas may be present at birth in various parts of the body. They often appear as a network of small, blood-filled capillaries near the surface of the skin, forming a flat red or purple birthmark (a 'strawberry' or 'raspberry' mark), which tends to disappear in childhood. The type of haemangioma known as a 'port-wine' stain tends to persist.

haematemesis the vomiting of blood. In newborn infants it may be a sign of HAEMORRHAGIC DISEASE or a result of swallowed maternal blood. Fetal and maternal blood may be distinguished by SINGER'S TEST.

haematinic 1. improving the quality of blood. 2. an agent that improves the quality of the blood, increasing the haemoglobin level and the number of erythrocytes; examples are iron preparations, liver extract and the B complex vitamins.

haematocele a collection of blood in a cavity. *Pelvic h.* a collection of blood in the pouch of Douglas, generally resulting from tubal abortion or rupture.

haematocolpos accumulation of blood in the vagina.

haematocrit *See* PACKED CELL VOLUME.

haematology the science dealing with the nature, functions and diseases of blood.

haematoma a localized collection of extravasated blood in an organ, space or tissue. Haematoma of the vagina, vulva or perineum may occur as a result of trauma during childbirth. Trauma to the fetus in labour may result in a cephalhaematoma, which is due to the rupture of small blood vessels between the skull and pericranium. It develops a few hours after birth and does not cross suture lines.

haematometra an accumulation of blood in the uterus.

haematopoiesis the formation and development of blood cells, usually taking place in bone marrow. Also may take place in the spleen, liver and lymph nodes; then called extramedullary haematopoiesis.

haematoporphyrin an iron-free derivative of haem, a product of the decomposition of haemoglobin.

haematosalpinx an accumulation of blood in the fallopian tube.

haematuria blood in the urine, due to injury, infection or disease of any of the urinary organs.

haemoconcentration loss of fluid from the blood into the tissues, as may occur in shock or dehydration.

haemodialysis a procedure used to remove toxic wastes from the blood of a patient with acute or chronic renal failure.

haemodilution an increase of plasma in the blood in proportion to the cells. This occurs normally in pregnancy, as the blood volume increases (see HYDRAEMIA), or in haemorrhage, when fluid is drawn from the tissues into the blood to maintain the volume of circulating blood.

haemoglobin a pigment contained in the red blood cells which enables them to transport oxygen round the circulation. It is a compound of the ferrous-iron containing pigment haem combined with the protein globin. Each haemoglobin molecule contains 4 atoms of ferrous iron, 1 in each haem group, and can unite with 4 molecules of oxygen. Oxygenated haemoglobin (oxyhaemoglobin) is bright red in colour; haemoglobin inbound to oxygen (deoxyhaemoglobin) is darker. *In utero* fetal haemoglobin HbF, which is formed in the liver and spleen, has an increased affinity for oxygen. When erythropoiesis shifts to the bone marrow in the first year of life, the adult haemoglobins HbA and HbA_2 begin to be produced.

haemoglobinopathy any haematological disorder due to alteration in the genetically determined molecular structure of haemoglobin, with characteristic clinical and laboratory abnormalities and often overt anaemia. The main haemoglobinopathies which complicate pregnancy are SICKLE CELL DISEASE and THALASSAEMIA.

haemolysin ANTIBODY with COMPLEMENT which releases haemoglobin from the red blood cells.

haemolysis the liberation of haemoglobin from the confines of the red blood cell. In excess, it can cause ANAEMIA and JAUNDICE. Some microbes such as the beta haemolytic streptococcus form substances called haemolysins that have the specific action of destroying red blood corpuscles. In a transfusion reaction or in HAEMOLYTIC disease of the newborn, incompatibility causes the red blood cells to clump together. The agglutinated cells eventually disintegrate, releasing haemoglobin into the plasma. Kidney damage may result as the haemoglobin crystallizes and obstructs the renal tubules producing renal shutdown and uraemia. Other haemolysins include snake venoms, and certain vegetable and chemical poisons.

haemolytic pertaining to, characterized by or producing HAEMOLYSIS. *H. disease of the newborn* a blood dyscrasia of the newborn characterized by haemolysis of erythrocytes usually due to incompatibility between the baby's blood and the mother's. The fetus has Rh-positive blood and its mother has Rh-negative blood. In Rh incompatibility the mother builds up antibodies against the cells of the fetus; these antibodies pass through the placenta, entering the fetal circulation. There they destroy the fetal erythrocytes very rapidly. To compensate for this rapid destruction of red blood cells, there is increased bone marrow production and early release of immature red blood cells (erythroblasts). The condition is therefore also known as erythroblastosis fetalis.

haemophilia an inherited disease of delayed clotting of the blood. It is manifested only in males, but transmitted by the female as a sex-linked recessive gene. Over 80% of all patients with haemophilia have haemophilia A, which is characterized by a deficiency of clotting factor VIII. Haemophilia B (Christmas disease), which affects about 15% of all haemophiliac patients, is caused by a deficiency of factor IX. Treatment aims to raise the level of the deficient clotting factor and maintain it in order to stop local bleeding.

Haemophilus a genus of pathogenic bacteria including *H. ducreyi*, the organism of soft chancre, and *H. influenzae*, associated with influenza.

haemopoiesis *See* HAEMATOPOIESIS.

haemoptysis the coughing up of blood from the lungs. It is distinguishable from vomited blood by its bright colour and frothy character.

haemorrhage an escape of blood from its vessels either externally or within the body. *Antepartum h.* bleeding before delivery, usually classified as any bleeding in pregnancy after 24 weeks' gestation. Causes are (a) *accidental h.* or abruption of a normally situated placenta, (b) bleeding from an abnormally situated placenta, i.e. placenta praevia, (c) incidental causes. *Cerebral h.* due to rupture of a cerebral blood vessel, may occur in pregnancy associated with any hypertensive condition, e.g. eclampsia, essential hypertension. *Concealed h.* bleeding in which the amount of blood loss revealed is much less than the actual amount; clinical signs are not in keeping with the measured blood loss. In the child, *intracranial h.*

occurs in difficult delivery as a result of a tear at the junction of the TENTORIUM CEREBELLI and FALX CEREBRI and the blood vessels they contain. *Intraventricular h.* occurs in small and preterm babies. *Petechial h.* subcutaneous haemorrhage occurring in minute spots. Sometimes seen in the newborn when the cord has been tightly around the neck, or following a difficult delivery. *See also* POSTPARTUM HAEMORRHAGE.

haemorrhagic characterized by haemorrhage. *H. disease of the newborn* a condition occurring in the first week of life. The haemorrhage is usually from the gut, showing as haematemesis or melaena. Bleeding can also occur from the umbilicus, puncture sites or internally, as haematuria. It is associated with an unusually low level of blood prothrombin. It is treated by the administration of vitamin K (phytomenadione 1 ml intramuscularly) and, if necessary, blood transfusion. It should be clearly differentiated from haemolytic disease of the newborn.

haemorrhoids piles. Varicose veins of the lower rectum and canal (internal), or around the anal orifice (external). They commonly enlarge and become painful during pregnancy, due to the relaxing effect of the high secretion of PROGESTERONE on the smooth muscle of the vein walls. Constipation, general increased vascularity and congestion increase the dilatation of the veins and cause discomfort. Symptomatic relief is obtained by applying local analgesic ointment or suppositories, especially if a mild laxative is also used to soften faeces. Vaginal delivery aggravates the condition by direct pressure from the fetal head, increasing venous congestion and stasis. During the puerperium they usually resolve spontaneously as hormone levels fall and medical or surgical treatment is not often thought necessary.

haemostasis the arrest of bleeding.

haemostatic any drug or other agent capable of arresting bleeding. Those which work by reason of their astringent qualities are called styptics.

hair analysis used as an adjunct to other tests in preconception care to assess nutritional status and detect the concentration of up to 18 metals. High levels of some metals such as lead may be associated with congenital abnormalities. Deficiencies of substances such as zinc can be treated with dietary advice and/or supplements.

hallucination a false perception in which the patient believes he/she sees, smells, hears, tastes or feels an object or person when there is no basis in the external environment for the belief. This condition is a PSYCHOSIS, and may be *organic*, resulting from bacterial toxins, drugs, thyrotoxicosis, *psychogenic* or *functional*, where there are no apparent changes in the central nervous system. Any stress, such as childbirth, can precipitate this condition in one who has an inherited susceptibility. *See also* PUERPERAL PSYCHOSIS.

halothane a colourless, non-flammable, volatile liquid whose vapour is inhaled to produce general ANAESTHESIA. Rarely used for obstetric anaesthesia as postpartum haemorrhage may result due to relaxation of the uterus. More than one halothane anaesthetic within a 6-month period has been known to lead to hepatic failure.

hamamelis witchazel, employed as an astringent, especially for haemorrhoids or oedema of the vulva.

hand presentation the hand may present in labour in uncorrected oblique lie with shoulder presentation and prolapse of an arm, or in COMPOUND PRESENTATIONS. On vaginal examination a hand may be distinguished from a foot by the ability of the thumb to abduct, the absence of the prominent heel and the digits being longer than toes.

handicap a disadvantage for a given individual, resulting from an impairment or a disability that limits or prevents the fulfilment of a role that is normal for that individual.

haploid having half the number of chromosomes characteristically found in the somatic (diploid) cells of an organism.

hard chancre syphilitic ulcer of the first stage. Contagious; may be seen on the labium.

hare lip *See* CLEFT LIP.

Hartmann's solution a solution containing sodium chloride, sodium lactate, and phosphates of calcium and potassium; used intravenously as a systemic alkalizer and as a fluid and electrolyte replenisher.

hashish extract from the hemp plant, *Cannabis sativa*, which is smoked or chewed for its euphoric effects. Also called marijuana. The effects of the drug in pregnancy are uncertain as it is commonly used in conjunction with smoking and alcohol consumption and adverse outcomes for mother or fetus are attributable to the combination of substances.

head circumference the head circumference of a well-flexed fetus is the suboccipitobregmatic which measures 33 cm, and of a deflexed head, the occipitofrontal, which measures 35 cm.

head fitting an attempt to fit the non-engaged fetal head into the brim of the maternal pelvis, whereby disproportion between the head and the brim may be excluded if the head can be made to engage on pressure. In all doubtful cases, X-ray pelvimetry provides much more accurate and detailed information about the pelvis.

headache pain in the head. A symptom of a great variety of disorders. Women often suffer headaches in the first trimester of pregnancy as a result of dilatation of the cerebral blood vessels due to the action of progesterone. Headache occurring during pregnancy should never be ignored as it may be associated with pre-eclampsia, though it is usually a late symptom. It is of particular significance if other prodromal signs of eclampsia are present, i.e. raised diastolic blood pressure, spots or flashes before the eyes, or epigastric pain. *Spinal h.* an occasional complication of epidural anaesthesia when the dura mater is inadvertently punctured resulting in the loss of cerebrospinal fluid. The headache may persist for about a week.

headbox a Perspex box placed over the baby's head into which additional oxygen can be administered.

Heaf test a form of tuberculin testing.

healing the restoration of structure and function of injured or diseased tissues. The healing processes include blood clotting, inflammation and repair.

health the World Health Organization (WHO) states that 'health is a state of complete physical, mental and social well-being and not merely the absence of disease or infirmity'.

health centre a centre placed strategically in the community, to provide the full range of primary health care, commonly focused around the general practitioner's services. It may also provide facilities for minor surgery.

health education various methods of education aimed at the prevention of disease. Midwives and health visitors have particular responsibilities and opportunities to promote good health, especially with mothers and young babies.

Health Education Authority a special health authority responsible for giving authoritative advice both nationally and locally on a wide range of health education issues through campaigns and publications (formerly the Health Education Council). Now an integral part of the health service and thus participates with other health authorities in planning health service policies and priorities.

health education officer an officer appointed to make health education resources available to the community.

Health and Safety at Work Act 1974 this Act came into force in 1975. It is comprehensive legislation dealing with the welfare, health and safety of all employers and employees, except domestic workers in a private house.

health visitor (HV) a registered nurse who has also obtained the health visitor's qualification following a year's full-time course in social and preventive medicine. The main area of responsibility for the health visitor is health education and preventative care of mothers and children under 5, although some specialize in preventative care of the elderly, the handicapped and other special groups. The midwife liaises with the health visitor when she transfers the mother and baby into her care between 10 and 28 days after delivery.

hearing test See AUDITORY RESPONSE CRADLE. A hearing test is peformed by the health visitor on all babies at 7 months of age.

heart the organ which pumps the blood into the arteries to be conveyed to every part of the body. The cardiac output is considerably increased in pregnancy, since (*a*) there is much growth in the size and circulation of the uterus, (*b*) the blood volume is considerably increased, (*c*) the metabolism is increased, and (*d*) the body weight increases. *H. disease in pregnancy* girls born with congenital heart disease now survive into adult life and may become pregnant, whereas previously mitral stenosis as a result of childhood rheumatic fever or chorea was the main form of heart disease presenting in pregnant women. Antenatal, labour and postnatal care is shared between the obstetrician and cardiologist, and these women should be delivered in a consultant maternity unit. There are four grades of heart disease, and during pregnancy the condition of the mother may deteriorate by at least one grade. *H. defects* disorders, some of which may be congenital. FALLOT'S TETRALOGY and PATENT DUCTUS ARTERIOSUS are examples of congenital heart defects. *H. failure* the inability of the heart to perform its function of pumping sufficient blood to assure a normal flow through the circulation. *H. murmur* any sound in the heart region other than normal heart sounds.

heartburn a burning sensation in the chest, caused by gastro-oesophageal regurgitation, i.e. regurgitation of stomach contents into the lower oesophagus. It is a very troublesome disorder in pregnancy, caused by the relaxation of the cardia of the stomach. Magnesium trisilicate and other alkaline mixtures give transient relief. Heartburn which is troublesome at night may be relieved if the woman sleeps propped up with sev-

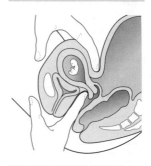

Hegar's Sign

eral pillows. Osteopathy, acupuncture or homoeopathy may be effective treatments.

heat shield a Perspex shield which may be placed over a low birth weight and/or sick baby in an incubator to prevent radiant and convective heat loss.

Hegar's dilators a series of graduated dilators used to dilate the cervix uteri.

Hegar's sign a test for pregnancy, not often used as it is uncomfortable for the woman, and now unnecessary for accurate diagnosis. It may be elicited between the 6th and 10th weeks of gestation when the embryo only occupies the upper part of the uterus. The lower part above the cervix is greatly softened and on bimanual examination almost allows the fingers to meet.

Hellin's law one in about 89 pregnancies ends in the birth of twins; one in 89^2, or 7921, in the birth of triplets; one in 89^3, or 704 969, in the birth of quadruplets. This is roughly correct as the incidence of spontaneous twin pregnancies in the UK is between 1 in 80 to 1 in 90, although infertility treatments have raised the rate of multiple pregnancies.

HELLP syndrome severe coagulation complication of pregnancy-induced hypertension (pre-eclampsia) characterized by Haemolysis, Elevated Liver proteins and Low Platelets. Diagnosed by biochemical blood tests for blood film, platelet levels and coagulation studies.

Heminevrin *See* CLOMETHIAZOLE EDISILATE.

hemiplegia paralysis of one side of the body.

hemisphere half a sphere. One of the two halves of the cerebrum.

heparin an anticoagulant formed in the liver and circulating in the blood. Injected intravenously it prevents the conversion of prothrombin into thrombin, and is used in the prevention and treatment of thrombosis. May also be administered subcutaneously, either intermittently or continuously. Rapidly excreted from the body. Protamine sulphate is used to counteract overdosage, but if used in excess, may itself act as an anticoagulant.

hepatic pertaining to the liver.

hepatitis inflammation of the liver. Usually due to a virus infection. There are two forms of viral hepatitis. *Virus A* causes infectious hepatitis which mostly affects children and young adults. It is usually a mild disease which occurs in epidemics and does not cause serious complications in pregnancy. *Virus B* causes serum hepatitis which affects all ages and is a serious complication of pregnancy. The disease is bloodborne and there is a serious risk of midwives and doctors contracting the infection if they have an abrasion which is a portal of entry for infected blood. The incubation period is 50 to 160 days and the disease is characterized by a low fever, malaise, marked anorexia, nausea, vomiting and jaundice. Bed rest in a single room with separate bathroom facilities is required. If the mother is bleeding or in labour, strict isolation and special precautions to prevent the spread of infection are carried out. Acute hepatic necrosis is a serious complication. The baby of a mother with hepatitis B should be given hepatitis B vaccine within 24 hours of delivery and it is repeated at 1 and 6 months of age. Infective jaundice is statutorily notifiable. Healthcare workers are now routinely offered vaccination against hepatitis B.

hepatomegaly enlargement of the liver.

hepatosplenomegaly enlargement of the liver and spleen.

herbal medicine a form of complementary or alternative medicine in which plants are used for their therapeutic properties. There are many herbal remedies which can effectively treat disorders in pregnancy and childbearing, but the mother should be advised to seek expert help as there are also many herbal preparations which are contra-indicated in pregnancy. Also called phytotherapy.

hereditary transmissible or transmitted from parent to offspring; genetically determined.

heredity the inheritance of physical and mental characteristics from the parents and ancestors by the offspring. The science of heredity is termed genetics. The hereditary characteristics are transmitted in the genes, many according to laws first described by Gregor Mendel, a Moravian monk. *See also* INHERITANCE.

hermaphrodite having the characteristics of both sexes. In the human subject partial development of both male and female sex organs may occur. True hermaphrodites are rare, PSEUDOHERMAPHRODITES relatively more common.

hernia a protrusion of peritoneum and other abdominal structures through a defect in the wall of the cavity. *Diaphragmatic h.* a protrusion into the thorax of any of the abdominal contents, e.g. stomach, gut. It may occur as a serious congenital malformation, in which case an emergency operation will be needed. *Femoral h.* protrusion, usually of a loop of bowel, through the femoral canal. It is more common in females. *Hiatus h.* protrusion of part of the stomach through the diaphragm into the thorax. This may be responsible for severe heartburn in pregnancy. *Inguinal h.* protrusion of bowel through the inguinal canal into the groin or scrotum. It is much commoner in males, and may be present at birth. *Umbilical h.* protrusion of bowel through the gap in the recti at the umbilicus. It is common in babies of African descent. It almost always heals spontaneously.

heroin a narcotic made from morphine. Used medicinally as an analgesic and abused illicitly for its euphoriant effects. The drug has a great capacity for inducing physical dependence and may be sniffed, smoked or injected subcutaneously or intravenously.

herpes an inflammatory skin eruption characterized by small vesicles. *H. gestationis* a skin eruption of unknown origin occurring occasionally in early or middle pregnancy and causing considerable irritation. *H. simplex* or *labialis*. 'Cold' sore on the face or lip, associated with head colds and fevers. *Genital h.* is usually caused by type 2 virus. Lesions appear on the cervix, vulva and surrounding skin in women and on the penis in men. Caesarean section is recommended for those who have clinical genital tract herpes within 2 weeks of delivery in order to prevent neonatal herpes. Congenital *h. simplex* is a very serious condition with a generalized vesicular rash. The baby dies from encephalitis. *H. zoster* shingles. An extremely painful condition caused by the virus of chickenpox, in which the eruption follows the course of a cutaneous nerve.

heterogeneous dissimilar. Made up of different characteristics.

heterosexual 1. pertaining to, characteristics of, or directed toward the opposite sex. 2. a person with erotic interests directed towards the opposite sex.

heterozygous carrying dissimilar genes. Used commonly to describe a man whose blood is Rhesus positive, but who may transmit to his children either Rhesus-positive or Rhesus-negative genes. cf. homozygous.

heuristic encouraging or promoting investigation; conducive to discovery.

hexachlorophene an antiseptic widely used in midwifery.

hiatus a space or gap. *H. hernia.* See HERNIA.

hibitane See CHLORHEXIDINE.

higher education institutions universities and colleges which provide academic programmes to diploma and degree level, including programmes of midwifery and nursing.

hilot See TRADITIONAL BIRTH ATTENDANT.

hindwaters in labour the amniotic fluid is divided into the fore- and hindwaters. When the well-flexed fetal head descends on to the cervix, it separates the small bag of amniotic fluid in front, the forewaters, from the remainder which surrounds the body, the hindwaters.

Hirschsprung's disease congenital absence of the parasympathetic nerve ganglia in the anorectum or proximal rectum, resulting in the absence of peristalsis in the affected portion of the colon and a consequent massive enlargement of the colon, constipation and obstruction. Severe cases require surgery. Called also aganglionic megacolon and congenital megacolon.

hirsute hairy.

histamine a chemical substance produced when tissue is injured. It is thought to be a factor in the causation of anaphylactic shock, which is characterized by dilatation and increased permeability of capillaries. Antihistamine drugs counteract some of these effects.

histogram a graph in which values found in a statistical study are represented by lines or symbols placed horizontally or vertically, to indicate frequency of distribution.

histology the visualization of the minute structure, composition and function of tissues and organs.

history taking a detailed synopsis of the woman's history and lifestyle, which is recorded by the midwife at the first appointment, and which forms the basis on which care is planned for the current pregnancy, labour and following childbirth. Questions are asked about the woman's personal and family medical, surgical and obstetric history, and information is obtained regarding the present pregnancy and lifestyle.

Hodge pessary a pessary which is used to maintain the position of the uterus following correction of a retroversion. See PESSARY.

Hogben test a pregnancy test, rarely used since the immunological tests were introduced. Injection of pregnancy urine into the dorsal lymph sac of the *Xenopus* toad. If gonadotrophic hormone is present in the urine, the toad will ovulate in about 8–15 hours after the injection. The test is then said to be positive for pregnancy.

holism a philosophy in which the person is considered as a functioning whole rather than as a composite of several systems.

holistic pertaining to totality, or to the whole. The client's physical, emotional, psychological, social and spiritual needs are recognized as interdependent and he or she is treated as a complete person, rather than focusing only on one problem or condition.

Homans' sign pain felt in the calf when the foot is dorsiflexed with the leg extended. It is a sign of deep vein thrombosis in the calf.

home birth *planned h.b.* women can choose to deliver their babies at home and receive care from the community midwife and general practitioner, or sometimes from an INDEPENDENT MIDWIFE. The midwife is legally obliged to provide appropriate care for any woman within her area of practice, even if the mother's wish for a home birth is against the advice of the midwife or doctor. *Unplanned h.b.* occurs when a baby who is intended to be born in hospital is born unexpectedly or prematurely at home, or where the pregnancy is concealed.

home help service a branch of the social services department, which provides domestic and housekeeping assistance to those in need. It is on either a short-term or long-term basis, and payment is according to means.

homeostasis a tendency of biological systems to maintain stability while continually adjusting to conditions that are optimal for survival. For instance, it is through homeostatic mechanisms that body temperature is kept within normal range, and nutrients are supplied to cells as needed, to give but two examples. The two basic homeostatic regulators are: 1. negative feedback controls; and 2. on–off switches, in which a response either does or does not occur. Hormonal secretions from the ENDOCRINE glands are typically regulated by the closed-loop feedback control systems, while responses of the nervous system are of the on–off type.

homoeopathy a form of complementary medicine in which treatment is by the administration of minute doses of substances which, in large quantities, would actually cause the symptoms they are intending to treat (often referred to as treating like with like). The remedy chosen must be matched exactly to the symptom picture of the individual. *See also* ARNICA.

homogeneous having the same nature or being of the same composition throughout.

homologous having the same structure or pattern.

homosexual 1. pertaining to the same sex. 2. an individual who is attracted to a person of the same sex.

homosexuality the attraction for and desire to establish a sexual relationship with a member of the same sex. Female homosexuality is known as lesbianism.

homozygous having a pair of genes which are the same. Used most commonly in midwifery in relation to the genotype of a man who is Rhesus positive. If homozygous, he can transmit only the Rhesus-positive genes to his offspring. All his children will be Rhesus positive even if the mother is Rhesus negative. cf. HETEROZYGOUS.

hookworm a parasitic roundworm that enters the human body through the skin and migrates to the intestines, where it attaches itself to the intestinal wall and sucks blood from it for nourishment. A large number of worms cause considerable blood loss and anaemia. The infection is found mainly in temperate regions where conditions are very insanitary, and in the tropics and subtropics. Shoes should be worn out of doors as the hookworm usually enters the body through the sole of the foot.

horizon a specific anatomical stage of embryonic development, of which 23 have been defined, beginning with the unicellular fertilized egg and ending 7 to 9 weeks later, with the beginning of the fetal stage.

hormone a chemical substance secreted into the blood stream by an endocrine gland, and exerting an effect on some other part of the body.

hospital delivery is advised for any woman whose medical condition is unfavourable, or whose previous or current obstetric history suggests potential problems in the forthcoming labour. The woman is, however, legally entitled to reject the advice to have her baby in hospital, and to request a HOME BIRTH.

hourglass constriction a constriction ring in the uterus, occurring during the third stage of labour, and imprisoning the placenta. An uncommon cause of retained placenta. It is relieved by the inhalation of amyl nitrite, or by anaesthesia. *See also* CONSTRICTION RING.

Housing Department a department of the local authority, responsible for providing housing.

Hourglass Constriction

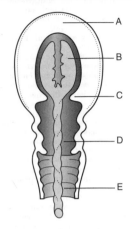

A, Upper uterine segment;
B, placenta; C, hourglass constriction; D, lower uterine segment; E, vagina.

human chorionic gonadotrophin (HCG) a hormone produced by the TROPHOBLAST. Pregnancy tests can detect its presence in the urine from 30 days after conception. The level is raised in multiple pregnancy and in cases of chorion carcinoma. It is thought to be one of the hormones responsible for nausea and vomiting in early pregnancy.

Human Fertilization and Embryology Act 1990 an amended version of the 1967 Abortion Act. Termination of pregnancy must be performed before 24 weeks of pregnancy by a registered medical practitioner, agreed with a second doctor that the woman or her family would suffer physical, mental or social trauma if the pregnancy were to continue, or if the baby is at risk of gross physical or mental abnormality. Termination of pregnancy may be performed at any time if there is serious risk to the mother's life if the pregnancy were to continue.

human immunodeficiency virus (HIV) a virus, commonly thought to have developed from a mutation of a virus found in monkeys, first identified in homosexual men in the early 1980s. In some African countries, such as Uganda and Kenya, the incidence amongst pregnant women is as high as 30%. In the UK those most at risk are recently arrived immigrants from areas such as Africa, particularly south of the Sahara, intravenous drug abusers, and women whose partners are bisexual or haemophiliacs. The virus is bloodborne and infects the T-cells and macrophages and other brain cells, eventually leading to severe deficiency of the autoimmune system. After a latent period of between 18 months and many years, the ACQUIRED IMMUNE DEFICIENCY SYNDROME develops and death will follow relatively quickly. It is not thought that pregnancy accelerates the progression of the disease in affected women but the virus may be transmitted to the fetus, either by transplacental transmission or as a result of trauma during delivery – for this reason, invasive investigations such as fetal blood sampling or the application of fetal skin electrodes should be avoided where possible. Caesarean section may reduce the risk of transmission, as may maternal administration of zidovudine (AZT). The virus can be transmitted during

117

breastfeeding and in developed countries is one of the few contraindications to breastfeeding; in developing and underdeveloped countries, the risk of transmission of HIV is probably exceeded by the risk of gastroenteritis from poor hygiene during the preparation of artificial feeds.

Screening tests for HIV are based on detection of the antibody to the virus, so that a woman found to be HIV positive will have been infectious for 12 weeks before the test becomes positive. Detailed counselling and advice is crucial for women requesting or requiring the test. Routine testing remains controversial although anonymous testing has been carried out in some centres for data regarding prevalence of the virus.

It is good practice for midwives at all times to work according to safety guidelines for the protection of themselves and others from contamination with blood products; special precautions in the event of known HIV-positive women may be necessary, but it is much more likely that a midwife may come into contact unknowingly with a woman with HIV or indeed hepatitis infection.

human placental lactogen (HPL) a hormone secreted by the placenta to aid growth and development of the breast. It is also thought to resemble growth hormone and to affect carbohydrate metabolism.

humerus the bone of the upper arm.

humid moist.

humidity the degree of moisture in the atmosphere.

Huntington's disease (chorea) a rare hereditary disease which appears in adulthood between the ages of 30 and 45 years. It is characterized by mental deterioration, speech disturbances and quick involuntary movements caused by degenerative changes in the cerebral cortex and basal ganglia. Total incapacitation and death ensue.

Hutchinson's teeth typical notching of the borders of the upper incisor teeth occurring in congenital syphilis.

hyaline resembling glass. *H. membrane* a protein material found in the alveoli of babies with hyaline membrane disease. This condition is also known as the respiratory distress syndrome (RDS) – a diagnosis of hyaline membrane disease can only be made on post mortem. The baby has increasing difficulty in breathing from birth, with expiratory grunting and rib and sternal recession. Babies who are preterm or born of diabetic mothers are particularly at risk. It is due to a lack of SURFACTANT in the lungs and is demonstrated at post mortem examination. It consists of fibrin with red cells, and necrosed protein and epithelial cells.

hyaluronidase an enzyme which can hasten the absorption of drugs into body tissues. It is found in the testes and is present in semen. The permeability of connective tissue is increased by its action and it disperses the cells of the corona radiata around the newly released ovum thereby facilitating entry of the spermatozoon and consequently conception.

hydatidiform mole vesicular mole. A benign neoplasm of the TROPHOBLAST, often the precursor of CHORIOCARCINOMA. It appears like a collection of hydropic vesicles. The incidence is 1 in 2000 pregnancies. Signs and symptoms of early pregnancy, particularly nausea and vomiting, are often severe, but no embryonic development occurs. The uterus must be evacuated surgically and the woman tested at intervals to ensure there is no regrowth of vesicles, which could progress to choriocarcinoma. She is usually advised to refrain from conceiving for 2 years.

hydraemia a modification of the blood in which there is an excess of plasma in relation to the cells. A degree of this is physiological in pregnancy.

hydralazine antihypertensive drug administered orally or intravenously. Contraindicated in early pregnancy and in women with tachycardia.

hydramnion, hydramnios excessive accumulation of amniotic fluid. *See* POLYHYDRAMNIOS *and* OLIGO-HYDRAMNIOS.

hydro- prefix signifying water or hydrogen.

hydrocele a swelling caused by accumulation of fluid, especially in the tunica vaginalis surrounding the testicles. It is very common in the newborn and usually disappears spontaneously.

hydrocephalus 'water on the brain'. An increased amount of cerebrospinal fluid distending the ventricles of the brain. A congenital malformation, severe degrees of which are incompatible with life, though in milder cases the child may survive and in many cases it can be treated by an operation in which cerebrospinal fluid is diverted from the ventricles into the blood stream. It may be recognized antenatally through an investigation of failure of the head to engage or persistent breech presentation or through observation of an unusually large fetal head. The most accurate method of diagnosis is serial cephalometry by ULTRASOUND.

hydrochloric acid chemical symbol, HCl. A strong acid. It is secreted into the gastric juice. Very acid gastric juice (pH less than 2.0), aspirated into the lungs, is the main cause of bronchospasm in MENDELSON'S SYNDROME.

hydrocortisone one of the hormones secreted by the adrenal cortex.

hydrogen a gas which combines with oxygen to form water (H_2O). Symbol H.

hydrogen ion concentration the proportion of hydrogen ions in the blood, whereby the pH of the blood is determined.

hydrogen ions hydrogen atoms carrying a positive electrical charge. Cations.

hydromeningocele protrusion of the meninges, containing fluid, through a defect in the skull or vertebral column.

hydromyelomeningocele a defect of the spine marked by a protrusion of the membranes and tissue of the spinal cord, forming a fluid-filled sac.

hydronephrosis a collection of urine in the pelves of the kidney, resulting in atrophy of the kidney structure, due to the constant pressure of the fluid, until finally, the whole organ becomes one large cyst. The condition may be (*a*) congenital, due to malformation of the kidney or ureter, or (*b*) acquired, due to any obstruction of the ureter by tumour or stone, or to back pressure from stricture of the urethra.

hydrops fetalis severe oedema of the fetus due to blood incompatibility, usually resulting in either STILLBIRTH or neonatal death.

hydrosalpinx distension of the fallopian tube by an aqueous fluid.

hygiene the science of health. *Communal h.* the maintenance of the health of the community by provision of a pure water supply, efficient sanitation, good housing, etc. *Personal h.* the cleanliness and care of the body and clothing.

119

hygroscopic readily absorbing moisture.

hymen a fold of skin, partly occluding the vaginal introitus in a virgin. The hymen is ruptured during sexual intercourse, leaving small tags of skin called *carunculae myrtiformes*. *Imperforate h.* membrane which completely occludes the vaginal orifice.

hyoscine (scopolamine) a drug with anti-salivary and amnesic properties.

hyper- prefix meaning 'excessive' or 'above normal'.

hyperbilirubinaemia an excess of bilirubin in the circulating blood.

hypercalcaemia abnormally high concentration of calcium in the blood. *Idiopathic h.* a condition of infants associated with vitamin D intoxication, characterized by elevated serum calcium levels, increased skeletal density, mental deterioration and nephrocalcinosis.

hyperdactyly the presence of supernumerary digits on the hand or foot.

hyperemesis excessive vomiting. *H. gravidarum* an uncommon serious complication of pregnancy, characterized by severe and persistent vomiting, the aetiology of which is not fully understood.

hyperglycaemia excess of glucose in the blood (adult normal 3.3–5.3 mmol/l; 60–95 mg/100 ml). Persistent hyperglycaemia is a sign of DIABETES MELLITUS.

hyperkalaemia an excess of potassium in the blood.

hypernatraemia an excessive concentration of sodium in the blood, usually diagnosed when the plasma sodium is above 150 mmol/l. It can occur if a baby has excessive salt in its feeds or if it becomes dehydrated. Convulsions can occur and can lead to brain damage. The condition can be prevented by giving low-sodium feeds, half or quarter normal strength, to a baby suffering from diarrhoea.

hyperphenylalaninaemia excess phenylalanine in the blood, as in phenylketonuria.

hyperplasia growth by multiplication of cells. Both hyperplasia and HYPERTROPHY occur in the uterus during pregnancy.

hyperprolactinaemia increased levels of prolactin in the blood; in women it is associated with infertility and may lead to galactorrhoea (excessive or spontaneous milk flow), and it has been reported to cause impotence in men.

hyperptyalism abnormally increased secretion of saliva.

hyperpyrexia excessively high body temperature, i.e. over 40°C (104°F).

hypertension abnormally high blood pressure. This may be a sign of any one of a number of diseases, e.g. acute or chronic nephritis, coarctation of the aorta; or it may be raised in an individual who is otherwise healthy, in which case it is termed *essential hypertension.* The cause of essential hypertension is not known, but it is a very common disease in the adult population and, unless treated and controlled, may lead to damage to the blood vessels in such vital organs as the heart, brain and kidneys. In pregnancy, a reading of 140/90 mmHg is regarded as the upper limit of normal, or a rise of 15–20 mmHg or more above the level recorded in the first trimester. Hypertensive diseases in pregnancy include pre-eclampsia and eclampsia which are induced by pregnancy, and pre-existing medical conditions such as essential hypertension and renal disease. The cause of pregnancy-induced hypertension is still unknown. In severe cases it is complicated by proteinuria and may develop into eclampsia which is characterized by epileptiform fits. The risk of mortality to both mother and fetus is then greatly increased.

hyperthyroidism thyrotoxicosis. Excessive activity of the thyroid gland resulting in a raised basal metabolic rate and, often, exophthalmos.

hypertonic 1. relating to hypertonia or to excessive tone or tension as in a blood vessel or muscle. *H. action of the uterus* is a type of abnormal uterine action in which the muscle tone is excessive. The contractions are extremely painful, the intermissions brief, with inadequate relaxation, labour is prolonged and exhausting to the mother and the fetus often becomes hypoxic. The mother should be under the care of an obstetrician. She will benefit from EPIDURAL ANALGESIA and intravenous oxytocin but if progress is not made she may need a caesarean section. cf. hypotonic. 2. applied to solutions which are stronger than physiological saline, e.g. hypertonic saline.

hypertrophy growth resulting from increase in the size of cells. *See also* HYPERPLASIA.

hyperventilation overbreathing, in which an excessive amount of carbon dioxide is removed from the blood. A transient respiratory alkalosis commonly results. Symptoms include 'faintness', palpitations or pounding of the heart, fullness of the throat and tetany, with muscular spasms of the hands and feet. This condition occasionally occurs when a woman is overbreathing in labour. Reassurance and a return to normal breathing is usually sufficient to rectify the situation.

hyperviscosity excessive viscosity of the blood. Occurs in conditions such as polycythaemia when the number of red blood cells is increased. Venesection to remove excess red cells may be necessary.

hypervolaemia abnormal increase in the volume of circulating fluid (plasma) in the body.

hypnosis a state of apparent deep sleep in which a person acts only under the influence of some external suggestion.

hypnotherapy a form of complementary medicine in which hypnosis is used to affect behavioural changes in the client. This is done by the induction of a trance-like state so that the person is more relaxed and open to suggestion and, if pertinent, long-forgotten memories may be brought back to the conscious mind. Conditions with a psychological component can therefore be treated, such as changing habitual behaviour, enuresis or severe anxiety states. Research has demonstrated its effectiveness as a means of altering the woman's perception of pain and discomfort in labour, and hypnotherapy has even been used as an alternative to general anaesthesia for caesarean section.

hypnotic an agent which produces sleep.

hypo- prefix meaning 'lacking in' or 'below normal'.

hypocalcaemia a low level of calcium in the blood. *Neonatal h.* can occur within 48 hours of delivery or between the 5th and 8th days of life. Convulsions may occur in the latter, especially in babies fed on unmodified cows' milk formula. The high phosphorus content in the formula contributes to this condition. Since the Report on Infant Feeding (HMSO, 1974), the majority of artificially produced milk is modified to make it as near to breast milk as possible. The condition is also a rare complication of EXCHANGE TRANSFUSION.

hypocapnia diminished carbon dioxide in the blood.

hypochondria morbid preoccupation or anxiety with one's health.

hypochondrium a region of the ABDOMEN.

hypochromic deficient in pigmentation of colouring, as with red blood cells if they are deficient in iron.

hypodactyly less than the usual number of digits on the hand or foot.

hypodermic beneath the skin. Applied to injections into the subcutaneous tissues. *H. syringe* a plastic or glass syringe, used for hypodermic injections.

hypofibrinogenaemia deficiency of fibrinogen in the blood. A rare but serious cause of postpartum haemorrhage, often associated with disseminated intravascular coagulation, severe abruptio placentae, amniotic fluid embolism and intrauterine death.

hypogastric arteries branches from the internal iliac arteries, which in the fetus pass out into the umbilical cord to carry deoxygenated blood to the placenta.

hypogastrium *See* ABDOMEN.

hypoglycaemia an abnormally low blood sugar. It may develop in a diabetic patient who is receiving insulin if insufficient carbohydrate is taken. *Neonatal h.* occurs when the blood glucose is less than 1.7 mmol/l in the baby at term and less than 1.2 mmol/l in low birth-weight babies. It may occur very soon after delivery in a baby of a diabetic (or gestational diabetic) mother, where it produces too much insulin (hyperinsulinaemia) for its extrauterine needs. It also may occur within 24–48 hours of delivery in a SMALL FOR GESTATIONAL AGE baby or any baby after severe ASPHYXIA, due to lack of GLYCOGEN in the liver. Fits or APNOEA may occur, when brain damage can ensue. Symptomatic hypoglycaemia may be prevented by early feeding and frequent screening with Dextrostix hourly during the first few days of life in babies at risk.

hypomagnesaemia abnormally low magnesium content of the blood, manifested chiefly by neuromuscular hyperirritability.

hypomenorrhoea menstruation at intervals longer than 1 month.

hyponatraemia deficiency of sodium in the blood; salt depletion. Hyponatraemia is present when the sodium concentration is less than 135 mmol/l. Symptoms include muscular weakness and twitching, progressing to convulsions if unrelieved.

hypopituitarism deficiency of secretion from the anterior lobe of the pituitary gland. It may follow severe postpartum haemorrhage, with failure of lactation and subsequent amenorrhoea and sterility. SHEEHAN'S SYNDROME.

hypoplasia underdevelopment of a part or organ. adj. *hypoplastic.*

hypoprothrombinaemia a lack of prothrombin in the blood. By lessening the clotting power of the blood, it tends to encourage bleeding. *See* HAEMORRHAGIC DISEASE OF THE NEWBORN.

hypospadias a malformation in which the urinary meatus opens upon the undersurface of the penis.

hypostatic pertaining to decreased movement. *H. pneumonia* may develop if an ill or elderly patient, or one with eclampsia, lies supine for long periods.

hypotension blood pressure below the normal range. *Postural h.* temporary fall in blood pressure when the patient stands up, resulting in dizziness and, occasionally, fainting. Common in pregnancy.

Mild Hypospadias

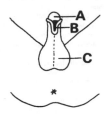

Severe Hypospadias

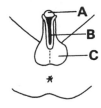

A, Glans penis; B, urethral orifice; C, scrotum.

hypotensive pertaining to low blood pressure. *H. drugs* are drugs which lower the blood pressure, e.g. hydralazine and bupivacaine, as used in epidural anaesthesia.

hypothalamus a part of the brain lying near the third ventricle. It controls the activity of the pituitary gland, the sympathetic and parasympathetic nervous system, food intake and temperature regulation, and possibly has other functions.

hypothermia a fall in the body temperature to subnormal levels. Produced artificially as an alterna-

tive or an adjunct to local or general anaesthesia. *Neonatal h.* the newborn baby may lose heat rapidly due to the large surface area of the body, especially if he/she is not adequately dried following delivery, and is worse in preterm infants who lack brown fat to help them maintain their temperature. Extreme chilling causes the baby to use up energy and oxygen, and if the temperature falls below 35°C, neonatal cold injury develops which may lead to death.

hypothesis any theory presented as a basis for argument or discussion.

hypothyroidism the condition produced by deficiency of thyroid secretion. In the child, cretinism; in the adult, myxoedema.

hypotonia deficient muscle tone, often applied to the abdominal and uterine muscles.

hypotonic describes solutions which are more dilute than physiological saline. *H. uterine action* weak, ineffective contractions with prolongation of labour unless intravenous oxytocin is used, when the contractions usually become normal. cf. hypertonic.

hypovolaemia an abnormally low circulating blood volume.

hypovolaemic pertaining to hypovolaemia. *H. shock*, or haemorrhagic shock, may occur following antepartum or postpartum haemorrhage. Emergency treatment is required to maintain an airway, administer oxygen and replace fluids intravenously. The volume of fluid required is estimated by the use of a central venous pressure line. The midwife is responsible for assisting with emergency treatment, maintaining contemporaneous records, keeping the woman as calm and undisturbed as possible and avoiding overheating of the mother.

hypoxaemia low oxygen tension in arterial blood; low P_{CO_2}.

hypoxia a diminished oxygen tension in the body tissues. *See also* ANOXIA.

hysterectomy removal of the uterus. *Abdominal h.* removal via an abdominal incision. *Pan-h.* an old term for removal of the uterus and adnexa. *Subtotal h.* removal of the body of the uterus only. *Total h.* removal of the body and cervix. *Vaginal h.* removal *per vaginam*. *Wertheim's h.* in addition to the uterus, fallopian tubes and ovaries, the parametrium, upper vagina, and all the local lymphatic glands are excised: a successful method of treatment of carcinoma of the cervix.

hysteria a psychoneurosis, with widely varied symptoms, but no organic disease.

hystero-oophorectomy excision of the uterus and one or both ovaries,

hystero-salpingectomy excision of the uterus and one or both of the uterine tubes.

hystero-salpingography radiography of the uterus and the uterine tubes after instillation of a contrast medium.

hysterotomy an incision into the uterus. An operation which consists of incision of the abdominal wall and the uterus in order to remove the ovum or evacuate the contents of the uterus before the 24th week of pregnancy and after 12 weeks.

iatrogenic induced by treatment.

ichthammol an ammoniated coal tar product, used in ointment form for certain skin diseases.

ichthyosis a rare congenital skin abnormality characterized by scaliness and desquamation of the skin of the whole body.

icterus jaundice. Yellow staining of the skin and mucous membranes resulting from an excess of bile pigments in the blood and in the tissues. *I. neonatorum* jaundice of the newborn. *I. gravis neonatorum* severe jaundice of the newborn, usually caused by Rhesus ISOIMMUNIZATION.

identical exactly alike. *I. twins* twins of the same sex developed from a single fertilized ovum. Also known as MONOZYGOTIC TWINS.

ideology 1. the science of the development of ideas. 2. the body of ideas characteristic of an individual or of a social unit.

idiopathic of unknown cause.

idoxuridine an analogue that prevents replication of DNA viruses; used topically in herpes simplex keratitis.

ileocaecal valve the valve at the junction of the ileum with the caecum.

ileum the last part of the small intestine, terminating at the caecum.

ileus paralysis of the wall of the gut, so that it is unable to propel food onward. A functional obstruction. An uncommon complication following caesarean section and other abdominal operations. *Meconium i. see* CYSTIC FIBROSIS.

iliac pertaining to the ilium. *I. crest* the crest of the hip bone. *I. fossa* a large shallow depression forming much of the inner surface of the ilium above the pelvic brim.

iliopectineal pertaining to the ilium and pubes. *I. line* the ridge which crosses the innominate bone from the sacroiliac joint to the *iliopectineal eminence*, a small protrusion marking the fusion of ilium and os pubis.

ilium the upper broad part of the innominate bone.

imaging the production of diagnostic images, e.g. radiography, ultrasonography or scintigraphy.

immature not mature. Not sufficiently developed.

immune protected against infectious diseases, foreign tissue, foreign non-toxic substances and other ANTIGENS. *I.-reactive trypsin (IRT) test* a blood test carried out for the diagnosis of cystic fibrosis.

immunity the resistance possessed by the body to infectious diseases, foreign tissues, foreign non-toxic substances and other ANTIGENS. Immunological responses in humans can be divided into two broad categories: humoral immunity, which takes place in the body fluids and is concerned with antibody and complement activities; and cell-mediated or cellular immunity, which involves a variety of activities designed to destroy or at least contain cells that are recognized by the body as alien and harmful. Both types of response are instigated by lymphocytes that originate in the bone marrow as stem cells and later are converted into mature cells having specific properties and functions. The two kinds of lymphocytes that are important to the establishment of immunity are T lymphocytes (T cells) and B lymphocytes (B cells). B lymphocytes mature into plasma cells that are primarily responsible for forming antibodies, thereby providing humoral immunity. Cellular immunity is dependent upon T lymphocytes, which are primarily concerned with a delayed type of immune response as occurs in the rejection of transplanted organs, defence against some slowly developing bacterial diseases, allergic reactions and certain autoimmune diseases. *Acquired i.* is produced specifically in response to an ANTIGEN. It involves a change in the behaviour of cells and in the production of antibody. Antibody is produced as a primary response, and after a short while the body becomes sensitized. The secondary response is produced more quickly and is more marked. *Active i.* this may be (*a*) natural, i.e. from infectious diseases, or (*b*) artificial, i.e. from injection of living or dead organisms or their products in the form of toxins and toxoids. *Passive i.* this may be: (*a*) natural, e.g. maternal immunoglobulin G (IgG) via the placenta which protects the infant from various infectious diseases for a few months, but undesirable antibodies such as anti-D immunoglobulin may also be transmitted to the fetus; or (*b*) acquired, e.g. the temporary immunity which follows the injection of antibodies of human (GAMMA GLOBULIN) or, more rarely, animal origin. *Natural or innate i.* is mainly non-specific. It is provided by intact cellular barriers of epithelium and by humoral substances such as COMPLEMENT and LYSOZYME. It is affected by genetic factors, age, race and hormone levels.

immunization rendering immune. *I. programme see* Appendix 14.

immunoglobulin antibody. A variety of chemical compound found mainly in GAMMA GLOBULIN. Immunoglobulins are major components of the humoral immune response system. They are synthesized by lymphocytes and plasma cells and found in the serum and in other body fluids and tissues. The 5 classes of immunoglobulin (Ig) are: IgA, IgD, IgE, IgG, and IgM. There are two types of IgA and both are known to have antiviral properties. Secretory IgA is present in non-vascular fluids such as colostrum and breast milk. IgD is found in trace quantities in serum. It serves as a B-lymphocyte surface receptor. IgE is called the reaginic antibody and may be increased in persons with allergy. IgG is the most abundant of the five classes of immunoglobulins and is the major antibody in the secondary humoral response of immunity. It is the only immunoglobulin to cross the placenta. IgM is principally concerned with the primary antibody response.

immunological pregnancy test urinary tests using red cells or latex particles covered with human chorionic gonadotrophin (HCG) rather than biological tests using animals such as mice, rabbits or toads. HCG antiserum is added to urine which, if the woman is pregnant, contains HCG. The HCG antibodies are therefore neutralized and when red cells or latex particles covered with HCG are added to the urine there is no agglutination. If the woman is not pregnant there will be agglutination because the HCG antibodies are not neutralized.

impacted driven into, as a wedge; lodged in a narrow strait, e.g. impacted shoulder presentation.

imperforate having no opening. *I. anus* a congenital malformation requiring surgical treatment.

impetigo blisters or raw patches over the skin, especially trunk and buttocks, usually caused by STAPHYLO-COCCI, more rarely by streptococci. In its severe form it is known as PEM-PHIGUS NEONATORUM and is highly contagious.

implant the introduction into the body tissues of drugs or tissue.

implantation the act of planting or setting in, e.g. of the fertilized ovum in the endometrium. *I. bleeding* sometimes called nidation or decidual bleeding. Vaginal bleeding at the time and from the site of embedding of the blastocyst. Because this coincides closely with the first missed menstrual period it may lead to an error in the calculation of the expected date of delivery.

implementation third stage of the process approach to midwifery care; preceded by ASSESSMENT and planning and followed by EVALUATION.

impotence absence of sexual power. The man is unable to achieve or maintain a penile erection of sufficient rigidity to perform sexual intercourse successfully. adj. *impotent*.

impregnate 1. to saturate or instil. 2. to render pregnant.

imprinting a species-specific, rapid kind of learning during a critical period of early life in which social attachment and identification are established.

in vitro within a glass, observable in a test tube, in an artificial environment.

Incarceration of a Retroverted Gravid Uterus

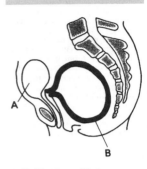

A, Bladder; B, gravid uterus.

in vitro **fertilization** fertilization of an ovum in laboratory conditions; the fertilized ovum is then replaced within the uterus of the woman; a form of infertility treatment.

in vivo within the living body.

incarcerated imprisoned. Held fast.

incarceration of the retroverted gravid uterus the term is applied to a retroverted pregnant uterus which has failed to correct its position spontaneously, and which has, by the 14th week of pregnancy, grown so large that it is now imprisoned under the sacral promontory, and cannot rise out of the pelvis. It may lead to acute retention of urine, abortion or, very rarely, SACCULATION OF THE UTERUS.

incest sexual activity between persons so closely related that marriage between them is legally or culturally prohibited.

incidence the number of particular events which occur in a population in a given period of time, e.g. the number of stillbirths per 1000 live births per annum.

incidental haemorrhage bleeding from the vagina which is due to extraplacental causes, such as cervical polyps or erosions, acute vaginitis and occasionally carcinoma of the cervix. It is uncommon, easily recognized by performing a speculum examination and rarely leads to dangerous haemorrhage. The treatment is that of the cause.

incompatibility the state of being incompatible, applied to blood or chemicals, etc.

incompatible mutually repellent. Unsuitable for combination.

incomplete abortion an abortion in which some part of the products of conception – usually the placenta – has been retained in the uterus. A cause of serious haemorrhage. *See* ABORTION.

incontinence inability to control excretory functions. *I. of urine* enuresis. *Stress i.* involuntary escape of urine due to strain on the orifice of the bladder, as in coughing, sneezing or laughing. *Faecal i.* may occur following childbirth if the woman sustains a third degree tear which involves the anal sphincter.

incoordinate lacking in harmony. *I. uterine action* failure of polarity, i.e. the ability of the upper uterine segment to contract and retract while the lower uterine segment contracts and dilates. This results in weak, ineffectual contractions, even though they may be frequent and regular, with delay in the first stage, and poor cervical dilatation which may be irregular. Oxytocic drugs are used to coordinate rather than accelerate uterine action.

incubate to place in an optimal situation for the development of living matter, by providing a suitable

temperature, humidity and oxygen concentration.

incubation, incubation period the time which elapses between invasion of the body by pathogenic bacteria and the clinical manifestation of the disease. Some common incubation periods are:

Chickenpox	14–15 days
Diphtheria	2–4 days
German measles	17–18 days
Measles	10–14 days
Mumps	14–28 days
Scarlet fever	2–4 days
Smallpox	10–14 days
Whooping cough	7–14 days

incubator 1. an apparatus for providing a suitable environment for low-birth-weight or sick babies. 2. a heated apparatus used to culture micro-organisms in a laboratory.

independent midwife a midwife who chooses to work in a self-employed capacity, either alone or in a partnership, and who contracts directly with the mothers for whom she cares. She should ensure that she has sufficient indemnity insurance and that her practice is contemporary, research-based and of the highest standards. She is personally accountable for her practice and is required to notify her intention to practise to the supervisor of midwives in each of the areas in which she works.

indigenous occurring naturally in a certain locality. *I. midwife see* TRADITIONAL BIRTH ATTENDANT.

indomethacin an anti-inflammatory, analgesic and anti-pyretic agent, used in arthritic disorders and degenerative bone disease. Also a prostaglandin inhibitor, thus reduces uterine activity. May also be used in neonates to treat patent DUCTUS ARTERIOSUS.

induction causing to occur. Used in reference to abortion, anaesthesia or labour. *I. of labour* this may be carried out when the life or health of the mother or fetus is in danger if the pregnancy continues. Indications for induction of labour include poor fetal growth or well-being, a maternal medical condition such as diabetes, hypertension, cardiac or renal disease, a poor obstetric history, or problems in the current pregnancy such as antepartum haemorrhage, breech presentation or postmaturity. The cervix is assessed for favourability using the BISHOP'S SCORE; a score of 6 or more indicates that conditions are favourable and therefore induction is likely to succeed; scores of below 6 indicate the need to deliver the baby by caesarean section. Labour may be induced using prostaglandin pessaries, amniotomy, or with intravenous syntocinon. *See also* BISHOP'S SCORE.

inertia sluggishness. *Uterine i.* better termed 'hypotonic uterine action'. Inability of the uterine muscle to contract efficiently. A common cause of prolongation of labour.

inevitable that which cannot be avoided. *I. abortion* the process of abortion at a stage when it is irreversible. *I. (unavoidable) haemorrhage see* PLACENTA PRAEVIA.

infant a young child from birth to 1 year of age. *I. feeding* breast and artificial feeding. *Preterm i.* one born before 37 weeks completed gestation.

infant mortality rate the number of registered deaths of infants under the age of 1 year for every 1000 live births registered in any given year.

infanticide the murder of an infant.

infantile paralysis POLIOMYELITIS.

infarct an area of necrosis in an organ caused by local ischaemia. In the placenta it is due to an obstruction to the local circulation caused by fibrin deposits in the INTERVILLOUS spaces, so that any VILLI in the area die from ischaemia. Infarcts occur in ABRUPTIO PLACENTAE and in hypertensive conditions such as pre-eclampsia. Initially in the acute phase they are seen as deep red infarcts, subsequently changing colour, through brown and yellow, to white infarcts, after about a week. If large areas occur, the fetus may die or be SMALL FOR GESTATIONAL AGE, with all its complications.

infarction the formation of an infarct. *Pulmonary i.* necrosis of the lung tissue, resulting from an embolus.

infection the invasion of tissues by pathogenic micro-organisms. There are several stages in the infectious process: 1. the causative agent, which must be of sufficient number and virulence or capable of destroying normal tissue; 2. reservoirs in which the organism can thrive and reproduce; 3. a portal through which the pathogen can leave the host, e.g. via the intestinal or respiratory tract; 4. a mode of transfer, e.g. the hands, air currents and FOMITES; 5. a portal of entry through which the pathogens can enter the body, e.g. through open wounds, the respiratory, intestinal and reproductive tracts; 6. susceptible host; not having any immunity to it, or lacking adequate resistance to overcome the invasion by the pathogens. The body responds to the invading organisms by the formation of ANTIBODIES and by a series of physiological changes known as inflammation. *Aerobic i.* infection caused by an AEROBE. *Airborne i.* infection by inhalation of organisms suspended in air on water droplets or dust particles. *Anaerobic i.* infection caused by an ANAEROBE. *Cross i.* infection transmitted between patients *Droplet i.* infection due to inhalation of respiratory pathogens suspended on liquid particles exhaled by someone already infected. *Endogenous i.* 1. that due to reactivation of organisms present in a dormant focus, as occurs in tuberculosis; 2. that caused by organisms present in or on the body. *Exogenous i.* that caused by organisms not normally present in the body but which have gained entrance from the body surface of others or from the environment. *Hospital acquired i.* those acquired during hospitalization. *Nosocomial i.* hospital-acquired infection. *Opportunistic i.* infection caused by a micro-organism which does not normally cause disease, but may do so when the woman's resistance is lowered, e.g. after severe postpartum haemorrhage. *Secondary i.* infection by a pathogen superimposed on an infection already present. *Sexually transmitted i.* infection transmitted by intimate contact with the genitals, mouth and rectum.

inferior longitudinal sinus venous sinus within the tentorium cerebelli which, with the superior longitudinal sinus, drains blood away from the head. Joins with the great vein of Galen and straight sinus at the confluens sinuum – a point which tears easily in situations where excess or rapid moulding of the fetal skull occurs and can lead to tentorial tears and intracranial haemorrhage; *see* FETAL SKULL.

infertility inability to conceive.

infestation animal parasites on or within the body.

infibulation the process of fastening, for example joining the edges of wounds with clasps during surgery. It is performed as part of FEMALE GENITAL MUTILATION in some areas of the world, when the labia are joined together to reduce the vestibular introitus.

infiltration the entrance and diffusion of some liquid. *I. analgesia* injection of lidocaine (lignocaine) into the tissues.

inflammation a series of changes in tissues indicating their reaction to injury, whether mechanical, chemical or bacterial, so long as the injury does not cause death of the affected part. The cardinal signs are: heat, swelling, pain, redness and loss of function. *Acute i.* the onset is sudden, the signs are marked and progressive. *Chronic i.* a form with slow progress and formation of new connective tissue.

influenza an acute epidemic virus infection of the respiratory tract. It is usually in the form of an acute general illness with fever, generalized aching, pain in the limbs and relatively minor respiratory symptoms. In severe cases pneumonia may follow, usually as a result of secondary bacterial infection.

infra- prefix meaning 'below'.

infundibulum a funnel-shaped structure. The fimbriated end of the fallopian tube.

infusion 1. The process of extracting the soluble principles of substances (especially drugs) by soaking in water. 2. treatment by the introduction of fluid into the body, e.g. dextrose or saline.

ingestion the introduction of food and drugs by the mouth.

inguinal relating to the groin. *I. canal* the channel through the abdominal wall, above POUPART'S LIGAMENT, through which the spermatic cord and vessels pass to the testicle in the male, and which contains the round ligament of the uterus in the female. *I. hernia, see* HERNIA.

inhalation the breathing of air, vapour or volatile drugs into the lungs. *I. anaesthesia* anaesthesia induced by the inhalation of drugs. *I. analgesia* nitrous oxide and oxygen inhaled from specially designed machines, and used for the relief of pain in labour. *See* ENTONOX.

inheritance transmission of characteristics or qualities from parent to offspring.

inhibition arresting or restraining.

inhibitor an agent which interferes with or inhibits a reaction.

iniencephaly a congenital malformation with herniation of the brain in the occipital region.

injection the act of introducing a liquid into the body by means of a syringe or other instrument. *Epidural i.* into the epidural space. *Intradermal i.* into the skin. *Intramuscular i.* into the muscles. *Intrathecal i.* into the theca of the spinal cord. *Intravenous i.* into a vein. *Subcutaneous i.* below the skin.

inlet (pelvic) the brim, the entrance to the true pelvis. *See* PELVIS.

innate inborn; present in the individual at birth.

inner cell mass the group of cells in the cavity of the blastocyst, from which the amniotic membrane and the fetus will develop.

innervation nerve distribution to an organ or part of the body.

innominate without a name. *I. artery* a branch of the arch of the aorta. *I. bone* the hip bone made up of the fused ilium, ischium and os pubis. *See* PELVIS.

inoculation introduction into the body of a protective substance, e.g. antitoxin or vaccine.

inquest a legal or judicial inquiry into some matter of fact. A *coroner's i.* is held in all cases of sudden or unexplained death in order to determine the cause.

insemination introduction of semen into the vagina or cervix. *Artificial i.*

insemination by other means than sexual intercourse.

insertion a point of attachment, e.g. of a muscle to a bone or of the cord to the placenta.

insidious a term applied to a disease or condition which develops almost imperceptibly.

insomnia inability to sleep.

inspection looking. Inspection forms a part of the antenatal abdominal examination: the midwife should observe the mother's abdomen for the size and shape, scars, STRIAE GRAVIDARUM, presence of the LINEA NIGRA, and any fetal movements.

inspiration drawing in the breath.

instillation pouring a liquid into a cavity drop by drop, e.g. into the eye.

instruments *see* Appendix 3.

insufficiency a state of inadequate function. *Placental i.* failure of the placenta to fulfil its function adequately. It is often associated with pre-eclampsia, essential hypertension, chronic nephritis, postmaturity and heavy smoking. The effect is to cause the fetus to be SMALL FOR GESTATIONAL AGE or even, in extreme cases, to die *in utero*.

insufflation the blowing of gas, fluid or powder into a cavity. *I. of the fallopian tubes* the blowing of carbon dioxide via the uterus into the fallopian tubes to test their patency. A dye, methylene blue, is now more often used for this purpose.

insulin the HORMONE produced in the islets of Langerhans in the pancreas, which regulates carbohydrate metabolism. Deficiency causes DIABETES MELLITUS. Various preparations of insulin are used in the treatment of diabetes. Overdosage of insulin leads to HYPOGLYCAEMIA.

integrated medicine contemporary term implying the integration of

131

complementary or alternative medicine into conventional health care.

Intention to Practise statutory requirement of all registered midwives intending to practise midwifery in a particular health board or trust. A designated form is completed annually or at any time when a midwife intends to provide midwifery care in a trust other than her usual.

inter- a prefix signifying 'between'.

interaction the quality, state or process of (two or more things) acting on each other. *Drug i.* the action of one drug upon the effectiveness or toxicity of another (or others).

intercellular between the cells, i.e. the tissue spaces.

intercostal between the ribs. *I. muscles* those of the chest wall.

intermittent having intervals or pauses. Not continuous, e.g. uterine contractions to allow fetal oxygenation.

intermittent mandatory ventilation (IMV) a method used to wean a baby from a ventilator by gradually reducing the ventilator pressure and then the respiratory rate settings.

intermittent positive pressure ventilation (IPPV) a form of respiratory therapy utilizing a VENTILATOR for the treatment of patients with inadequate breathing. Very small babies, or those with severe respiratory distress syndrome, may require virtually all the work of breathing to be done for them. The indications for mechanical ventilation of babies include severe apnoea, a Po_2 of less than 5 kPa despite a high concentration of oxygen in inspired air and a Pco_2 greater than 12 kPa associated with acidosis which fails to respond to treatment. Some paediatricians now ventilate all very-low-birthweight babies for 24 hours or so in the absence of frank respiratory distress because it is thought to prevent the development of the condition and to avoid such complications as intraventricular haemorrhage. The complications of mechanical ventilation of small babies include pneumothorax, infection, bronchopulmonary dysplasia and retinopathy of the lens due to high oxygen and possibly carbon dioxide levels.

internal os the opening through which the cavity of the cervix communicates with the cavity of the body of the uterus.

internal version usually internal podalic version. Turning the child by intrauterine manipulation to make the breech present. A manoeuvre once frequently and now occasionally practised during labour to convert the fetus from an oblique to a longitudinal lie or to correct a brow presentation. It consists of inserting a hand into the uterus, grasping one of the child's feet and, with the help of abdominal manipulation, bringing the foot through the cervix to stabilize the presentation.

International Code of Marketing of Breast Milk Substitutes See WHO INTERNATIONAL CODE OF MARKETING OF BREAST MILK SUBSTITUTES.

intersex a person having an abnormality in the sex chromosomes, the gonads, the sex hormones or the genitalia. *See* KLINEFELTER'S SYNDROME *and* TURNER'S SYNDROME.

interspinous between the (ischial) spines. *See* PELVIS.

interstitial pertaining to a space in the body.

intertrigo an erythematous skin eruption occurring on apposed surfaces of the skin, such as the folds of the groin and armpit. It is caused by moisture, warmth, friction, sweat retention and infectious agents.

Good hygiene and the application of a talcum powder containing zinc oxide is the usual treatment.

intervillous between (chorionic) villi. The intervillous spaces allow maternal arterial blood to flow and cascade round the terminal villi of the placenta when gaseous exchange and transport of amino acids, glucose, minerals and vitamins take place.

intestine that part of the alimentary canal which extends from the stomach to the anus. *Small i.* the first 7 m (20 ft) from the pylorus to the caecum, consisting of the duodenum, jejunum and ileum. *Large i.* this is 2 m (6 ft) in length and consists of the caecum, vermiform appendix, ascending, transverse, descending and pelvic colon and rectum. The canal completes the process of digestion and eliminates waste matter.

intra- prefix signifying 'within'.

intracellular within a cell. *I. organisms* those which invade cells, e.g. the gonococcus. *I. fluid* the fluid within the cells of the body.

intracranial within the cranium. *I. membranes* the MENINGES covering the brain. A vertical fold in the midline between the cerebral hemispheres forms the falx cerebri. This joins posteriorly a horizontal fold, the tentorium cerebelli, which separates the cerebellum and cerebrum. The membranes contain blood vessels (sinuses) and undue pressure or trauma during delivery may cause tearing of the membranes and sinuses leading to cerebral haemorrhage. *I. pressure* the pressure exerted by the cerebrospinal fluid within the subarachnoid space and ventricles of the brain. It can be measured by monitoring pressure within the cerebral ventricles.

Intracranial Membranes and Sinuses

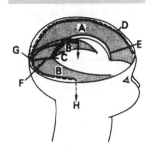

A, Falx cerebri; B, tentorium cerebelli; C, great cerebral vein; D, superior longitudinal sinus; E, inferior longitudinal sinus; F, straight sinus; G, confluens sinuum; H, lateral sinuses leaving skull as internal jugular veins.

---

intragastric within the stomach. *I. tube feeding* artificial feeding, usually by nasogastric tube.

intramuscular within or into muscle.

intrapartum literally, within parturition, i.e. labour: the time between onset of the first stage of labour and completion of the third stage.

intraperitoneal within the peritoneal cavity. By *i. transfusion* it is possible to introduce sufficient Rhesus-negative red cells to replace some of the haemolysed Rhesus-positive cells to prolong the intrauterine life of the affected fetus.

intrauterine within the uterus. *I. contraceptive device (IUCD)* a mechanical device inserted into the uterine cavity for the purpose of contraception. Their mode of action is not

133

fully understood but they increase tubal motility, render the endometrium less favourable for implantation and may also increase prostaglandin production, thereby increasing the likelihood of expulsion of the conceptus. *I. death* death of the fetus *in utero*. Generally used to refer to a death during pregnancy rather than one during labour. *I. growth retardation (IUGR)* poor fetal growth due to placental insufficiency and leading to a baby who is SMALL FOR GESTATIONAL AGE, or in severe cases, stillborn. *I. transfer* transfer of a pregnant mother to a maternity unit with facilities for a neonatal intensive care, usually a woman in very preterm labour.

intravascular within a vessel, usually a blood vessel. *I. coagulation* clotting of blood within the circulation. *See* DISSEMINATED INTRAVASCULAR COAGULATION.

intravenous within a vein.

intraventricular haemorrhage (IVH) a serious cerebral haemorrhage which occurs in preterm infants below 34 weeks of gestation. It begins on the lateral wall of the ventricle of the brain and causes periods of APNOEA and death. It is now the most common lethal condition in very-low-birthweight infants (VLBW). It can be diagnosed by COMPUTED TOMOGRAPHY (CT) but more conveniently with a portable REAL-TIME ultrasound scanner.

intrinsic relating to a quality of a structure or substance, which is inherent within itself.

introitus the entrance to any cavity of the body. *I. vaginae* the entrance to the vagina.

intubation the introduction of a tube. *Endotracheal i.* introduction of a tube or catheter into the trachea. A doctor or midwife may intubate the trachea of an asphyxiated infant, with the aid of a direct-vision laryngoscope, and insufflate with oxygen or air at a controlled pressure.

intussusception prolapse of one part of the intestine into the lumen of an immediately adjacent part, causing intestinal obstruction. May occur during the first year of life.

inverse reverse of the normal.

inversion of the uterus a rare condition in which the uterus is partly or completely turned inside out. *Acute i.* occurs in the third stage of labour (a) as a result of attempting CREDÉ'S EXPRESSION, when the uterus is relaxed; (b) by traction on the umbilical cord when the uterus is relaxed and the placenta not completely separated; and (c) spontaneously. It causes extreme shock. Replacement should be undertaken as quickly as possible.

involuntary independent of the will.

involution returning to normal size after enlargement, e.g. the uterus after labour. Immediately after labour the uterus weighs about 0.9 kg, 1 week later it weighs 0.45 kg and at the end of the puerperium (6–8 weeks) it weighs only about 60 g. The length is reduced from about 17.5 cm to about 7.5 cm. This process is due to ischaemia and AUTOLYSIS of muscle fibre following withdrawal of oestrogen and stimulation of protein synthesis. The soluble end-products are removed by the blood stream. The thrombosed uterine blood vessels also disappear by autolysis and new vessels form. The placental site contracts rapidly at first, then more slowly, and disappears by the 6th or 7th week. *See also* SUBINVOLUTION.

iodide a compound of iodine.

iodine a non-metallic element with a distinctive odour, obtained from seaweed. *Tincture of i.* is the preparation most commonly used. Radioactive iodine is used to evaluate thyroid activity. *See also* ISOTOPE.

ion an electrically charged atom or group of atoms formed when an electrolyte dissolves in water. Hydrogen ions carry a positive charge; hydroxyl ions a negative charge. The hydrogen ion concentration of a fluid determines its reaction, expressed as its pH.

iridology a form of diagnostic technique, used in complementary medicine, in which the irises of the eyes are thought to reflect all other areas of the body. Each part of the iris is considered to relate to an area of the body; by identifying changes in the iris it may be possible to diagnose problems elsewhere in the body.

iris the coloured part of the eye made of two layers of muscle, the contraction of which alters the size of the pupil.

iritis inflammation of the iris, causing pain, photophobia, contraction of the pupil and discoloration of the iris.

iron a metallic element, which is an important constituent of haemoglobin. Iron compounds ingested in food are converted for use in the body by the action of the hydrochloric acid produced in the stomach. This acid separates the iron from the food and combines with it in a form that is readily assimilated by the body. Vitamin C enhances absorption of iron. The administration of alkalis hampers iron absorption. The amount of new iron needed every day by an adult is 15 mg. Iron deficiency anaemia is a common problem, especially in pregnancy as a result of increased demands on the mother's blood. Iron-rich foods are advised and, if necessary, iron supplements prescribed.

ischaemia local insufficiency of blood supply.

ischial pertaining to the ischium.

ischiocavernosus muscle muscle extending from the ischium of the pelvis to the clitoris or penis, aiding in their erection.

ischiococcygeus muscle muscle extending from the pelvis ischium to the coccyx; the posterior portion of the levator ani muscle.

ischium the lower posterior part of the innominate bone of the pelvic girdle.

isoimmunization immunization within the species. This occurs in a Rhesus-negative woman if Rhesus-positive cells from her fetus pass into her circulation via the placenta, causing sensitization and then antibody production (anti-D), to these red cells. When the antibody enters the fetal circulation, HAEMOLYSIS occurs.

isolation the separation of an infected person from those not infected.

isometric maintaining, or pertaining to, the same length; of equal dimensions.

isoniazid an antibacterial compound used in treatment of tuberculosis.

isotonic of the same strength or tension. *I. solution* is of the same osmotic pressure as the fluid with which it is compared. Normal, or physiological, saline is isotonic with blood plasma.

isotope an element having the same atomic number, that is the number of protons in the nucleus, but a different number of NEUTRONS. This leads to instability, often with emission of radioactivity, making even minute quantities identifiable with a Geiger counter.

isoxsuprine hydrochloride a beta-adrenergic stimulant used as a vasodilator in peripheral vascular disease and cerebrovascular insufficiency. Used intravenously to arrest preterm labour by relaxing the myometrium.

ispaghula oral laxative which works by increasing faecal mass.

isthmus *See* UTERUS.

J

Jacquemier's sign blueness of the lining of the vagina seen from the early weeks of pregnancy due to increased blood supply.

jaundice yellow discoloration of the skin, sclerotics and mucous membranes, due to an excess of bile pigments in the blood and tissues. It may be (a) *haemolytic*, when the bile pigment is derived from the haemoglobin of haemolysed red blood cells, or (b) *obstructive*, when the bile pigment is present as a constituent of bile. Jaundice may occur in pregnancy from severe HYPEREMESIS GRAVIDARUM, severe pre-eclampsia or eclampsia and acute liver atrophy. It can also be due to coincidental causes such as infective hepatitis, serum hepatitis or drugs. Though rare, these are dangerous conditions, and a midwife observing jaundice during pregnancy in any circumstances should consult a doctor. *Breast milk j.* elevated unconjugated bilirubin in some breastfed infants due to the presence of a steroid in the breast milk which inhibits glucuronyl transferase conjugating activity. *Infectious j.* 1. infectious hepatitis. 2. leptospiral jaundice. *Physiological j.* mild icterus neonatorum during the first few days of life. The newborn baby no longer requires the high levels of circulating fetal haemoglobin which assisted in intrauterine oxygenation and the excess red blood cells need to be broken down (haemolysed) into fat soluble bilirubin. This must then be conjugated into water soluble bilirubin in order to be excreted. A liver enzyme, glucuronyl transferase, is required for this process, but due to the relative immaturity of neonatal hepatic function, the process is sometimes delayed. Bilirubin accumulates in the blood and leaks into the tissues, causing a yellow staining of the skin and sclerae. Treatment is rarely necessary unless the serum bilirubin remains high, when phototherapy may be used to reduce the level of unconjugated bilirubin and so avoid the danger of KERNICTERUS.

jejunum the portion of the small intestine from the duodenum to the ileum.

jelly a soft, coherent, resilient substance; generally a colloidal semi-solid mass. *Contraceptive j.* a non-greasy jelly used in the vagina for prevention of conception. *Petroleum j.* a purified mixture of semi-solid hydrocarbons obtained from petroleum. *Wharton's j.* the soft, jelly-like intracellular substance of the umbilical cord, which insulates the vein and arteries, preventing occlusion and fetal hypoxia.

joint an articulation. The junction of two or more bones. The primary function of a joint is to provide motion and flexibility to the human frame.

joule (J) the international (SI) unit which measures the energy of food, and is replacing CALORIES. One joule = 4.2 calories.

jugular concerning the neck. *J. veins* these are three in number, the *anterior, external* and *internal* jugular veins, and are responsible for carrying blood away from the head.

justominor pelvis a small gynaecoid pelvis; all the diameters are reduced but are in proportion.

juxta- word element meaning situated near, adjoining.

juxtaposition apposition; a placing side by side or close together.

K

Kahn test a blood test to detect syphilis.

kalaemia the presence of potassium in the blood.

kalium potassium (symbol K).

kanamycin a broad-spectrum antibiotic effective against many Gram-negative bacteria, and some Gram-positive and acid-fast bacteria.

kaolin China clay used as a dusting powder and for poultices.

Kaposi's sarcoma a multi-focal metastasizing, malignant reticulosis with angiosarcoma features, involving chiefly the skin. Kaposi's sarcoma is a major feature of AIDS, particularly in homosexuals.

karyo- word element meaning nucleus.

karyotype the chromosomal constitution of the cell nucleus; by extension, photomicrograph of chromosomes arranged in numerical order.

Kegel exercises specific exercises named after Dr Arnold H. Kegel, a gynaecologist who first developed the exercises to strengthen the pelvic–vaginal muscles as a means of controlling stress incontinence in women. All women of reproductive years should be encouraged to practise pelvic floor exercises several times daily, and as often as ten times daily in the puerperium. The exercise consists of tightening the vaginal, pelvic floor and rectal muscles. Effectiveness of the exercise can be tested occasionally by attempting to control/stop the flow of urine during micturition. However, women should be strongly discouraged from regularly practising the exercise during micturition as this may cause urinary reflux into the ureters and predispose to urinary tract infection.

keloid overgrowth of a fibrous tissue in a scar.

keratin a tough protein which forms the base of all horny tissues.

keratitis inflammation of the cornea.

kernicterus nuclear jaundice. Yellow staining of the kernel cells in the basal ganglia of the brain, occurring in infants with severe jaundice, particularly that caused by Rhesus ISOIMMUNIZATION. It is manifested by signs of irritability, fits and athetoid movements of the arms. It may be fatal, or the child may survive but be left with some mental or neurological defect. It may develop in any newborn child in whom the unconjugated serum bile pigment rises above 350 μmol/l (20 mg/100 ml) or lower in preterm or seriously ill babies. Infants in whom kernicterus is a danger are treated by one or more replacement transfusions or by phototherapy to prevent development of kernicterus.

Kernig's sign sign of meningitis. When the thigh is supported at right angles to the trunk, the patient is unable to straighten the leg at the knee joint.

ketoacidosis state of electrolyte imbalance with ketosis and lowered blood pH.

ketone bodies acetone, acetoacetic acid and β-hydroxybutric acid; except for acetone (which may arise spontaneously from acetoacetic acid), they are normal metabolic products of lipids and pyruvate within the liver, and are oxidized by muscles; excessive production leads to urinary excretion of these bodies, as in diabetes mellitus. Called also acetone bodies.

ketonuria the presence of ketones in urine.

ketosis the condition in which ketones are formed in excess in the body. In starvation or in uncontrolled DIABETES MELLITUS, there is a great increase in fatty acid metabolism, and impaired or absent carbohydrate metabolism, which results in greatly increased production of ketone bodies. The production of ketone bodies is reduced to the normal low level and the ketoacidosis is reversed when adequate carbohydrate metabolism is restored. The client with ketosis often has a sweet or 'fruity' odour to her breath which is produced by acetone.

key worker a person (commonly a social worker) designated as coordinator for action where several people are involved in the care of a person or family. The key worker is also responsible for calling a CASE CONFERENCE.

kick chart more properly, a movement chart. A chart on which the mother herself records fetal movements in a given period of time. Evidence of 10 movements a day is considered acceptable. The mother may be advised to call the midwife or doctor if she does not experience 10 fetal movements per day. However, as this is a subjective assessment, it is usually combined with other tests of fetal well-being.

kidneys two bean-shaped organs, situated near the lower thoracic and upper lumbar vertebrae and behind the peritoneum. The kidney consists of a cortex and medulla, and is made up of about one million nephrons. The functions of the kidneys are: 1. to maintain the water balance and solute content of the body, thus maintaining the osmotic pressure; 2. to keep the plasma pH constant between 7.35 and 7.45; and 3. to excrete waste products, especially nitrogen from protein metabolism; to regulate the blood pressure via the renin–angiotensin–aldosterone mechanism. The kidneys respond to ischaemia by secreting a proteolytic enzyme called RENIN. This acts on a plasma protein (renal substrate) in the blood to produce ANGIOTENSIN I. A converting enzyme from the lungs converts angiotensin I to II, which causes widespread vasoconstriction, increases peripheral resistance and raises the blood pressure. Angiotensin II also effects an increase in blood pressure through its influence on sodium and water retention, by increasing the secretion of aldosterone from the adrenal cortex.

Kielland's forceps See KJELLAND'S FORCEPS.

kilo- the prefix indicating 'one thousand', e.g. kilogram (kg) 1000 grams, kilometre (km) 1000 metres, kilopascal (kPa) 1000 pascals, kilocalorie (kcal) 1000 calories.

Kjelland's forceps obstetric forceps with a sliding lock and no pelvic curve, designed to apply to the fetal head, whatever its position in the pelvis. The head may then be rotated to an occipitoanterior position with the forceps before it is extracted.

Klebsiella a genus of Gram-negative bacteria.

Klebs–Loeffler bacillus the bacillus of diphtheria.

Kleihauer test a microscopic test to detect fetal cells in the maternal circulation, usually done immediately after delivery so that, if the mother is Rhesus-negative and the fetus Rhesus-positive, anti-D immunoglobulin may be given to prevent ISOIMMUNIZATION.

Klinefelter's syndrome an example of intersex. A male with one or more extra X chromosomes. The genitalia appear normal until puberty, when the testes fail to descend and the man is consequently infertile. Development of the breasts also occurs.

Klumpke's paralysis paralysis of the lower arm and hand, resulting in wrist-drop. It is due to injury to the lower part of the BRACHIAL PLEXUS, the eighth cervical and first dorsal nerves. It may occur when bringing down extended arms in a breech labour, or by applying undue traction when releasing the anterior shoulder in a vertex delivery.

knee presentation a type of breech presentation in which one or both knees lie below the buttocks.

Kocher's forceps artery forceps used at birth to clamp the umbilical cord before separation; may also be used for artificial rupture of the membranes; see Appendix 3.

Konakion See PHYTOMENADIONE.

Koplik's spots small, irregular, bright red spots on the buccal and lingual mucosa, with a minute bluish white speck in the centre of each; they are pathognomonic of beginning measles.

Korotkoff's method a method of finding the systolic and diastolic blood pressure by listening to the sounds produced in an artery while the pressure in a previously inflated cuff is gradually reduced. The method was first described by Korotkoff, a Russian surgeon in 1905. *Korotkoff 1* is the onset of clear rhythmical tapping as the cuff is deflated and represents the systolic pressure. *Korotkoff 2* is a murmur or swishing sound. *Korotkoff 3* is a crisper, more intense tapping. *Korotkoff 4* is muffled and low-pitched and in pregnancy may be easier to record than *Korotkoff 5*. *Korotkoff 5* is the absence of sound which in adolescents and adults usually represents the diastolic pressure. During pregnancy some muffled tapping may be heard down to 0 when the cuff is fully deflated. It is important for midwives to be aware of local practices for the recording of diastolic pressure.

kraurosis vulvae dryness and atrophy of the vulva.

kwashiorkor a condition occurring in babies and young children due to severe protein deficiency. Symptoms include oedema, impaired growth and development, distension of the abdomen (pot belly), pathological liver changes and pigmentation changes of skin and hair.

kyphosis posterior curvature of the spine; humpback.

L

labetalol hydrochloride an alpha and beta-adrenergic receptor blocker used in the treatment of hypertension. May be given orally or by intravenous infusion.

labial pertaining to the lips or labia.

labile unstable. Liable to variation. *L. hypertension* a term used in reference to a woman whose blood pressure is variable between normal and an appreciably higher level.

labium a lip. *L. majus pudendi* the large fold of flesh surrounding the vulva. *L. minus pudendi* the lesser fold within. pl. *labia.*

labour parturition or childbirth. *Normal l.* occurs spontaneously at term with a vertex presentation of a singleton fetus and is completed within 24 hours without trauma to mother or fetus. Physiology depends on the interaction between the uterine action, maternal pelvis and the fetus. During the *first stage* effacement and dilatation of the cervix occur; contractions are fundally dominant; POLARITY in the uterus facilitates contraction and RETRACTION in the upper uterine segment and contraction and dilatation in the lower uterine segment. The *second stage* commences when the cervix uteri is fully dilated and involves delivery of the fetus from the birth canal. The *third stage* involves separation and expulsion of the placenta and membranes and the control of haemorrhage. *Obstructed l.* a rare condition in which there is an insuperable barrier to the passage of the fetus, so that despite good uterine action, there is no advance of the presenting part. This may be because the mother's pelvis is contracted, or the available space is occupied by a mass such as a tumour, or due to fetal malpresentation, malposition or abnormality such as hydrocephalus. There is a high risk of uterine rupture, especially in a multiparous woman, and fetal death. The mother is in severe pain and distress, with a raised pulse rate and temperature, oliguria and ketonuria. On abdominal examination the uterus appears 'moulded' around the fetus; it feels continuously hypertonic and fetal parts cannot be felt. With adequate midwifery and obstetric care the condition is largely preventable and is rarely seen in the UK but may present in areas of the world where good care is not available. Pain, dehydration and shock should be treated and caesarean section should be performed. If this is not possible, manipulative or destructive procedures are undertaken to extricate the fetus in order to save the mother's life. *Precipitate l.* one in which the entire process of labour is completed in under two hours. Uterine action is extremely powerful and the mother may be unaware of it. There is a danger to the mother of haemorrhage and uterine inversion, and to the fetus of trauma and birth injury due to the rapid delivery and moulding

Physiological Changes in the Cervix During the First Stage of Labour

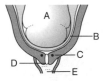

Cervix uneffaced

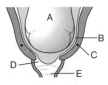

Cervix effaced
and partly dilated

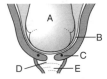

Cervix partly effaced

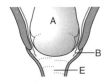

Cervix fully dilated

A, Fetal head; B, membranes; C, internal os; D, external os; E, vagina.

of the head. *Preterm l.* labour occurring after the 24th week of pregnancy and before full term. *Spontaneous l.* that which occurs without being artificially induced or accelerated. *Spurious l.* contractions which occur without any change in the state of the cervix, so that there is no progress towards delivery. Also called false labour.

laceration tear. *Perineal l. see* PERINEAL.

lacrimal pertaining to tears. *L. ducts* minute openings at the inner end of each eyelid, which convey the fluid into the nose by the nasolacrimal duct to mix with the secretions of the nose. *L. glands* small bodies situated in the orbital cavity at the upper and outer surface of each eyeball, the function of which is to provide the fluid (tears) which keeps the conjunctiva moist and free from infection by LYSOZYME, except in the neonate.

lactalbumin the main protein in human milk. It is easily digested by the baby.

lactase an enzyme produced by the cells of the small intestine, which splits LACTOSE into the MONOSACCHARIDES GLUCOSE and GALACTOSE.

lactation the secretion of milk by the breasts. *L. period* the period during which a child is suckled. *See* Figure, p. 145.

Third Stage of Labour

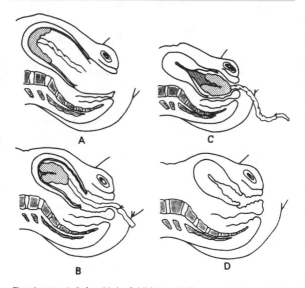

The placenta. A, Before birth of child; B, partially separated immediately after birth; C, completely separated; D, contraction and retraction of uterus after expulsion.

lacteals the lymphatics of the intestine which absorb split fats.

lactic acid an acid formed in the body during hypoxia. It is the main acid which appears in the blood of an asphyxiated baby, and accounts for the high ACIDAEMIA. The acid may also be produced in the gut by fermentation of lactose through the action of bacilli.

lactiferous conveying milk.

Lactobacillus acidophilus Döderlein's bacillus. A Gram-positive bacillus (*see* GRAM STAIN), which is a normal inhabitant of the vagina during childbearing years. It converts glycogen to lactic acid, which inhibits the growth of other organisms; it is also found predominating in the stools of breastfed babies.

Physiology of Lactation

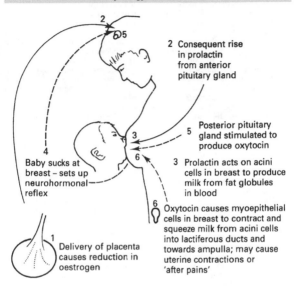

2 Consequent rise in prolactin from anterior pituitary gland

5 Posterior pituitary gland stimulated to produce oxytocin

4 Baby sucks at breast – sets up neurohormonal reflex

3 Prolactin acts on acini cells in breast to produce milk from fat globules in blood

6 Oxytocin causes myoepithelial cells in breast to contract and squeeze milk from acini cells into lactiferous ducts and towards ampulla; may cause uterine contractions or 'after pains'

1 Delivery of placenta causes reduction in oestrogen

lactoferrin the iron-binding protein found in human milk. It has a powerful bacteriostatic effect on ESCHERICHIA COLI.

lactogen any substance that enhances lactation. *Human placental l. (HPL)* a hormone secreted by the placenta, which disappears from the blood immediately after delivery. It has lactogenic, luteotrophic and growth-promoting activity, and inhibits maternal insulin activity during pregnancy.

lactoglobulin a globulin occurring in milk.

lactose milk sugar, a DISACCHARIDE. *L. intolerance* this can cause diarrhoea in the neonate, as the lactose may not be split if there is not sufficient LACTASE. It can be treated by giving milk which does not contain lactose, but another sugar. It should not be confused with GALACTOSAEMIA.

lactosuria lactose in the urine. Lactose reduces Benedict's solution, and lactosuria must be distinguished from glycosuria by further tests. Lactosuria often occurs in the lactation period, and occasionally at the end of pregnancy. It is not significant.

lactulose an oral laxative; may take up to 48 hours to take effect.

laked describes blood when haemoglobin has separated from the red blood cells.

LaLeche League an organization formed in 1957 for the purpose of helping women to breastfeed.

Lamaze method a method of preparation for natural childbirth developed by the French obstetrician Fernand Lamaze, and based on the Russian psychoprophylactic technique of training the mind and body for the purpose of modifying the perception of pain during labour and delivery.

lambda the posterior fontanelle of the skull, so-called from its resemblance to the Greek letter lambda (λ).

lambdoidal suture the suture between the occipital bone and the two parietal bones.

Lancefield classification the classification of haemolytic streptococci into groups on the basis of serological action.

Landsteiner's classification a classification of blood groups in which they are designated O, A, B and AB, depending on the presence or absence of agglutinogens A and B in the erythrocytes; called also international classification.

Langerhans' islets collections of specialized cells in the pancreas, producing insulin which controls carbohydrate metabolism. Disease of the islet cells causes DIABETES MELLITUS.

Langhans' cell layer cytotrophoblast. The inner layer of the TROPHOBLAST.

lanolin wool fat used as a basis for ointments.

lanugo the fine hair covering the fetus *in utero*. Most of it has disappeared by the time the child is born at term.

laparoscope an instrument for examination of the peritoneal cavity.

laparoscopy examination of the interior of the abdomen by means of a LAPAROSCOPE.

laparotomy exploratory opening of the abdominal cavity.

Largactil *See* CHLORPROMAZINE.

laryngoscope an endoscopic instrument for inspecting the larynx and vocal cords and aiding the insertion of an endotracheal tube.

larynx the organ of the voice, situated at the upper end of the trachea. It has a muscular and cartilaginous frame, lined with mucous membrane. Across it are spread the vocal cords of elastic tissue. The space between the cords is termed the glottis.

laser a device that transfers electromagnetic radiation of various frequencies into an extremely intense, small and nearly non-divergent beam of monochromatic radiation in the visible region, with all the waves in phase; from light amplification by simulated emission of radiation. Capable of mobilizing immense heat and power when focused at close range, it is used as a tool in surgery, in diagnosis and in physiological studies.

Lasix *See* FUROSEMIDE.

last menstrual period (LMP) the date of the first day of the last normal menstrual period needs to be ascertained in order to estimate the probable date of delivery. The midwife should check that the date given by the mother refers to vaginal bleeding which occurred at the expected interval after the previous period, and which lasted the normal number of days, as the mother may mistake a small amount of blood loss at the time of implantation as a normal menstrual period.

latent hidden; not manifest. *L. period* a seemingly inactive period as in the early part of the first stage of labour.

lateral relating to the side.

'laughing gas' NITROUS OXIDE.

lavage washing out a cavity. *Colonic l.* of the colon. *Gastric l.* of the stomach.

lavender oil a highly concentrated aromatherapy oil used by some midwives who have been trained in its use, to aid perineal healing and to ease discomfort during labour and after delivery. It should not be used in conjunction with epidural anaesthesia due to its hypotensive action. Contraindicated until late pregnancy as it is thought to be an EMMENAGOGUE.

laxative a medicine that loosens the bowel contents and encourages evacuation. A laxative with a mild or gentle effect on the bowels is also known as an aperient; one with a strong effect is referred to as a cathartic or a purgative. It can be dangerous to use purgatives in pregnancy because they may stimulate uterine activity and thereby bleeding.

lead professional the 'CHANGING CHILD-BIRTH' REPORT (1993) recommended that every pregnant woman should be cared for by one professional who takes the principal responsibility for her care, although other professionals may also be involved. The lead professional may be the midwife, consultant obstetrician or general practitioner obstetrician depending on the mother's needs and wishes.

learning difficulty contemporary term for mental handicap. Also known as learning disability. Children who suffer cerebral palsy as a result of birth injury may have learning difficulties, as will those with congenital chromosomal disorders such as Down's syndrome.

Leboyer method a method of childbirth advocated by a French doctor, Leboyer. He is especially concerned with the baby being born gently and quietly. The room is darkened for the delivery, and the baby born in quietness and lifted on to its mother's abdomen; the baby is then put into a warm bath. It is claimed that the baby will cry less and become a more contented child and adult because the shock of delivery is minimized.

lecithin a complex molecule of protein and fatty acid which is found in the alveoli of the lung. SURFACTANT is a lecithin and helps to keep the lungs open. The lecithin which is produced in the fetal lung flows out into the amniotic fluid, where it can be measured to give an indication of fetal maturity. *L./sphingomyelin ratio* lecithin, but not sphingomyelin, is produced in greater quantities as pregnancy progresses. Therefore the ratio increases with fetal lung maturity. A ratio of 2 or more indicates that there is little or no risk of respiratory distress in the neonate. Abbreviated L/S ratio.

Lee–Frankenhauser plexus nerve network consisting of the third and fourth sacral, hypogastric and ovarian nerves and relating to the cervical area of the uterus.

Leeds test screening test, similar to the BART'S TEST, which aims to identify women at higher than normal risk of carrying a fetus with Down's syndrome. Also called the *Triple Plus test*. Blood is taken and analysed for alpha-fetoprotein, unconjugated oestriol and human chorionic gonadotrophin, plus additional markers such as neutrophil alkaline phosphatase. Women at low risk are those with less than a 1:250 chance of having an affected baby. Those with more than a 1:250 risk level are offered further diagnostic tests such as amniocentesis.

leiomyoma smooth muscle tumour (fibroids), commonly occurring in the uterus.

length an expression of the longest dimension of an object, or of the measurement between its two ends. The internationally accepted (SI) unit of length is the metre (m). *Crown–heel l.* the distance from the crown of the head to the heel in embryos, fetuses and infants; the equivalent standing height in older persons. *Crown–rump l.* the distance from the crown of the head to the breech in embryos, fetuses and infants; the equivalent of sitting height in older persons. Measured by B-mode ultrasound during the first 14 weeks of pregnancy to assess fetal maturity; accurate to within 3 to 4 days.

lesion an injury, would or morbid structural change in an organ. Used as a general term for a local morbid condition.

'let down' reflex the neurogenic process which stimulates the release of milk from the breasts, for example, when the mother hears her baby crying.

leucine naturally occurring essential amino acid, vital for infant growth and for adult nitrogen equilibrium.

leucocyte a white blood corpuscle.

leucocytosis an increase in the number of leucocytes in the blood, usually as a response to infection.

leucopenia decreased number of leucocytes in the blood.

leucorrhoea a white, mucoid, non-irritating vaginal discharge. The glands of the cervix normally secrete a certain amount of mucus-like fluid that moistens the membranes of the vagina. The discharge is frequently increased at the time of ovulation, before a menstrual period and throughout pregnancy. It is also

stimulated by sexual excitement. It should be white, inoffensive and non-irritating. Otherwise infections should be suspected and investigations carried out.

leukaemia an uncommon malignant blood disease. It is characterized by a marked increase in abnormal leucocytes. It is accompanied by a reduced number of erythrocytes and blood platelets, resulting in anaemia and increased susceptibility to infection and haemorrhage.

levallorphan an analogue of levorphanol, which acts as an antagonist to analgesic narcotics.

levator a muscle which raises a part.

levator ani a broad sheet of muscle, which forms the principal part of the pelvic floor.

levonorgestrel progestin used in combination with an oestrogen as an oral contraceptive.

libido sexual desire.

Librium *See* CHLORDIAZEPOXIDE.

lidocaine (lignocaine) hydrochloride (Xylocaine) a drug used for infiltration analgesia and nerve block. Up to 1% solution may be used by midwives for infiltration of the perineum, prior to performing episiotomy and perineal repair.

lie the relation of the long axis of the fetus to the long axis of the mother's uterus. Normally these are parallel and the lie is said to be longitudinal. Abnormally, the fetus lies across the mother's uterus, the lie is transverse or oblique and, unless this is corrected, labour will become obstructed.

ligament a tough fibrous band of tissue connecting bones or supporting internal organs. The ligaments which support the uterus are (a) *transverse cervical* or *cardinal l.*, (b) *pubocervical l.* and (c) *uterosacral l.* The *round ligaments* extend from the cornua of the uterus to the labia majora. The *broad ligaments* are folds of peritoneum, adjacent to that of the uterus and covering the fallopian tubes so they are not true ligaments.

ligation the process of applying a ligature.

ligature a thread, usually of catgut, nylon or wire, used for tying blood vessels.

light for dates *See* SMALL FOR GESTATIONAL AGE BABY.

lightening the relief experienced in the late stages of pregnancy when the presenting part sinks into the pelvis and the fundus ceases to press on the diaphragm, usually shortly after 36th week in nulliparae and just before or after the onset of labour in multiparae.

linea a line. *L. alba* the tendinous area in the centre of the abdominal wall into which the transversalis and part of the oblique muscles are inserted. *L. nigra* the pigmented line which often appears, during pregnancy, on the abdomen between the umbilicus and pubis, at times extending up to the ensiform cartilage. Pigmentation is due to increased pituitary gland production of melanocytic hormone. The line fades after delivery when hormone levels decrease.

lint a loosely woven cotton fabric, one side of which is fluffy, and the other smooth, used for surgical dressings.

lipase an ENZYME, present in pancreatic juice, which splits fat into fatty acids.

lipid one of a group of fatty substances that are insoluble in water but soluble in alcohol or chloroform. An important part of the diet. Normally present in body tissues.

Lippe's loop an intrauterine contraceptive device.

liquor amnii the fluid which fills the amniotic sac surrounding the fetus. The composition is similar to that of intracellular fluid: about 99% water, containing proteins, fats and carbohydrates, sodium and potassium in solution, with debris consisting of desquamated fetal epithelial cells, vernix caseosa, lanugo and various enzymes and pigments. Its functions are: (*a*) it acts as a shock absorber; (*b*) it allows unhindered growth; (*c*) it distributes pressure evenly over the whole fetus; (*d*) it permits the free movement necessary for muscle function; and (*e*) it prevents diminution of the placental site. The volume is approximately 1 litre at 37–38 weeks' gestation, but this diminishes by nearly half at term. *See also* AMNIOCENTESIS.

Listeria a genus of Gram-negative bacteria. It produces upper respiratory tract disease, septicaemia and encephalitic disease. Transmitted by consumption of infected unpasteurized dairy produce, or by direct contact with infected animals or contaminated soil. Newborn infants, pregnant women, elderly people and the immunosuppressed are more susceptible to infection.

lithopaedion a dead fetus that has become petrified owing to lime salt deposition. This occurs only in a fetus that has undergone extrauterine development and so is very rare.

lithotomy position the woman lies on her back with thighs and legs flexed and abducted and held in place with lithotomy poles. This position is adopted for forceps or breech delivery and for perineal suturing. Care should be taken when lifting the woman's legs into or out of the stirrups, that both legs are lifted together (preferably by two people, one on each side) to avoid possible hip dislocation due to laxity of the joint under the influence of relaxin and progesterone.

149

litmus paper blotting paper impregnated with litmus, a pigment which is used to ascertain the reaction of fluids. Blue litmus is turned red by acids and red litmus is turned blue by alkalis.

litre a measure of volume, 1000 ml or about 35 fl. oz.

live birth an infant who is born alive.

liver the large wedge-shaped gland situated in the right hypochondrium and epigastrium. It is essential to life. Its chief functions are: (*a*) formation of bile; (*b*) production of plasma proteins except GAMMA GLOBULINS; (*c*) storage of carbohydrates as glycogen, iron and vitamins A, D, E and K; (*d*) regulation of metabolism of fat, protein and carbohydrate; (*e*) detoxication of drugs and other substances; (*f*) the formation and destruction of ERYTHROCYTES; (*g*) production of PROTHROMBIN; and FIBRINOGEN; (*h*) heat production; and (*i*) phagocytic action on bacteria.

livid cyanotic. The blueness is associated with venous congestion and an inadequate supply of oxygen.

lobe a section of an organ, separate from neighbouring parts by fissures.

lobule a small segment or lobe, especially one of the smaller divisions making up a lobe. adj. *lobular*.

local authority the local government.

local supervising authority (LSA) local organization, usually the regional health authority, responsible for monitoring midwifery practice within its area. This is done by the appointment of supervisors of midwifery, facilitating their education and training and enabling communication with the supervisors, developing systems to ensure eligibility to practise of each midwife working within the area and, where necessary, suspending from practice any midwife who is felt to have

acted in an unsafe or negligent manner. The LSA has a nominated officer who must be a practising midwife, to carry out its functions. *See also* SUPERVISOR OF MIDWIVES.

lochia the discharges from the uterus following childbirth or abortion, consisting of blood from the placental site, shreds of decidua, shed vaginal epithelial cells and, at first, debris from the uterus, e.g. liquor amnii, vernix caseosa and meconium. *L. alba* (whitish) contains white blood cells and mucus. *L. rubra* (red) is largely fresh and then staler blood. *L. serosa* (pinkish) contains fewer red and more white cells. Lochia may be expected to continue for 2–3 weeks or possibly rather longer. Red, profuse lochia should raise the suspicion of subinvolution or infection. An offensive odour is indicative of infection. *Sing.* lochium.

locked twins the condition of twins with their bodies and heads so placed that neither can be born naturally; a rare cause of obstructed labour.

locus place; site; in genetics, the specific site of a gene on a chromosome.

longitudinal study investigation that involves making observations of the same group at sequential time intervals. Valuable for studying human development or change. May also be used to observe change over time within an organization.

lordosis exaggeration of the normal forward curve of the lumbar spine. A moderate degree is common in pregnancy due to musculoskeletal laxity caused by relaxin and progesterone. Poor posture exacerbates the problem and advice should be given regarding posture, exercises and relaxation. The weight of the uterus pulls the body forwards and, to compensate this, the woman leans backwards, thus throwing extra strain on the relaxed sacroiliac joints and causing backache.

Lövset's manoeuvre a manoeuvre whereby the fetal shoulders are delivered when the arms are extended during breech labour. It consists in rotating the fetus through a half circle, keeping the back uppermost, so as to bring the posterior arm into an anterior position below the symphysis pubis, where it can be delivered. The fetus is then rotated a half circle in the reverse direction and the second arm is similarly delivered.

low-birth-weight baby any baby weighing 2.5 kg or less at birth. Low-birth-weight babies may be: 1. preterm, if born before 37 completed weeks of pregnancy; or 2. small for gestational age, if the birth weight is below the tenth centile for gestational age. Some babies are both preterm and small for gestational age.

lower uterine segment the part of the UTERUS lying between the vesicouterine peritoneal fold superiorly and the junction of the uterus and cervix inferiorly.

lubricant a cream, jelly or similar substance applied to the hands, gloves or instruments in order to make them slippery and to facilitate manipulations.

lumbar pertaining to the loins. *L. puncture* introduction of a hollow needle into the subarachnoid space, usually between the 4th and 5th lumbar vertebrae, to withdraw cerebrospinal fluid. This may be carried out for diagnostic purposes, to relieve pressure or to introduce drugs.

lumbosacral relating to both lumbar and sacral vertebrae or regions.

lumen the space inside a tube.

lumpectomy the surgical excision of only the local lesion (benign or malignant) of the breast.

lungs a pair of conical organs of the respiratory system. Consisting of an arrangement of air tubes (bronchi and bronchioles), terminating in air spaces (alveoli); they occupy most of the thoracic cavity. The lungs supply the blood with oxygen inhaled from the outside air, and they dispose of waste carbon dioxide in the exhaled air, as a part of the process known as respiration.

lupus chronic skin disease with many different manifestations.

luteal pertaining to the CORPUS LUTEUM.

lutein the yellow pigment in the corpus luteum.

luteinizing hormone a hormone secreted by the anterior cells of the pituitary gland acting, with follicle-stimulating hormone, to cause ovulation of mature follicles and secretion of oestrogen by thecal and granulosa cells of the ovary; it is also concerned with formation of the corpus luteum. In the male, it stimulates development of the interstitial cells of the testes and their secretion of testosterone.

luteotrophin prolactin.

lymph a body fluid, derived from the fluid in the tissue spaces and carried in lymphatic vessels back to the blood stream. It is similar in composition to tissue fluid. Lymph nodes occur at intervals in the course of the lymphatic vessels. Their function is to act as a filter.

lymphatics vessels carrying lymph.

lymphocytes white blood cells, formed mainly from the lymphoid tissue in the bone marrow and thymus.

lymphoedema condition in which the intercellular spaces contain abnormal amounts of lymph due to obstruction of lymph drainage.

lyse to cause disintegration of a cell or substance.

lysin a cell-dissolving substance present in blood serum.

lysis 1. a gradual decline, e.g. of a fever. 2. a breaking down, as in haemolysis; a breaking down or destruction of red blood cells.

lysozyme an antibacterial (Gram-positive) agent present in all tissues and secretions, particularly in tears and breast milk.

lytic cocktail a combination of chlorpromazine, promethazine and pethidine, which can be used in the treatment of severe pre-eclampsia and eclampsia. Promethazine and pethidine only may be used. It induces deep sleep, aids muscular relaxation and lowers the blood pressure. Less commonly used now.

M

maceration the process of softening a solid by means of soaking. Maceration occurs when a dead fetus is retained in the uterus for more than 24 hours. It is characterized by discoloration, softening of tissues, peeling of the fetal skin and eventual disintegration of a fetus retained in the uterus after its death. It indicates that a stillbirth has been dead *in utero* before the commencement of labour, and may lead to disseminated intravascular coagulation.

Mackenrod's ligaments the transverse or cardinal ligaments that support the uterus in the pelvic cavity.

macro- prefix meaning 'large'.

macrocyte an abnormally large red blood corpuscle found in the blood in megaloblastic anaemia of pregnancy due to folic acid deficiency.

macronutrient essential nutrient with daily requirement over 100 mg, e.g. calcium, phosphorus, magnesium, potassium, sodium, chloride.

macrophage any of the large, mononuclear highly phagocytic cells derived from monocytes that occur in the walls of blood vessels and in loose connective tissue. They are components of the reticuloendothelial system and become actively mobile when stimulated by inflammation; they also interact with lymphocytes to facilitate antibody production.

macroscopic discernible with the naked eye.

magnesium an element. Symbol Mg. A bluish white metal. Minute quantities are essential to life, being required for the activity of many enzymes, especially those concerned with oxidative phosphorylation. It is found in intra- and extracellular fluids and is excreted in urine and faeces. The normal serum level is approximately 1 mmol/l. Magnesium deficiency causes irritability of the nervous system with tetany, vasodilation, convulsions, tremors, depression and psychotic behaviour. *M. sulphate* a saline purgative (Epsom salts). Used to control convulsions of eclampsia, and has been found to be more effective than either diazepam or phenytoin. Now recommended by WHO for treatment of eclampsia. Administered intravenously; blood levels must be monitored regularly to ensure they remain in the range 2–4 mmol/l. Toxicity leads to loss of maternal reflexes, muscle paralysis, respiratory and cardiac arrest. *M. trisilicate* an antacid powder used in the treatment of dyspepsia, peptic ulcer and heartburn, and to reduce the acidity of the gastric contents prior to general anaesthesia, particularly during labour to reduce risk of MENDELSON'S SYNDROME.

magnetic resonance imaging (MRI) an imaging technique based on the NUCLEAR MAGNETIC RESONANCE properties of the hydrogen nucleus. Cross-sectional images in any plane may be obtained and the images may represent one or more of several properties.

maintenance order a court order requiring a person to give a regular payment to someone for whom he/she has a responsibility, e.g. a father of a child.

mal- a prefix meaning 'bad', 'wrong', or 'ill'. *Grand m.* a generalized convulsive seizure attended by loss of consciousness. *See also* EPILEPSY. *Petit m.* momentary loss of consciousness without convulsive movements. *See also* EPILEPSY.

malabsorption impaired intestinal absorption of nutrients. *M. syndrome* a group of disorders marked by subnormal intestinal absorption of dietary constituents, and thus excessive loss of nutrients in the stool.

malacia softening of tissues. *Osteomalacia* softening of bone tissue, one effect being deformity of the pelvic bones. It is uncommon in developed countries.

malaise a feeling of general discomfort and illness.

malar pertaining to the malar bone of the face or the region adjacent to it.

malaria tropical infection contracted from mosquito bites and leading to the presence of protozoan parasites in the red blood cells. Periodic bouts of fever, sweating, chills and rigors may occur over several years. Prophylactic medication should be taken before, during and after travelling to any affected area of the world.

male reproductive system consists of two testes (A). These are contained within the scrotum (B) and have the sperm formed within them. A fine tubular system, the epididymis (C), collects the sperm which are then conveyed by a long tube, the vas deferens (D). This passes along the inguinal canal to run by the bladder, for the sperm to be stored in the sem-

Male Reproductive System

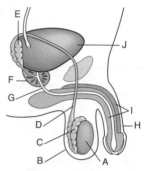

A, Testes; B, scrotum;
C, epididymis; D, vas deferens;
E, seminal vesicle; F, prostate
gland; G, urethra; H, penis;
I, erectile tissue; J, bladder.

inal vesicles (E). When ejaculation occurs, the prostate gland (F) adds fluid to the sperm, which are then passed into the urethra (G) inside the erect penis (H). At intercourse the sperm are deposited in the posterior fornix of the VAGINA.

malformation an anatomical abnormality. Often a deformity, either congenital or acquired.

malignant tending to become progressively worse and to result in death; having the properties of anaplasia, invasiveness and metastasis; said of tumours.

malnutrition the condition in which nutrition is defective in quantity or quality.

Malpighian body the glomerulus and Bowman's capsule of the kidney.

malposition misplaced situation of any organ or part in relationship to neighbouring structures or parts. The term is applied to a fetus with its occiput directed towards one or other posterior quadrant of the pelvis.

malpractice any professional misconduct, unreasonable lack of skill or fidelity in professional duties, or illegal or immoral conduct. Malpractice is one form of negligence, which in legal terms can be defined as the omission to do something that a reasonable person would do, or the doing of something that a reasonable and prudent person would not do. In midwifery malpractice results in injury, unnecessary suffering, or death of the mother or baby.

malpresentation any presentation of the fetus other than the vertex. It may be a breech, face, brow or shoulder presentation. Failure to diagnose the condition can lead to serious complications including obstructed labour, uterine rupture, fetal or maternal death.

maltase a sugar-splitting enzyme which converts maltose to glucose. Present in pancreatic and intestinal juice.

maltose a sugar (disaccharide) formed when starch is hydrolysed by amylase.

mamma the breast.

mammal a member of a division of vertebrates, including all that possess hair and suckle their offspring.

mammary pertaining to the breasts.

mammilla the nipple.

mammography radiography of the breast with or without injection of an opaque substance into its ducts. Simple mammography, without the use of contrast medium, is a routine screening procedure for the diagnosis of cancer and other disorders of the breast.

Manchester operation amputation of the cervix, with anterior and posterior colporrhaphy.

mandelic acid a keto acid used as a urinary antiseptic in nephritis, pyelitis, and cystitis.

mandible a horseshoe-shaped bone forming the lower jaw.

mania mental disorder characterized by exaltation and acceleration of all mental processes, often culminating in violence. It may follow childbirth.

manic-depressive psychosis a mental illness characterized by mania or endogenous DEPRESSION. The attacks may alternate between mania and depression or the woman may just have recurrent attacks of either mania or depression.

manipulation using the hands in a skilful manner, such as in changing the position of the fetus.

mannitol a sugar alcohol occurring widely in nature, especially in fungi; an osmotic diuretic used for forced diuresis and in cerebral oedema. Not recommended for use in pregnancy. Used when acute tubular necrosis presents following postpartum haemorrhage. Should never be added to whole blood.

manoeuvre similar to manipulation. A procedure carried out with the hands, e.g. to facilitate delivery or to speed the placenta. *See* LÖVSET'S M. *and* MAURICEAU–SMELLIE–VEIT MANOEUVRE.

manometer an instrument for measuring the pressure or tension of liquids or gases. *See* SPHYGMOMANOMETER.

Mantoux reaction reaction to the *Mantoux test*, which consists of an intradermal injection of old tuberculin to determine susceptibility to tuberculosis. A weal developing in hours indicates a positive reaction. This signifies that a previous infection has conferred some degree of immunity.

155

manual with the hand. *M. removal of the placenta* introducing a hand into the uterus to remove a retained placenta. The midwife working in isolated areas with no medical aid available may be required to perform this procedure in an emergency. Antiseptic cream is applied to the gloved hand which is introduced into the vagina and followed up the umbilical cord to the uterus and placenta, whilst supporting the uterus through the abdominal wall with the other hand. After finding a separated edge of the placenta the remainder is peeled off the uterine wall and withdrawn. Bimanual compression may be required to control bleeding. The risk of shock is greater when the procedure is performed without anaesthetic.

maple syrup urine disease a genetic disorder involving deficiency of an enzyme necessary in the metabolism of branched-chain amino acids, marked clinically by mental and physical handicap, feeding difficulties and a characteristic odour of urine.

marasmus severe malnutrition and weight loss in babies associated with a form of protein-calorie deficiency, but usually with retention of appetite and mental alertness. It is considered to be related to KWASHIORKOR.

Marcain *See* BUPIVACAINE.

Marfan's syndrome an hereditary disorder of connective tissue characterized by abnormal length of the extremities, especially of the fingers and toes, subluxation of the lens, congenital anomalies of the heart and other deformities.

marijuana, marihuana a preparation of the leaves and flowering tops of *Cannabis sativa*, the hemp plant, which contains a number of pharmacologically active principles. Hashish, also derived from the hemp plant, is obtained from the clear resin secreted by the flowering tops of the plant and is thought to be more potent than marijuana. Both drugs are used for their euphoric properties and are 3 or 4 times more potent when smoked and inhaled than when ingested. Its possession is illegal in many countries, including the UK. There is some evidence that marijuana increases the risk of miscarriage and birth defects.

marrow the soft, organic, sponge-like material in the cavities of bones. Its chief function is to manufacture erythrocytes, leucocytes and platelets. The bone marrow is occasionally subject to disease, as in aplastic anaemia, which may be caused by the destruction of the marrow by chemical agents or excessive X-ray exposure. Other diseases that affect the bone marrow are leukaemia, pernicious anaemia, myeloma and metastatic tumours.

massage systematic therapeutic stroking or kneading of the body. Therapeutic massage can aid relaxation, stimulate the circulation and excretory processes and lower the blood pressure. Some women like to receive massage during labour, although not all women like to be touched at this time; gentle circular massage of the abdomen can be helpful in easing discomfort in labour, as touch impulses reach the brain before pain impulses. *See also* EFFLEURAGE. *Cardiac m.* intermittent compression of the heart by pressure applied over the sternum (closed cardiac massage) or directly to the heart through an opening in the chest wall (open cardiac massage).

mast cells large connective tissue cells found in heart, liver and lungs. Contain granules which release heparin, serotonin and histamine in response to inflammation or allergy.

mastitis inflammation of the breast. Puerperal mastitis is an infection resulting usually from the presence of staphylococci and occasionally streptococci, which usually enter through cracked nipples. A wedge-shaped area of the breast becomes tender, red and warm and the woman feels generally unwell. The condition responds quickly to antibiotic treatment. Delay in treatment may lead to the development of an abscess which needs to be incised and drained.

MAT B1 maternity certificate, signed by midwife or doctor, confirming expected date of delivery. The woman must present this form in order to claim financial and employment benefits related to pregnancy.

materia medica the science of the source and preparation of drugs used in medicine. *Homoeopathic m.m.* resources detailing the actions and effectiveness of homoeopathic remedies after they have been thoroughly tested on healthy volunteers, and used by homoeopaths to determine precisely the most appropriate remedy for the client.

maternal pertaining to the mother. *M. mortality* death due to pregnancy or childbearing, the commonest causes of which are hypertensive and haemorrhagic disorders. *M. mortality rate* number of maternal deaths due to pregnancy and childbearing per 1000 registered live and stillbirths. The CONFIDENTIAL ENQUIRY into maternal deaths details all those which have occurred in the United Kingdom, and is published triennially.

maternity pertaining to childbearing. *M. Alliance* charity comprising various maternity related organizations concerned with campaigning for improved conditions for mothers and babies. It provides education, undertakes and supports research and publishes numerous books and leaflets. *M. benefits see* Appendix 12 for summary. *M. care assistant* auxiliary practitioner who is not a midwife but who is specifically trained to assist mothers and midwives.

Maternity Services Liaison Committee local committees set up to serve the interests of consumers of the maternity services through increased two-way communication between representatives from the obstetric, paediatric, anaesthetic and midwifery staff and prospective and retrospective users of the services, including members of the Community Health Council.

matrix the intercellular substance of a tissue, as bone matrix, or the tissue from which a structure develops, as hair or nail matrix.

Matthews Duncan expulsion of placenta the placenta is expelled maternal side first at the end of the third stage of labour. There is rather more bleeding and the placenta was probably lying lower in the uterus than in the SCHULTZE EXPULSION.

maturation ripening or developing. In biology, a process of cell division during which the number of chromosomes in the germ cell is reduced to one-half the number characteristic of the species.

Mauriceau a famous French male midwife. *M.–Smellie–Veit manoeuvre* a method of delivering the aftercoming head in a breech delivery. Flexion is increased, and jaw and shoulder traction applied. This method allows for better control over the delivery of the head than does the BURNS–MARSHALL TECHNIQUE in cases where forceps delivery is not possible.

Maxolon *See* METOCLOPRAMIDE.

mean an average; a numerical value intermediate between two extremes.

measles a highly infectious disease caused by a virus; called also rubeola or morbilli. Routine immunization with live attenuated vaccine (in combination with mumps and rubella vaccines) is given in the UK at 1 year.

meatus an opening or passage. *Auditory m.* the opening leading into the auditory canal. *Urinary m.* where the urethra opens to the exterior.

mechanism of labour the sequence of movements whereby the fetus adapts itself to pass through the maternal passages during the process of birth.

meconium the material present in the fetal intestinal tract, which is passed per rectum during the first few days of life. It is greenish black in colour and contains bile pigments and salts, mucus, intestinal epithelial cells and, usually, liquor amnii. *M. aspiration* the inhalation of liquor containing meconium, which can occur in babies who have been hypoxic *in utero*, especially those who are growth-retarded. *M. ileus* gross distension of the bowel with inspissated meconium found in CYSTIC FIBROSIS.

median situated in the median plane or in the midline of a body or structure. *M. nerve* a nerve that originates in the brachial plexus and innervates muscles of the wrist and hand. *M. plane* an imaginary plane passing longitudinally through the body from front to back and dividing it into right and left halves.

mediastinum 1. a median septum or partition. 2. the mass of tissues and organs separating the sternum in front and the vertebral column behind, containing the heart and its large vessels, trachea, oesophagus, thymus, lymph nodes and other structures and tissues. It is divided into anterior, middle, posterior and superior regions.

medical herbalism See HERBAL MEDICINE.

medicine 1. any drug or remedy. 2. the art and science of the diagnosis and treatment of disease and the maintenance of health. 3. the non-surgical treatment of disease.

Medicines Act 1968 established an administrative and licensing system to control the sale and supply of medicines to the public, retail pharmacies and the packing and labelling of medicinal products.

Medicines (Prescription Only) Order 1983 schedule 3, parts I and III of this order detail the medicines, normally only available on prescription issued by a doctor, which may be supplied to midwives who have notified their intention to practise for use in their practice. These include analgesics, oxytocics, sedatives and drugs for neonatal resuscitation.

medium 1. an agent by which something is accomplished or an impulse is transmitted. 2. a substance providing the proper nutritional environment for the growth of micro-organisms; also called culture medium.

medroxyprogesterone acetate (Depo-Provera). A single dose intramuscular contraceptive, effective for 12 weeks. May be given to women following rubella vaccination or to a woman whose partner has had a vasectomy. There is a risk of heavy bleeding if used before the 5th postnatal week.

medulla the central or inner portion of an organ. *M. oblongata* the lowest part of the brain-stem, lying between the pons varolii and the spinal cord. It is the seat of the vital centres, i.e. the cardiac, respiratory and vasomotor centres.

mega (M) word element meaning 'large'; used in naming units of measurement to designate an amount of 10^6 (one million) times the size of the unit to which it is joined, as in megacuries (10^6 curies).

megalo- a prefix meaning 'great'.

megaloblastic anaemia an anaemia which occurs in pregnancy, in which immature red cells circulate in the blood. It is due to a deficiency of folic acid. Women who are epileptic and on long-term administration of PHENYTOIN may become folic acid deficient.

megaloblasts large nucleated immature red blood cells, normally present in the bone marrow.

meiosis the process by which the germinal epithelium in either ovary or testis gives rise to a gamete containing only one CHROMOSOME from each pair. This number is called the haploid and is 23 in humans; the normal number is the diploid, and is 46 in humans.

melaena the presence of dark, altered blood in the stools. It occurs in haemorrhagic disease of the newborn and may be accompanied by HAEMATEMESIS.

melanin dark pigment found in hair, choroid coat, etc. It is sometimes deposited in malignant tumours. Increased pigmentation occurs during pregnancy due to the presence of raised melanocytic hormone levels and results in the LINEA NIGRA, darkening of the areolae of the nipples and, in some women, facial CHLOASMA.

melanocyte-stimulating hormone (MSH) a peptide from the anterior pituitary that influences the formation or deposition of melanin in the body.

membrane a thin tissue covering the surface of certain organs and lining the cavities of the body. *Mucous m.* contains secreting cells, and lines all

cavities connected directly or indirectly with the skin. *Fetal membranes*, the CHORION and AMNION.

menarche the first sign of menstruation.

Mendel's laws the pattern, first demonstrated by Gregor Mendel, a Moravian monk, whereby inherited characteristics are transmitted, some being dominant and others recessive.

Mendelson's syndrome this occurs when even a small volume of acid gastric juice is inhaled during general anaesthesia. The midwife may be asked by the anaesthetist to apply CRICOID pressure as a preventative measure. It causes marked irritation of bronchi and alveoli, giving severe bronchospasm and pulmonary oedema. The signs are extreme dyspnoea, cyanosis and tachycardia. It may lead to hypotension and death.

meninges the membranes covering the brain and spinal cord. There are three: the dura mater, arachnoid and pia mater.

meningitis inflammation of the meninges.

meningocele a congenital deformity of the fetus, characterized by protrusion of the meninges through the skull or spinal column, appearing as a cyst filled with cerebrospinal fluid. *See also* SPINA BIFIDA.

meningoencephalocele hernial protrusion of the meninges and brain substance through a defect in the skull.

meningomyelocele hernial protrusion of the meninges and spinal cord through a defect in the vertebral column.

meniscocyte a sickle cell.

menopause the normal cessation of menstruation. *Artificial m.* a cessation induced by operation or irradiation.

menorrhagia an excessive menstrual discharge.

Endometrial and Follicular Changes During the Menstrual Cycle (from Weller B. 2000 Baillière's Nurses' Dictionary, Baillière Tindall, p. 140, with permission)

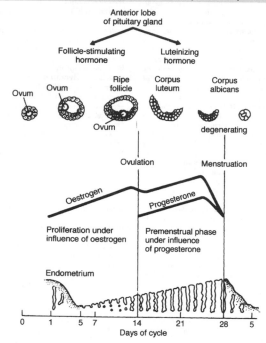

menses menstruation.

menstrual pertaining to menstruation. *M. cycle* the series of events which occurs in the endometrium between the the 1st day of one menstrual period and the 1st day of the next, normally 28 days. Menstrual bleed-

ing occurs on day 1 as a result of a fall in progesterone levels, and normally lasts 4–5 days, during which the endometrium is shed down to the basal layer. In the secretory phase which follows, increasing oestrogen levels from the pituitary gland act on the ovary to stimulate one of the Graafian follicles to mature while at the same time the endometrium is thickening in anticipation of receiving a fertilized ovum. Once the follicle has ripened (usually 14 days *before* the next period) it bursts to release the ovum (ovulation) which begins its journey along the fallopian tube towards the uterus. At the same time progesterone levels now rise and, should fertilization take place, are maintained to assist the embedding and development of the embryo. If conception does not occur the ovum passes to the uterus and a fall in hormone activity causes the thickened endometrium to be shed with the ovum and some blood. Changing hormone levels also cause the ruptured uterine follicle to degenerate, when it becomes known as the corpus luteum.

menstruation a discharge of blood from the uterus, at approximately 4-week intervals commencing at puberty and lasting until the menopause.

mental 1. pertaining to the mind. 2. pertaining to the chin.

mentoanterior with the chin directed anteriorly in the pelvis. Similarly, mentolateral and mentoposterior.

mentum the chin; the denominator in face presentation.

meptazinol a newer narcotic analgesia claimed to cause less respiratory depression than pethidine. It has a relatively quick onset of action but a short duration of action of 2–4 hours. Nausea and vomiting are quite common side-effects.

Meptid *See* MEPTAZINOL.

mercury an element. Symbol Hg. A heavy liquid metal. It is used in thermometers because it expands with heat, and in SPHYGMOMANOMETERS because it is much heavier than water, so a short tube only is needed to record a wide variation in pressure.

meridian an imaginary line. In traditional Chinese medicine it refers to the energy lines throughout the body along which are situated the points for acupuncture or acupressure.

mesentery a membranous fold attaching various organs to the body wall, especially the peritoneal fold attaching the small intestine to the dorsal body wall. adj. *mesenteric*.

mesoderm cells lying between ectoderm and entoderm cell layers in the embryo, from which are developed bone, muscle, heart, blood, blood vessels, gonads, kidneys and connective tissues.

mesosalpinx the peritoneum covering the fallopian tubes.

mesovarium a fold of peritoneum connecting the ovary to the broad ligament.

meta-analysis analysis and evaluation of the results of all accessible trials on the same subject.

metabolism the process of life, by which tissue cells are broken down by combustion (catabolism) and new protein is built up from the end products of digestion (anabolism). *Basal m. See* BASAL METABOLIC RATE. *Inborn error of m.* a genetically determined biochemical disorder in which a specific enzyme defect produces a metabolic block that may have pathological consequences at birth, as in phenylketonuria, or in later life.

metastasis the transfer of disease from one organ to another not directly connected with it. pl. *metastases*. A growth of malignant cells or pathogenic micro-organisms distant from the primary site.

metatarsum the part of the foot between the ankle and the toes, its skeleton being the 5 bones (metatarsals) extending from the tarsus to the phalanges.

methadone hydrochloride a synthetic compound with pharmacological properties qualitatively similar to those of morphine and heroin. May be prescribed for drug addicts in pregnancy as a maintenance drug.

methicillin-resistant *Staphylococcus aureus* (MRSA) strain of *S. aureus* which is resistant to 'methicillin-like' antibiotics. People carry the organism in the nose or on skin without exhibiting symptoms. Spread by direct contact. Treatment is not normally necessary but severe cases are given vancomycin intravenously.

methohexitone sodium an intravenous anaesthetic.

methotrexate folic acid antagonist used as an anti-neoplastic agent; it is also used in the treatment of psoriasis.

methyldopa a hypotensive drug, sometimes used in essential hypertension in pregnancy. It is known to cross the placenta, but there is no evidence that it affects the fetus.

metoclopramide drug which increases gastric action. Used to treat nausea and vomiting, and heartburn.

metopic suture the frontal suture.

metra the uterus.

metra-, metro- word element meaning 'uterus'.

metre (m) the Système International (SI) unit which measures length and distance; the equivalent of 39.371 inches.

metritis inflammation of the uterus.

metronidazole (Flagyl) an antimicrobial drug effective for anaerobic infections, especially *Trichomonas vaginalis*.

metropathia haemorrhagica a disease characterized by painless excessive menstrual and intermenstrual bleeding and failure of ovulation,

hence failure of corpus luteum development.

metrorrhagia haemorrhage from the uterus independent of menstruation.

metrostaxis persistent slight haemorrhage from the uterus.

Michel's clips small metal clips for closing skin wounds.

miconazole an antifungal agent used topically for dermatophytic infections such as athlete's foot or vulvovaginal candidiasis, orally for candidiasis of the mouth and gastrointestinal tract, and systemically by intravenous infusion for systemic fungal infections.

micro- 1. prefix meaning 'small', of microscopic size. 2. the prefix indicating 'one-millionth', e.g. microgram (μ), one-millionth of a gram.

microbe a micro-organism, especially a pathogenic bacterium. adj. *microbial, microbic*.

microcephaly possessing an abnormally small head. A microcephalic infant has markedly ossified skull bones and is always mentally subnormal.

microcytic having unusually small cells. *See* ANAEMIA.

micrognathia an unusually small mandible or lower jaw, with a receding chin. *See* PIERRE–ROBIN SYNDROME.

Microgynon 30 combined oral contraceptive pill containing oestrogen and progesterone. *See* ETHINYL-ESTRADIOL.

Micronor a proprietary contraceptive pill composed only of progesterone, used (*a*) during breastfeeding and (*b*) for patients with a risk of thrombosis or who suffer severe side-effects from pills containing oestrogen.

micro-organism a minute living organism, animal or vegetable (such as a virus or bacterium), visible under a microscope.

microphage a small phagocyte; an actively mobile neutrophilic leucocyte capable of phagocytosis.

micturition the act of passing urine.

midwife 'a person who, having been regularly admitted to a midwifery education programme, duly recognized in the country in which it is located, has successfully completed the prescribed course of studies in midwifery and has acquired the requisite qualifications to be registered and/or legally licensed to practise midwifery. She [or he] must be able to give the necessary supervision, care and advice to women during pregnancy, labour and the postpartum period, to conduct deliveries on her [or his] own responsibility and to care for the newborn and the infant. The care includes preventative measures, the detection of abnormal conditions in mother and child, the procurement of medical assistance and the execution of emergency measures in the absence of medical help. She [or he] has an important task in health counselling and health education, not only for the patients, but also within the family and the community. The work should involve antenatal education and preparation for parenthood and extends to certain areas of gynaecology, family planning and child care. She [or he] may practise in hospitals, clinics, health units, domiciliary conditions or in any other service.' Definition adopted by the International Confederation of Midwives, and International Federation of Gynaecologists and Obstetricians in 1972 and 1973, respectively, following amendment of the definition formulated by the World Health Organization.

midwifery dealing with childbirth. Midwifery is the art and science of caring for women undergoing *normal* pregnancies, labours and puerperia; OBSTETRICS is the medical science and art of caring for women with *abnormal* pregnancies, labours or postnatal periods.

miliaria a cutaneous condition with retention of sweat, which is extravasated at different levels in the skin; called also prickly heat or heat rash.

military attitude attitude of the fetus which is neither flexed nor extended.

milk the secretion of the mammary gland. The average composition of cows' and human milk, as a percentage, is:

	Cows' milk	Human milk
Protein	3.5	1.5
Fat	4.5	3.5
Carbohydrate	4.0	7.0
Mineral salts	0.75	0.2
Water	87.3	87.8

These percentages in human milk, particularly of fat, vary according to the time of day and the time during a feed. *Pasteurized m.* may be prepared in two ways: (*a*) high temperature short time (HTST), where the milk is held at 73°C for 15 seconds and then cooled quickly; or (*b*) where the milk is kept at 63–66°C for 30 minutes then rapidly cooled and bottled. *Sterilized m.* this has been heated to 100°C for 15 minutes to render it free from bacteria. *Tuberculin-tested m.* milk from cows certified free from tuberculosis and subject to strict bacteriological tests.

milk flow mechanism, milk ejection reflex this occurs about 30–40 seconds after the baby takes the AREOLA of the breast between its jaws. Oxytocin is released from the posterior lobe of the pituitary in response to the nervous stimulation, which causes contraction of the MYOEPITHELIAL CELLS so that milk is driven out of the ALVEOLI into the ducts and lacteal sinuses, so becoming available to the baby.

milli- the prefix indicating 'one-thousandth', e.g. milligram (mg) one-thousandth of a gram, millilitre (ml) one-thousandth of a litre, millimetre (mm) one-thousandth of a metre.

Milton a proprietary antiseptic consisting of a standardized 1% solution of electrolytic sodium hypochlorite. It is used especially for the sterilization of babies' feeding bottles.

mineral any naturally occurring non-organic homogeneous solid substance. There are 19 or more minerals forming the mineral composition of the body, of which at least 13 are essential to health. These minerals are supplied in a mixed and varied diet of animal and vegetable products.

Minilyn a contraceptive pill of oestrogen and progesterone combined.

Minovlar, Minovlar ED proprietary contraceptive pills containing oestrogen and progesterone.

miscarriage ABORTION. The expulsion of the fetus before the 24th week of pregnancy, i.e. before the fetus is legally viable, the fetus not being born alive.

missed abortion failure of pregnancy in which all the products of conception are retained *in utero*; the woman may or may not suffer vaginal bleeding. Usually due to a blighted ovum such as a CARNEOUS MOLE. Evacuation of the uterus by vacuum extraction, dilatation and curettage or prostaglandins is necessary.

Misuse of Drugs Act 1971 came into effect in 1973, to control the possession and supply of certain drugs. Narcotic drugs such as papaveretum (Omnopon), cocaine, morphine, diamorphine and those which affect the central nervous system (e.g. LSD and amfetamines) are included.

mitosis the normal process of cell multiplication, where nuclear division occurs, with each chromosome dividing into two, so that two identical cells are formed. cf. MEIOSIS.

mitral shaped like a mitre. *M. incompetence* a term which describes a defective mitral valve, usually the result of scar tissue following endocarditis. *M. regurgitation* the result of mild endocarditis, when the valve is puckered and closes imperfectly. *M. stenosis* a more serious condition in which fibrous tissue causes a narrowed orifice. Both regurgitation and stenosis may be present together. Mitral stenosis is the commonest cardiac lesion occurring in childbearing women. *M. valve* the bicuspid valve between the left atrium and left ventricle of the heart. *M. valvotomy* cutting into, and therefore widening, the narrowed mitral valve, performed to relieve mitral stenosis.

mittelschmerz abdominal or pelvic pain occurring between menstrual periods, and possibly related to ovulation.

mobile epidural a low concentration of bupivacaine, sometimes combined with an opiate, is administered into the epidural space by a 'patient-controlled epidural analgesic system' (PCEAS) pump to enable the mother to be mobile during labour, although pain relief may not be as complete as with conventional epidural anaesthesia. The midwife should remain in attendance and monitor the mother's respiratory rate, when opiates are used, in addition to normal observations.

Mogadon See NITRAZEPAM.

mole a dead and degenerate ovum.

molecule the smallest particle of an element or compound consisting of a varying number of atoms. Water, as seen from the symbol H_2O, has a molecule consisting of two hydrogen atoms and one oxygen atom.

mongolian blue spot a smooth, brown to greyish blue naevus consisting of an excess of melanocytes sometimes found at birth in the sacral region. This is found in babies of African and Asian parents and sometimes in those of Mediterranean origin. It usually disappears during childhood.

mongolism *See* DOWN'S SYNDROME.

Monilia a former name for the genus of fungi now known as *Candida*. *Candida albicans* is the common cause of thrush in infants, and of monilial vaginitis. Particularly common in pregnant women.

moniliasis candidiasis.

Monitor an adaptation for the UK of the USA Rush Medicus system of assessing quality of nursing care. It consists of 'checklists' for quality leading to a scoring system. The closer the score to 100% the better the care being given. The master list has over 200 criteria which are divided into 4 categories based on patient dependency levels.

monoamine an amine containing only one amino group. *M. oxidase inhibitors (MAO inhibitors)* substances that inhibit the activity of monoamine oxidase, increasing catecholamine and serotonin levels in the brain; they are used as antidepressants and antihypertensives. Pethidine should not be given to women receiving amino oxidase inhibitors as these drugs potentiate the action of pethidine about 10 times, thus the combination is highly dangerous.

monoclonal derived from a single cell. *M. antibodies* are derived from a single clone of cells. All the antibody molecules are identical and will react with the same antigenic site.

monosaccharide the simplest form of sugar, e.g. dextrose, glucose.

monozygotic pertaining to or derived from a single zygote (fertilized ovum). *M. twins* (sometimes termed uniovular) develop from one ovum and one spermatozoon which divide. They are the same sex, there is one placenta and one chorion, but two amniotic sacs. Developmental abnormalities are more common in monozygotic twins than DIZYGOTIC. *See also* MULTIPLE PREGNANCY.

mons veneris the area covered with hair over the pubes in a woman.

Montgomery's glands or tubercles sebaceous glands around the nipple, which enlarge during pregnancy.

morbid diseased, or relating to diseased parts.

morbidity relating to morbid.

moribund dying.

morning sickness *See* NAUSEA *and* VOMITING.

Moro reflex in response to any sudden movement or noise nearby, a normal newborn child will quickly extend his/her arms and bring them together again. Variously called the 'embrace' or 'startle' reflex. Absence of the Moro reflex is noted in sick and preterm babies.

morphine sulphate the principal alkaloid obtained from opium, and given hypodermically as an analgesic. Can be given only on medical orders. Used in cases of severe pain, e.g. placental abruption. May cause respiratory depression.

mortality death. *M. rate* death rate of a given population, e.g. maternal, neonatal or infant mortality rates.

morula the fertilized ovum, about 4 days after fertilization when it resembles a small mulberry.

mosaicism a condition in which a person has several different types of cell within his/her body. An example is mosaicism for Down's syndrome. Here the individual may have some cells with 47 chromosomes.

motor nerves those which convey an impulse of motion from a nerve centre to a muscle.

mould a fungus, e.g. *Penicillium*.

moulding the process of overriding of the cranial bones at the sutures and fontanelles whereby the fetus adapts itself to the pelvis through which it is passing. The head is squeezed to a different shape, with alteration to various diameters. In normal moulding the head is well flexed with suboccipitobregmatic and biparietal diameters presenting and as the bones overlap these diameters are decreased, while the one at right angles (i.e. mentovertical) is slightly lengthened. Moulding which is abnormal in direction, excessive in amount, or extremely rapid may cause tearing of the falx cerebri and tentorium cerebelli, leading to intracranial haemorrhage and possible death.

movements (fetal) See 'QUICKENING'.

moxibustion a technique used in traditional Chinese medicine such as acupuncture. It involves the use of moxa sticks made from the herb, mugwort, which acts as a heat source when held over appropriate ACUPUNCTURE points. The procedure has been successfully used to turn breech presentations to cephalic.

mucoid resembling mucus.

mucopolysaccharidosis gargoylism. A serious inborn error of metabolism. There are several types, but in all of them mucopolysaccharide builds up within the body. The children look ugly and have large spleens, difficulty in joint movements and mental retardation.

Moulding

A

B

C

D

The unmoulded head is indicated by the heavy line; A, moulding in the occipitoanterior position; B, moulding in the persistent occipitoposterior position; C, face moulding; D, brow moulding.

mucopurulent containing mucus and pus.

mucosa mucous membrane.

mucous pertaining to or secreting mucus. *M. membrane see* MEMBRANE.

mucoviscidosis *See* CYSTIC FIBROSIS.

mucus the viscid secretion of mucous membranes.

müllerian duct either of the paired embryonic ducts developing into the vagina, uterus and uterine tubes in the female, and becoming largely obliterated in the male. Called also paramesonephric duct.

multicultural an adjective relating to a society, a community or country consisting of a number of different cultural and/or ethnic groups.

multidisciplinary involving two or more professional disciplines.

multifactorial 1. of, or pertaining to, or arising through the action of, many factors. 2. in genetics, arising as a result of the interaction of several genes.

multigravida a pregnant woman who has previously had more than one pregnancy. *Grande m.* a pregnant woman who has had 4 or more previous pregnancies. *See also* MULTIPARA. adj. *multigravid.*

multipara a woman who has borne more than one VIABLE infant. adj. *multiparous.* pl. *multiparae.*

multiple pregnancy a pregnancy of more than one fetus. Twin pregnancy is relatively common, occurring in England about once in 80 pregnancies. The incidence of triplet pregnancy is said to be about 1 in 80^2, i.e. 1 in 6400; and that of quadruplet pregnancy 1 in 80^3, i.e. 1 in 512 000 although this formula is not as reliable as previously due to the increased incidence of multiple pregnancies as a result of infertility treatments. The condition is suspected if, on examination, the uterus appears large for the gestation, if more than two fetal poles are palpated or if the fetal head feels small for the uterine size; it is confirmed on ultrasound scan. Physiological disorders of pregnancy, particularly pressure symptoms, are exacerbated, and complications such as hypertension, anaemia, preterm labour and malpresentations are more likely to occur. Where possible the mother should be delivered in a consultant obstetric unit with an attached neonatal unit.

multivariate analysis analysis of data collected on several different variables but all having relevance to the study. Data analysis indicates the effect of each of these variables and their interaction.

mumps a communicable paramyxovirus disease that attacks one or both of the parotid glands. Occasionally the submaxillary glands are also affected. Immunization in the first 2 years of life (with measles and rubella – MMR) is recommended.

Munro Kerr's manoeuvre *see* HEAD FITTING.

murmur an auscultatory sound, particularly a periodic sound of short duration of cardiac or vascular origin. May be associated with disease or abnormality.

muscle a bundle of long, slender cells, or fibres, that have the power to relax and contract and hence to produce movement. Uterine muscle, the myometrium, also has the power of retraction, whereby the muscle fibres retain some of the shortening of the fibres that occurs with contractions. This property of retraction assists in the progressive passage of the fetus down the birth canal.

muscular dystrophy a group of genetically determined, painless, degenerative myopathies that are progressively crippling because muscles are gradually weakened and eventually atrophy. *Duchenne m. d.* a sex-linked recessive disease carried by the woman and passed on to 1 in 2 of her sons. The disease gradually develops in childhood. Probes are now available which allow certain genes to be isolated from the DNA; thus some genetically determined diseases affecting the fetus such as Duchenne muscular dystrophy can be detected in pregnancy.

mutation a change in form or other characteristic. In genetics a change in a gene from parent to offspring.

myasthenia muscular debility or weakness. *M. gravis* an autoimmune disease manifested by a syndrome of fatigue and exhaustion of the muscles that is aggravated by activity and relieved by rest. The weakness ranges from being very mild to being life-threatening. The disease characteristically affects the ocular and other cranial muscles, tends to fluctuate in severity, and responds to cholinergic drugs.

mycobacterium a Gram-positive bacterium (*see* GRAM STAIN) distinguished by acid-fast staining, e.g. *M. tuberculosis.*

myocardium the middle and thickest layer of the heart wall, composed of cardiac muscle. adj. *myocardial.*

myoepithelial cells branched contractile epithelial cells which curve round each ALVEOLUS in the breast tissue. *See also* MILK FLOW MECHANISM, BREAST *and* LACTATION.

myoma a benign tumour of muscle tissue.

myomectomy removal of a myoma – usually referring to a uterine tumour as in the case of fibroids.

myometrium the uterine muscle.

myxoedema hypothyroidism. A disease caused by a lack of thyroid hormones being secreted by the thyroid gland. Marked by oedematous swelling of face, limbs and hands; dry and rough skin; loss of hair; slow pulse; subnormal temperature; slowed metabolism, and mental dullness. It is treated with preparations of thyroid gland. Congenital hypothyroidism causes CRETINISM.

N

Naboth's cysts (follicles) cyst-like formations due to occlusion of the lumina of glands in the mucosa of the uterine cervix causing them to be distended with retained secretion. Called also nabothian cysts or follicles.

Naegele's pelvis a very rare abnormal pelvis which is asymmetrical due to a congenital failure of one sacral ala to develop fully.

Naegele's rule a rule for calculating the estimated date of labour: subtract 3 months from the first day of the last normal menstrual period and add 7 days.

naevus a birthmark; a circumscribed area of dilated superficial blood vessels.

nalorphine a drug, related to morphine, previously used in asphyxia neonatorum but now replaced by NALOXONE.

naloxone (Narcan) the specific antidote to a narcotic drug. It may be administered to an asphyxiated neonate if the mother has been given a narcotic such as pethidine recently in labour. The usual neonatal dose is 0.01 mg/kg of estimated body weight. Occasionally a larger dose is given to the mother if delivery is judged to occur at a time when pethidine previously administered will be at its most effective. The baby should be observed for respiratory difficulties for the first 24 hours after birth.

nano- the prefix indicating 'one-thousand-millionth', e.g. nanogram (ng) one-thousand-millionth of a gram.

napkin rash any rash which occurs in the area usually covered by the napkin. There are several types, the most common being ammoniacal dermatitis. This is not likely to occur in the neonatal period, but later produces erythema and vesicles. Other causes are thrush, napkin psoriasis and perianal erythema.

Narcan *See* NALOXONE.

narco- a prefix denoting 'stupor'.

narcosis a state of unconsciousness produced by a narcotic drug.

narcotic 1. a drug that produces narcosis. 2. a drug that produces insensibility or stupor. Medically the term narcotic includes any drug that has this effect. By legal definition, however, the term refers to habit-forming drugs, e.g. opiates such as morphine and heroin, and synthetic drugs such as pethidine. Narcotics can be legally obtained only with a doctor's prescription. The sale or possession of narcotics for other than medical purposes is strictly prohibited by the Misuse of Drugs Act 1971.

nares the nostrils. *Posterior n.* the opening of the nares into the nasopharynx. sing. *naris.*

nasal pertaining to the nose.

Naseptin combination preparation containing chlorhexidine and neomycin, a nasal cream for the treatment of staphylococcal infections.

nasogastric tube a tube of soft rubber or plastic that is inserted through the nostril and into the stomach. The tube is inserted for the purpose of instilling liquid food or other substances, or as a means of withdrawing gastric contents.

nasojejunal feeding a method in which a silicone-coated catheter is passed through the nose into the jejunum, to provide sufficient nutrition to a sick baby on a ventilator or receiving CONTINUOUS INFLATING PRESSURE (CIP) by mask or nasal tube. It is used to prevent the dangers of aspiration with a nasogastric tube feed.

nasopharynx the part of the pharynx above the soft palate.

National Care Standards Commission body established to undertake registration and inspection of private maternity hospitals and clinics in England. From 2002, replaced local health authority responsibility for this process.

National Childbirth Trust (NCT) a charitable organization concerned with education for pregnancy, birth and parenthood, with over 300 branches and groups in the UK. Primarily through these local groups, it runs antenatal classes, breastfeeding counselling and postnatal support.

National Health Service (NHS) the NHS was established in 1948 to provide free accessible health care to all. Numerous reorganizations have occurred since then. Budgeting and organization of health services is dependent on the local population and an element of market economy has been introduced in an attempt to improve standards of care for patients and clients.

National Institute for Clinical Excellence (NICE) special health authority with responsibility for assessing clinical and cost effectiveness of new and existing health technologies, and providing guidance to the NHS on their adoption.

National Service Frameworks (NSFs) templates or blueprints for care in major service areas. Developed nationally by NICE; used locally by the NHS Executive and other healthcare organizations to review and reshape local service provision.

National Vocational Qualifications (NVQ) a national, government-supported system of training and education for vocational work, based on 5 levels of skills and knowledge, taught and assessed in the workplace.

natural childbirth approach to labour and delivery advocating avoidance of medical interference and technology, as well as analgesia in labour, and encouraging both parents to participate in and share the experience of childbirth. Also termed active birth.

naturopathy a complementary form of health care involving diet, fasting, detoxification, exercise, hydrotherapy and positive thinking.

nausea a sensation of sickness with inclination to vomit. A common physiological disorder of early pregnancy which normally resolves by about the 14th week. The cause is not fully understood, but could be associated with the hormonal or metabolic changes of early pregnancy. *See also* VOMITING.

navel the umbilicus.

Necator a genus of HOOKWORM.

necro- prefix meaning 'dead'.

necrobiosis degeneration and death of tissue. Uterine fibroids may undergo this process in the middle trimester. The treatment is rest in bed and the administration of analgesic drugs.

necropsy a post-mortem examination.

necrosis death of tissue.

necrotizing enterocolitis an inflammatory disease of the bowel of the neonate which is associated with septicaemia. It is thought to be due to bacteria proliferating in the bowel and penetrating the bowel wall at points where it has suffered ischaemic damage. Oedema, ulceration and haemorrhage of the bowel wall are found and may progress to perforation and peritonitis. Babies at risk of this condition include those with a history of asphyxia, respiratory distress, hypoglycaemia, hypothermia or cardiovascular disease. The condition is treated with parenteral nutrition, antibodies and, in cases of perforation, surgery.

negligence in law, the failure to do something that a reasonable person of ordinary prudence would or would not do in a certain situation. Negligence may provide the basis for a law suit when there is a legal duty, as the duty of a midwife or doctor to provide reasonable care to clients, and when negligence results in damage to the client.

Neisseria gonorrhoeae the microorganism which causes GONORRHOEA. It is difficult to culture outside the human body.

nem a unit of nutrition equivalent to the nutritive value of 1 g of breast milk.

neo- prefix meaning 'new'.

neomycin a broad-spectrum antibiotic; used as an intestinal antiseptic.

neonatal pertaining to the first 4 weeks after birth. *N. mortality rate* the number of deaths of infants up to 4 weeks old per 1000 live births in a year.

neonate a newborn child up to 4 weeks old.

neonatology branch of paediatric medicine dealing with disorders of the newborn infant.

neoplasm any new growth, e.g. a tumour.

nephrectomy excision of a kidney.

nephritis inflammation of the kidneys. *Acute n.* a kidney lesion which may follow a streptococcal infection such as scarlet fever or tonsillitis, characterized by pain in the lumbar region, pyrexia and oedema. Renal function is impaired, the urine contains albumin, blood and casts of the renal tubules, but little urea, while the blood urea rises. Most patients recover completely, while some develop chronic nephritis. *Chronic n.* renal function is permanently impaired and the patient has oedema, proteinuria and often hypertension, with a raised blood urea. *N. in pregnancy* a woman with severe nephritis is often infertile. If pregnant, she is more prone to abort and to develop PRE-ECLAMPSIA and all its complications, so needs frequent and specialized care during the antenatal period.

nephron the glomerulus, Bowman's capsule and the tubule system which is the functioning unit of the kidney. Each kidney contains about one million nephrons.

nephropathy any disease of the kidneys.

nephrosis any renal disease.

nephrotic syndrome any kidney disease, especially disease marked by purely degenerative lesions of the renal tubules. The disease may follow acute nephritis and is marked by excessive accumulation of fluid in the body, due to a great loss of protein in the body and decreased serum albumin. Diuretics, a high protein diet, possibly steroids and, recently, the possible administration of immunosuppressive drugs are the methods of treatment.

nerve a bundle of nerve fibres enclosed in a sheath called the epineurium. Its function is to transmit impulses between any part of the body and a nerve centre. *Motor (efferent) n.* conveys impulses causing movement from a nerve centre to a muscle. *N. fibre* the prolongation of the nerve cell, which conveys the impulse to or from the part which it controls. *Sensory (afferent) n.* conveys sensations from an area to a nerve centre. *Vasomotor n.* either dilator or constrictor to blood vessels.

nerve block a block by local analgesic drugs, to impulses passing along nerves, e.g. EPIDURAL ANALGESIA.

nervous 1. pertaining to, or composed of, nerves. 2. unduly excitable. *N. breakdown* a common term used to describe any type of mental illness that interferes with a person's normal activities. Can be used to describe any of the mental disorders. *N. system* the organ system which, along with the endocrine system, correlates the adjustments and reactions of an organism to internal and environmental conditions. It has 2 main divisions: the central nervous system, composed of the brain and spinal cord; and the peripheral nervous system, which is subdivided into the voluntary and autonomic systems.

neural tube defect a structural anomaly of the brain or spinal cord causing anencephaly or spina bifida. In anencephaly there is absence of the cranium, thus the brain tissue is exposed and the condition is incompatible with life. A defect of the posterior laminae and spinous processes of one or more vertebrae may present clinically as a hairy patch or dimple on the midline of the infant's back and requires no treatment (spina bifida occulta); if the defect allows herniation of the meninges (meningocele) surgery is required; herniation of both meninges and spinal cord (meningomyelocele) is a serious condition which requires

expert assessment to decide whether operative treatment is possible and likely to improve the quality of life. Many of these babies have other defects and complications which are incompatible with life.

neuritis inflammation of a nerve.

neuroblast embryonic nerve cell.

neuroblastoma malignant tumour of immature nerve cells, most often occurring in children.

neurohormonal pertaining to nerves and hormones, and particularly to their coordination. *N. reflex* the physiology of LACTATION involves a process in which nerves and hormones work in harmony to control the 'LET DOWN' REFLEX.

neuromuscular pertaining to nerves and muscles, and particularly to their coordination. *N. harmony* a term used to describe the relationship between the upper and lower segments of the uterus when the woman is in labour i.e. efficient uterine action occurs when the upper uterine segment contracts and RETRACTS and the lower segment and cervix contracts and dilates.

neuron, neurone nerve cell; any of the conducting cells of the nervous system, consisting of a cell body, containing the nucleus and its surrounding cytoplasm, and the axon and dendrites. *N. thermal environment* environmental temperature in which energy losses and oxygen consumption required to maintain body temperature within normal limits will be minimal.

neurosis a functional disturbance of the nervous system characterized by emotional instability but without any obvious structural change in the nerve substance.

neutral neither acid nor alkaline. A hydrogen ion concentration (pH) of 7 is neutral.

neutron a neutral particle found with protons in the nucleus of an atom.

Neville Barnes forceps obstetric forceps for operative vaginal delivery; these forceps have axis traction handle attachments to allow downward traction of a high head into the pelvis. These attachments are not used now and the forceps are used for low-cavity deliveries. *See* Appendix 3.

niacin a water-soluble vitamin of the B complex found in various animal and plant tissues, especially liver, yeast, bran, peanuts, lean meats, fish and poultry. It is required for the synthesis of some enzymes.

nicotine a very poisonous alkaloid. The nicotine in tobacco, though small in amount, can cause indigestion, increase in blood pressure and dull the appetite. It also acts as a vasoconstrictor.

nidation the embedding of the fertilized ovum in the endometrium of the uterus.

nipple the small conical projection in the centre of the AREOLA of the breast which gives outlet to the milk from the breast. The tip of the nipple contains 15–20 small depressions that are the openings of the lactiferous ducts. *Accessory n.* a rudimentary nipple anywhere in a line from the breast to the groin. *Retracted n.* one that is drawn inwards; may be a sign of breast cancer.

nitrazepam a hypnotic and sedative drug used to treat insomnia with early morning wakening.

nitrofurantoin an antibacterial agent used in the treatment of urinary tract infection. May produce neonatal haemolysis if given to the mother at term.

nitrogen an element. Symbol N. A gas which forms nearly 80% by volume of atmospheric air. A constituent of all protein foods and substances.

nitrous oxide N_2O. Laughing gas. A general anaesthetic inducing a brief spell of unconsciousness, and used largely for dental operations. With oxygen it is used extensively as an anaesthetic. With 50% oxygen it relieves pain without producing loss of consciousness, and this mixture, self-administered by inhalation, is used to relieve pain in labour. The gases are premixed in a single blue and white cylinder with a simple valve, tubing and face mask in the Entonox apparatus, which is approved by the Nursing and Midwifery Council for use by midwives. The gas is excreted via the lungs. Side-effects include giggling, loss of control and nausea.

node a small mass of tissue in the form of a swelling, knot or protuberance, either normal or pathological. adj. *nodal*.

nodule a small boss or node that is solid and can be detected by touch.

non-accidental injury (NAI) the variety of injury caused to a 'battered baby'. There may be fractures of bones, especially of the skull, with intracranial haemorrhage and other physical injuries. The term also includes the giving of poisons and dangerous drugs, sexual abuse, starvation and any other form of physical assault. The parents or other persons looking after the child, are usually responsible for inflicting the injuries. These cases need careful investigation and handling.

non-maleficence the concept in the healthcare services of the duty to avoid harm to the interests of others.

non-shivering thermogenesis the use of brown adipose tissue by the neonate to produce heat in times of cold stress. Brown fat is stored in the mediastinum, around the nape of the neck, between the scapulae and around the kidneys and suprarenal glands.

non-specific urethritis (NSU) common sexually transmitted disease, due to a variety of organisms. *Chlamydia trachomatis* causes 40% of cases.

noradrenaline (norepinephrine) a catecholamine which is the neurotransmitter of most sympathetic postganglionic neurons and also of certain tracts in the nervous system. It is released from the adrenal medulla in response to sympathetic stimulation, primarily in response to hypotension. It produces vasoconstriction, an increase in heart rate, and elevation of blood pressure.

norethisterone progesterone-only contraceptive pill, useful for mothers who are breastfeeding.

Noriday a proprietary contraceptive pill composed of progesterone alone and therefore suitable for use while breastfeeding.

Norinyl a proprietary combined oestrogen and progesterone contraceptive pill.

normoblasts immature nucleated red blood cells normally remaining in the bone marrow until maturity, but released into the circulation in certain anaemias.

normotensive having a normal blood pressure.

notifiable a term applied to certain transmitted diseases, the occurrence of which must be statutorily notified to the Director of Public Health in the health authority. Notification is the doctor's responsibility. A midwife suspecting any notifiable disease should immediately inform a doctor. Notifiable diseases include infective jaundice, leptospirosis, scarlet fever, whooping cough, measles, smallpox, diphtheria and tuberculosis. Ophthalmia neonatorum remains notifiable but puerperal pyrexia, notifiable for many years, is no longer so.

notification *See* INTENTION TO PRACTISE.

notification of birth *See* BIRTH, NOTIFICATION OF.

nucha the nape of the neck.

nuchal back of the neck. *N. scanning* ultrasound scan performed at 11–13 weeks' gestation to measure the thickness of the skin at the back of the fetal neck as an indicator of possible Down's syndrome.

nuchal displacement a complication of breech labour, when an arm is displaced behind the child's neck.

nuclear family parents and their children living together in a household without members of the extended family such as grandparents, aunts and uncles living with them, or in the same locality.

nuclear magnetic resonance a phenomenon exhibited by atomic nuclei having a magnetic moment, i.e. those nuclei that behave as if they are tiny bar magnets. When disturbed from equilibrium by a radiofrequency pulse their alignment changes but, at the termination of the pulse, the nuclei return to their position of equilibrium. Signals elicited can be analysed and used for chemical analysis (NMR spectroscopy) or for imaging (MAGNETIC RESONANCE IMAGING; MRI).

nucleic acids extremely complex, long-chain compounds of high molecular weight that occur naturally in the cells of all living organisms. They form the genetic material of the cell and direct the synthesis of protein within the cell. There are 2 major classes of nucleic acids: DEOXYRIBONUCLEIC ACID (DNA) *and* RIBONUCLEIC ACID (RNA).

nucleus the essential part of a cell containing the chromosomes, its division being essential for the formation of new cells. *Basal n.* group of nerve cells in the brain which, in severe jaundice in the newborn, may become stained with bilirubin, causing KERNICTERUS.

nullipara a woman who has never given birth to a viable child. She may, however, have been pregnant previously, but had either a miscarriage or termination of pregnancy. adj. *nulliparous*.

nurse 1. a person who is qualified in the art and science of nursing, and meets certain prescribed standards of education and clinical competence. 2. to provide services that are essential to, or helpful in the promotion, maintenance or restoration of, health and well-being. 3. to nourish at the breast. *Registered n.* in the UK, one whose name is on the Register held by the Nursing and Midwifery Council.

nursery, day a nursery for children under school age, for working mothers – especially those who are unsupported or parents who are sick. Provision is made, under the National Health Service Act 1977, by the local authority social services department. Day nurseries may also be run by private or voluntary bodies, provided they are registered and supervised by the local authority. *N. school* schools for children between the ages of $2\frac{1}{2}$ and 5 years provided by the local education authority. There are a limited number of places available in nursery schools and thus priority is given to children with special needs.

Nursing and Midwifery Council (NMC) Regulatory organization, designated by statute to regulate the nursing, midwifery and health visiting professions in the UK in order to protect the public. Replaced the UK Central

Council (UKCC) in 2002. Responsible for quality assurance of education programmes leading to registration and recordable qualifications. Maintains registers of practitioners. Publishes professional conduct rules and other documents to guide professional practice. *See also* Appendix 15.

nutrition the process by which food is assimilated into the body in order to nourish it. Nutrition is particularly concerned with those properties of food that build sound bodies and promote health. Good nutrition means a balanced diet containing adequate amounts of the essential nutritional elements that the body must have to function normally. The essential ingredients of a balanced diet are proteins, vitamins, minerals, fats and carbohydrates. The body can manufacture sugars from fats, and fats from sugars or proteins, depending on the need, but it cannot manufacture proteins from sugars and fats. *N. therapy* a form of complementary therapy in which not only the quantity and quality of food eaten is known to have effects on the body, but also the absorption, assimilation and utilization of the nutrients. Nutritional status may also be affected by biochemical individuality and by environmental factors.

nylon a synthetic material of exceptional strength, used for sutures.

nystagmus involuntary, rapid, rhythmic movement (horizontal, vertical, rotatory, or mixed, i.e. of 2 types), of the eyeball.

Nystan *See* NYSTATIN.

nystatin an antibiotic effective in the treatment of superficial fungal infections, e.g. candidiasis. May be administered orally or in the form of vaginal pessaries.

O

obesity excessive development of fat throughout the body; increase in weight beyond that considered desirable with regard to age, height and bone structure. Obesity can affect physical and mental health. In pregnancy, complications such as hypertension are more common in obese women.

oblique slanting. *See* PELVIS, diameters of the. *O. lie* an abnormal lie in which the long axis of the fetus lies between the oblique diameters of the pelvis. It may progress to a shoulder presentation and an obstructed labour with the risk of prolapse of the cord or a fetal arm, ruptured uterus, haemorrhage and death of the fetus or even the mother.

oblongata *See* MEDULLA OBLONGATA.

observation register a register of children whose development may be adversely affected by problems occurring during the fetal or neonatal period. They should be carefully followed up by the health visitor, general practitioner and special paediatric department.

observational study an epidemiological study of events without the intervention of the investigator.

obstetric pertaining to obstetrics. *O. conjugate* the pelvic diameter extending from the sacral promontory to the upper inner border or the symphysis pubis. It measures approximately 11 cm and is the first narrow strait through which the fetal head has to pass. *Emergency o. unit* an emergency team from a consultant maternity unit comprising obstetrician, midwife and, if required, anaesthetist and/or paediatrician, who go out by ambulance to emergencies in the home or small maternity hospitals. They take emergency equipment such as O-negative blood, equipment for blood transfusion, operative delivery, manual removal of the placenta, anaesthesia (if required) and resuscitation of both mother and baby. After treatment the mother is transferred to hospital in the ambulance. *O. history* information about all previous pregnancies, and abortions, including details of labours, the puerperia and infants which is taken and recorded when a woman books with her midwife or doctor for a subsequent pregnancy. *O. pulsar* an appliance used for transcutaneous electrical nerve stimulation (TENS). *O. shock* collapse associated with childbirth owing to circulatory failure which occurs most commonly as a result of haemorrhage, or trauma such as acute inversion of the uterus, or septicaemia caused by Gram-negative organisms.

obstetrician a person skilled in the art and practice of obstetrics. In the UK, an obstetrician commonly deals with abnormal pregnancies, labours and puerperia, thus differing from a midwife, who is an expert in the care of women with normal pregnancies, childbirth and puerperia.

obstetrics the branch of medicine dealing with pregnancy, labour and the puerperium.

obstipation intractable constipation.

obstructed labour a state in which it is mechanically impossible for the child to be born. There is no advance of the presenting part despite strong uterine contractions. Obstruction most commonly occurs at the brim of the pelvis but may occur at the outlet, e.g. deep transverse arrest in an android pelvis. Good midwifery care should identify risk factors so that the complications of obstructed labour can be avoided. In the advanced state the mother is in great distress, looks anxious and ill and has tachycardia, pyrexia, ketonuria and oliguria. There may be vomiting and persistent abdominal pain. The uterus appears 'moulded' around the fetus; on palpation it is continuously hard and fetal parts cannot be felt. Fetal death from anoxia occurs and thus fetal heart sounds are absent. BANDL'S RING can be seen as a ridge running obliquely around the abdomen and marks the junction between the grossly thickened upper segment and the dangerously thinned and overdistended lower uterine segment. Vaginal examination may reveal hot, dry, oedematous vaginal walls, a high presenting part with excessive caput succedaneum and a thick 'curtain' of cervix hanging around and below it. A multiparous woman is in imminent danger of death from uterine rupture and exhaustion; a primigravid uterus may develop secondary uterine inertia. Medical aid should be summoned urgently and intramuscular pethidine administered to relieve pain; intravenous fluids are commenced to combat shock and dehydration and blood is taken for cross-matching.

Caesarean section should be performed immediately wherever possible whether the fetus is alive or dead; in isolated areas it may be necessary to undertake a fetal destructive operation as the only means of emptying the uterus and saving the mother's life, although this also carries risk of rupturing the thinned overstretched lower uterine segment.

obturator anything that closes an opening. *O. foramen* the opening in the anterolateral aspect of the pelvic os innominatum closed by fascia and muscle.

occipital relating to the occiput.

occipitoanterior when the back of the fetal head, the occiput, is to the front of the mother's pelvis as it comes through the birth canal.

occipitolateral the fetal occiput is to the side of the mother's pelvis as it enters the brim, either on the right or the left side; also termed occipitotransverse. Good uterine contractions usually encourage the head to turn to the occipitoanterior position as it reaches the resistance of the pelvic floor.

occipitoposterior the fetal occiput is directed towards the right or left sacroiliac joint of the mother's pelvis. This is the commonest of all mechanical difficulties occurring during labour. It may be caused by an abnormal maternal pelvic shape such as an android or anthropoid pelvis; the fetal attitude is often a military (erect) one or deflexed and occurs in about 10% of all pregnancies. Diagnosis is made by abdominal examination in which the abdomen may appear flattened below the umbilicus and a high deflexed fetal head is palpated with limbs felt over a large area on both sides of the midline and fetal heart sounds heard in the middle and over the flank.

Vaginal examination reveals a high head with the bregma lying anteriorly or centrally. The condition presents risks of prolonged labour, difficult delivery and infection, together with fetal hypoxia and intracranial haemorrhage from the upwards moulding of the fetal skull. In the majority of cases the fetal head will flex as it meets the pelvic floor, so that it makes a long rotation to an occipitoanterior position and delivery follows normally. Where the head remains persistently posterior, labour is prolonged, painful and difficult, and there is a risk of cord prolapse. In the second stage DEEP TRANSVERSE ARREST may occur, requiring Kjelland's forceps delivery or the head is born FACE-TO-PUBES.

occiput the back of the head. The area extending from the lambdoidal suture to the nape of the neck.

occlusive cap a rubber cap which covers the cervix and mechanically obstructs the entrance of spermatozoa, thus used as a means of contraception. It should be used in conjunction with a spermicidal agent to increase its effectiveness.

occult obscure or hidden from view. *O. blood test* examination, microscopically or by a chemical test, of a specimen of faeces, urine, gastric juice, etc. to determine the presence of blood not otherwise detectable.

ocular pertaining to the eye.

oedema an excess of fluid, either because an excess is formed or because there is a failure of absorption. It may first be recognized by excessive weight gain only (occult oedema), then by pitting on pressure. It may be physiological, as in pregnancy, where the pregnant uterus presses on the pelvic veins, or in varicose veins. Approximately 50% of women develop mild ankle

Oesophageal Atresia with Tracheo-oesophageal Fistula

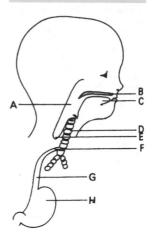

A, Pharynx; B, palate; C, tongue; D, trachea; E, oésophageal atresia; F, tracheo-oesophageal fistula; G, distal oesophagus; H, stomach.

oedema towards term, which is normal unless accompanied by other signs and symptoms, e.g. hypertension. In the puerperium, ankle oedema often worsens temporarily, as the kidneys are unable to cope immediately with excretion of the excess fluid as a result of the autolytic process of INVOLUTION. PATHOLOGICAL oedema occurs with chronic renal disease, PRE-ECLAMPSIA, ECLAMPSIA, severe heart disease, severe anaemia and malnutrition.

Pitting o. severe oedema in which pressure leaves a persistent depression in the tissues.

oesophageal pertaining to the oesophagus. *O. atresia* absence of the opening of the oesophagus. May occur in the baby of a pregnancy complicated by POLYHYDRAMNIOS. As the baby will be unable to swallow its saliva, this will come out of the mouth continuously as clear mucus. Any baby showing this sign must have a stiff tube passed via the mouth to ensure that the oesophagus is patent, as soon after delivery as possible. Any delay increases the mortality from the corrective operation. This condition is almost always accompanied by TRACHEO-OESOPHAGEAL FISTULA.

oesophagus the canal which extends from the pharynx to the stomach. It is about 22.5 cm (9 in) long in the adult.

oestradiol (estradiol) one of the ovarian hormones; the most potent naturally occurring OESTROGEN in humans.

oestriol (estriol) an ovarian hormone; a relatively weak human oestrogen.

oestrogen a generic term used to describe any hormone with OESTROGENIC activity, including oestradiol, oestriol and oestrone. It can be produced by the ovary, the adrenal gland and, in small amounts, the testis, and fetoplacental unit. Oestrogens are responsible for female secondary sexual characteristic development, and during the menstrual cycle act on the female genitalia to produce an environment suitable for fertilization, implantation and nutrition of the early embryo. During pregnancy oestrogens stimulate the growth of the uterus and the duct system of the breasts. They are also responsible for water and electrolyte retention, for the suppression of ovulation and inhibition of lactation in pregnancy.

oestrogenic producing secondary sex characteristics in a female at puberty, and some changes during the menstrual cycle and pregnancy, particularly development of the ducts in the breast and the uterine muscle.

oestrone (estrone) an OESTROGEN isolated from urine in pregnancy, the human placenta, and also prepared synthetically.

olfaction the sense of smell.

olfactory pertaining to the sense of smell.

oligaemia deficiency in volume of the blood.

oligohydramnios deficiency in the amount of amniotic fluid. It is associated with fetal malformations, e.g. renal agenesis and limb deformities and intrauterine growth retardation of the fetus.

oligomenorrhoea scanty menstruation.

oligospermia deficiency of spermatozoa in the semen.

oliguria diminished secretion of urine. It may be associated with impaired renal function following severe abruptio placentae, severe postpartum haemorrhage, severe pre-eclampsia or eclampsia.

ombudsman a person appointed to receive complaints about unfair administration. The officer in the National Health Service, appointed as 'ombudsman' or Health Service Commissioner, investigates complaints about failures in the health services. He is not able to pass judgement on clinical matters.

omentum fold of peritoneum extending from the stomach to adjacent abdominal organs.

omnivorous eating both plant and animal foods.

Omnopon *See* PAPAVERETUM.

omphalocele umbilical hernia.

omphalus the umbilicus.

onco- word element meaning 'tumour', 'swelling', 'mass'.

oncology the sum of knowledge regarding tumours; the study of tumours.

onych(o)- word element meaning 'the nails'.

onychia inflammation of the nail bed.

oöblast a primitive cell from which an ovum ultimately develops.

oöcyte the immature ovum.

oöphor(o)- word element meaning 'ovary'.

oöphorectomy removal of an ovary.

oöphoritis inflammation of an ovary.

oöphorosalpingectomy surgical removal of an ovary and its associated fallopian tube.

operant conditioning a form of behaviour therapy in which a reward is given when the subject performs the action required of him or her. The reward serves to encourage repetition of the action.

operculum the plug of mucus which fills the cervical canal during pregnancy and is shed at the beginning of labour. *See* 'SHOW'.

ophthalmia neonatorum any purulent discharge from the eyes of an infant within 21 days of birth. The causes of severe ophthalmia may be the GONOCOCCUS, *E. coli* or the staphylococci, but now is more commonly due to CHLAMYDIA TRACHOMATIS. Blindness can occur if the infection is gonococcal. It is therefore a condition NOTIFIABLE to the Director of Public Health.

ophthalmic pertaining to the eye.

ophthalmoscope an instrument for inspecting the interior of the eye.

opiate a class of drugs including: 1. the naturally occurring opiates, all of which are derived from the opium poppy. This group includes opium and its alkaloids (morphine and codeine); 2. the semi-synthetic opiates, including heroin and various other preparations; 3. the synthetic opiates, including methadone, pethidine and phenazocine; 4. the narcotic antagonists which, when used in conjunction with an opiate, block its effects but, when used alone, have opiate-like properties. Naloxone is an important exception, being an opiate antagonist but having no narcotic properties. The opiates have powerful analgesic and narcotic effects, and also produce both drug tolerance and drug dependence.

opium a substance derived from poppy juice and used to relieve pain. *Alkaloids of o.* morphine and codeine. *Tincture of o.* laudanum.

opportunistic 1. denoting a microorganism which does not ordinarily cause disease but becomes pathogenic under certain circumstances. 2. denoting a disease or infection caused by such an organism.

opsonin any substance which coats bacteria and so makes them more easily phagocytosed. Antibody is therefore an opsonin.

optic pertaining to vision.

oral pertaining to the mouth. *O. contraceptive pill* 1. the combined oral contraceptive pill contains both oestrogen and a synthetic form of progesterone and has a very low failure rate, 0.1–1 per hundred women years (HWY), i.e. the number who would become pregnant if 100 women used the method for one year. 2. the progestogen only pill is usually prescribed for breastfeeding women, for those over the age of 35 years and in other selected cases when the combined pill is contraindicated. The failure rate is 0.3–5 per HWY.

orbit the bony cavity containing the eyeball.

orbital ridge the bony rim of the orbit.

orchi(d)(o)- word element meaning 'testis'.

orchidopexy operation to release an undescended testis and place it in the scrotum.

orchitis inflammation of a testis.

organ a part of the body which performs a particular function.

organic pertaining to the structure of an organ.

organism an individual animal or plant.

organogenesis the origin or development of organs.

orgasm the apex and culmination of sexual excitement.

orifice any opening in the body.

oropharynx the part of the pharynx between the soft palate and the upper edge of the epiglottis.

-orrhaphy suffix meaning 'repair' or 'suturing', e.g. perineorrhaphy.

orthostatic standing erect. *O. albuminuria* albuminuria occurring when the individual is upright, but not after rest in bed.

Ortolani's test one method of diagnosing CONGENITAL DISLOCATION OF THE HIP. A 'click' or popping sensation is felt on reversing the movements of abduction and rotation of the hip while the child is lying with knees flexed.

os 1. a bone. *O. calcis* the heel bone or calcaneum. *O. innominatum* nameless bone. The right and left innominate bones articulate with the sacrum to form the pelvic girdle. 2. a mouth or opening. *External o.* the opening of the cervix into the vagina. *Internal o.* the junction of the cervical canal and cavity of the uterus. *O. uteri* the opening or the uterus into the vagina which dilates progressively as labour advances.

Osiander's sign pulsation of the uterine arteries through the lateral fornices which can be detected on examination *per vaginam* in early pregnancy. This is one of the signs which may assist in the diagnosis of pregnancy.

osmolality the concentration of a solution in terms of osmoles of solutes per kilogram of solvent. *Serum o.* a measure of the number of dissolved particles per unit of water in serum. Used in assessing status of hydration. *Urine o.* a measure of the number of dissolved particles per unit of water in the urine.

osmosis the passage of a solvent through a semi-permeable membrane into a more concentrated solution. The process of osmosis and the factors that influence it are important clinically in the maintenance of adequate body fluids and in the proper balance between volumes of extracellular and intracellular fluids.

osmotic pressure the power of a fluid, dependent on its molecular content, to draw another fluid towards it.

ossification the formation of bone. *O. centres* the appearance of these on X-ray at the distal end of the fetal femoral epiphysis between 35 and 40 weeks' gestation, and the proximal tibial epiphysis at 37–42 weeks may be helpful in determining fetal maturity if other methods are unsuitable or not available. *See also* ULTRASOUND. *Centres of o.* on the fetal head include frontal bosses, the occipital protuberance and the parietal eminences. The BIPARIETAL DIAMETER, normally 9.5 cm at term, is measured on ultrasound between the parietal eminences.

osteoblasts cells which mature and form bone.

osteogenesis the formation of bone. *O. imperfecta* an inherited condition of extreme fragility of the bones, in which spontaneous fractures are liable to occur. The gene is dominant.

osteomalacia adult rickets. A disease characterized by painful softening of bones. Due to gross vitamin D deficiency.

osteomyelitis inflammation of bone, localized or generalized, due to a pyogenic infection. It may result in bone destruction, in stiffening of joints if the infection spreads to the joints, and, in extreme cases occurring before the end of the growth period, in the shortening of a limb if the growth centre is destroyed.

osteopathy a system of medicine in which manipulation of the musculoskeletal system is used to restore structural and functional balance within the body. Once considered a form of complementary medicine, it is now recognized as a complete system of medicine in its own right. It can be particularly effective in treating disorders of pregnancy, assisting the mother in labour and for postnatal problems. *See also* CRANIOSACRAL THERAPY.

otitis inflammation of the ear. *O. externa* of the external ear. *O. media* infection of the middle ear, which occasionally occurs in newborn babies. *O. interna* labyrinthitis.

-otomy suffix meaning 'cutting into', e.g. hysterotomy, incision into the pregnant uterus.

ounce (oz.) a measure of weight in both the avoirdupois and the apothecaries' system. *Fluid o.* a unit of liquid measure of the apothecaries' system, being 8 fluid drams, or the equivalent of 29.57 ml.

outlet a means or route of exit or egress. *Pelvic o.* the inferior opening of the pelvis; literally that bounded by the ischial spines, lower border of the symphysis pubis and the sacrococcygeal joint.

output the yield or total of anything produced by any functional system

of the body. *Cardiac o.* the effective volume of blood expelled by either ventricle of the heart per unit of time (usually volume per minute); it is equal to the stroke output multiplied by the number of beats per the time unit used in the computation. *Fluid o.* the amount of urine passed, usually measured in comparison to oral fluid intake.

outreach clinic a clinic, for example an antenatal clinic, which is situated at some distance from the main maternity department, perhaps in a smaller hospital, general practitioner's surgery or public building such as a village hall, to enable clients and patients to access consultant care without having to make a long or inconvenient journey to the hospital.

ova plural of ovum.

ovarian pertaining to an ovary *O. cyst* a tumour of the ovary containing fluid. *O. pregnancy* a fertilized ovum developed in the ovary. *O. vein syndrome* obstruction of the ureter due to compression by an enlarged or varicosed ovarian vein; typically the vein becomes enlarged during pregnancy, the symptoms being those of obstruction or infection of the upper urinary tract. The right side is usually affected.

ovariotomy usually taken to mean removal of an ovary but, literally, incision of an ovary.

ovary one of a pair of glandular organs in the cavity of the female pelvis, attached to the posterior fold of the broad ligament near the fimbriated end of the fallopian tube. Their function is the production of ova and of the hormones (oestrogens and progesterone) which cause various changes in the body at the time of puberty and during pregnancy.

oviduct a passage through which ova leave the maternal body or pass to an organ communicating with the exterior of the body.

oviferous producing ova.

ovulation the process of liberating an ovum from the ovary by rupture of a Graafian follicle. Normally, in an adult woman, ovulation occurs at intervals of about 28 days and alternates between the 2 ovaries. Usually only 1 ovum is produced, but occasionally ovulation produces 2 or more ova which, if fertilized, may result in multiple births, such as twins or triplets.

ovum an egg. The reproductive cell of the female. pl. *ova*.

oxidase any of a class of enzymes that catalyse the reduction of molecular oxygen independently of hydrogen peroxide.

oxidation a process of combining with oxygen.

oxprenolol a beta-blocking drug used in the treatment of angina, hypertension and cardiac arrhythmias.

oxygen an element. Symbol O. A colourless, odourless gas, essential to life. It constitutes 21% of the atmosphere. In combination with hydrogen, it forms water; by weight, 90% of water is oxygen. Oxygen is essential in sustaining all kinds of life. Among the higher animals, it is obtained from the air and drawn into the lungs by the process of respiration. For therapeutic purposes it is stored in black and white cylinders. CYANOSIS is a sign of lack of oxygen (hypoxia). ANOXIA is the commonest cause of neonatal death. There are many predisposing causes, most of which are aggravated by labour, when the fetal heart beat may alter because of the acidaemia resulting from the hypoxia (fetal distress). In an asphyxiated baby, oxygen is used during resuscitation by ventilation through an endotracheal tube. When nursing the neonate, very careful monitoring of oxygen concentration is necessary, preferably by serial measurements of the Po_2 or visually by watching skin colour, to ensure that the amount of oxygen given is sufficient to prevent brain damage, but not so much as to cause retinopathy of prematurity leading to blindness in the preterm infant.

oxyhaemoglobin haemoglobin combined with molecular oxygen, the form in which oxygen is transported in the blood.

oxytetracycline a broad-spectrum antibiotic of the tetracycline group.

oxytocic term applied to any drug which stimulates contractions of the uterus in order to induce or accelerate labour.

oxytocin a hormone secreted from the posterior lobe of the pituitary gland, which causes stimulation (i.e. contraction) of the uterine myometrium. Oxytocin also causes milk to be expressed from the alveoli into the lactiferous ducts during suckling. Synthetic oxytocin (Syntocinon) may be administered intravenously to induce or augment labour, or intramuscularly or intravenously to contract uterine muscle after delivery of the placenta, and to control postpartum haemorrhage. Synthetic oxytocin may also be combined with ergometrine to produce SYNTOMETRINE.

P

pack 1. a large swab used to control abdominal contents during operation, or to control bleeding in any wound. 2. a tampon.

packed cells fresh blood for transfusion, from which a proportion of the plasma has been removed to facilitate cell haemolysis. Given when it is necessary to replace blood cells without overloading the circulation with fluid.

packed cell volume (PCV) the percentage of blood cells to PLASMA. The normal PCV is about 45%.

paediatrician a specialist in the study of infant and child in health and disease.

paediatrics that branch of medicine dealing with the care of babies and children.

paedophilia abnormal fondness for children; sexual activity of adults with children. adj. *paedophiliac*.

pain suffering and distress, caused by stimulation of specialized nerve endings. All receptors for pain stimuli are free nerve endings of groups of small myelinated or unmyelinated nerve fibres abundantly distributed in the superficial layers of the skin and in certain deeper tissues. Following stimulation, nerve endings in the skin transmit nerve impulses along sensory nerve fibres to the spinal cord. They then travel upward along the sensory pathways to the thalamus, which is the main sensory relay station of the brain. The conscious perception of pain probably takes place in the thalamus and lower centres; interpretation of the quality of pain is probably the role of the cerebral cortex. *P. in labour* this is caused by contractions of the upper uterine segment which first dilate the cervix and then expel the fetus through the birth canal. This pain is felt intermittently in the lower abdomen and back, occurring with increasing frequency and intensity as labour proceeds. At the same time pain may be felt in the sacral region. This originates in the cervix and if it is severe it indicates that the cervix is not relaxing well and labour may be abnormal. *See also* GATE CONTROL THEORY OF PAIN.

palate the roof of the mouth. *Hard p.* in front, is of bone. *Soft p.* continues from it, and is of muscle. *See also* CLEFT PALATE.

palliative an agent which relieves, but does not cure disease.

palpation examination by touch; the application of the fingers with light pressure to the surface of the body for the purpose of determining the condition of the parts beneath in physical diagnosis. *See* ABDOMINAL EXAMINATION *and* VAGINAL EXAMINATION.

palpitation abnormally rapid beating of the heart of which the person is conscious.

palsy paralysis. *Bell's p.* facial paralysis due to lesion of the facial nerve, resulting in characteristic facial distortion. *Cerebral p.* a persisting qualitative motor disorder appearing before age 3. *Erb's p.* a limp inwardly rotated arm with half-closed hand turned outwards; caused by damage to the upper roots of the brachial plexus. *Klumpke's p.* paralysis of the hand and wrist drop; caused by damage to the 8th cervical and 1st thoracic nerve roots.

Panadol *See* PARACETAMOL.

pancreas a racemose gland about 15 cm (6 in) long, lying behind the stomach, with its head in the curve of the duodenum and its tail in contact with the spleen. It secretes digestive juice, which enters the duodenum by the pancreatic duct which joins the common bile duct. The pancreas also secretes the hormone INSULIN from the islets of Langerhans.

pancreatic duct the main excretory duct of the pancreas, which usually unites with the common bile duct before entering the duodenum at the major duodenal papilla.

pancuronium a neuromuscular blocking agent used as a muscle relaxant during surgery, or during mechanical intermittent positive pressure ventilation, when it has been shown to prevent pneumothorax in babies actively expiring against ventilator inflation.

pandemic an epidemic spreading over a wide area.

panhysterectomy total hysterectomy, i.e. removal of the body and cervix of the uterus.

Papanicolaou test (smear) a simple test used most commonly to detect cancer of the uterus and cervix; often called the smear test. Malignant epithelia shed their surface cells more rapidly than normal cells. A blunt wooden spatula (Ayre's spatula) is passed through the cervix and rotated 360° near the internal os to scrape off surface cells. These cells are transferred on to a glass slide and examined microscopically.

papaveretum (Omnopon) an analgesic drug; a mixture of opium alkaloids.

papilla a small nipple-like eminence. pl. *papillae*.

papilloma a benign tumour derived from epithelium. *P. virus* a sexually transmitted infection causing anogenital warts (condylomata acuminata). It is associated with an increased incidence of cervical carcinoma. *Laryngeal p.* a rare condition in the neonate due to infection acquired during vaginal delivery.

papule a small solid raised elevation of the skin.

papyraceous like paper. *Fetus papyraceus* may very rarely occur early in a multiple pregnancy when one fetus dies and becomes flattened. It is discovered at delivery.

para used to describe a woman who has produced one or more VIABLE offspring. adj. *parous*. Numerals designate the number of viable infants delivered by the mother, a NULLIPARA being para 0, a woman who has delivered one baby being para 1 or a PRIMIPARA and a woman who has delivered more than one baby being para 2, 3, 4 etc. or a MULTIPARA. All babies delivered over the 24th week of gestation and all live births are counted in the number. Thus, stillbirths are counted, but miscarriages and terminations are not: these are usually identified by adding +1 after the number designating viable deliveries, e.g. para 3^{+1}.

para- prefix meaning 'near', e.g. parametrium; connective tissue near the uterus.

paracentesis puncture of the wall of a cavity in order to draw off fluid. *P. uteri* amniocentesis. Puncture of the abdominal and uterine wall to gain access to the uterine cavity in pregnancy. *See* POLYHYDRAMNIOS.

paracervical block infiltration of LEE–FRANKENHAUSER PLEXUS with local anaesthetic performed through the lateral fornices to relieve the pain of cervical dilatation in labour. Effective for up to 3 hours. Inadvertent injection into the uterine artery which is in close proximity to the plexus may cause fetal bradycardia and possibly intrauterine fetal death.

paracetamol an oral analgesic and antipyretic drug commonly used instead of aspirin for relief of moderate pain and reduction in fever. Acute paracetamol overdosage can cause severe and potentially fatal hepatic necrosis.

paraesthesia disorder of sensation, e.g. a feeling as of 'pins and needles'. It may occur with the CARPAL TUNNEL SYNDROME and is occasionally felt in the feet following epidural analgesia.

paraldehyde a powerful hypnotic, sedative and anticonvulsant drug, quick in action and generally safe, but having a strong and unpleasant smell.

paralysis palsy. Failure of function of a nerve, especially of a motor nerve, and therefore failure or impairment of the muscles (voluntary or involuntary) supplied by the affected nerves. *Facial p. see* BIRTH INJURY. *Infantile p.* POLIOMYELITIS. *See also* ERB'S PARALYSIS *and* KLUMPKE'S PARALYSIS.

paralytic pertaining to or affected by paralysis.

paramedical, paramedic having some connection with or relation to the science or practice of medicine; adjunctive to the practice of medicine in the maintenance or restoration of health and normal functioning. The paramedical services include physiotherapy, and occupational and speech therapy, etc., and the services

of social workers. Some ambulance service personnel who have received specialist training to perform certain procedures normally carried out by doctors are now also called paramedics.

parametric 1. situated near the uterus; parametrial. 2. pertaining to or defined in terms of a parameter.

parametritis inflammation of the PARAMETRIUM; pelvic cellulitis.

parametrium the pelvic connective tissue surrounding the lower part of the uterus and filling in the spaces between it and the related organs.

paranoia a mental disorder characterized by well-systematized delusions of persecution, illusions of grandeur, or a combination of both. adj. *paranoiac*. It is a chronic disease that develops over months and years and for which usually there is no cure.

paranoid 1. resembling paranoia. 2. paranoiac.

paraplegia paralysis of the legs and, in some cases, the lower part of the body. adj. *paraplegic*. Paraplegia is a form of central nervous system paralysis, in which the paralysis affects all the muscles of the parts involved.

parasite a plant or animal which lives within or upon another living organism, termed the host, upon which it satisfies all its needs without compensation.

parasympathetic nervous system part of the autonomic NERVOUS SYSTEM; post-ganglionic fibres are distributed to the heart, smooth muscles, and glands of the head and neck, and the thoracic, abdominal and pelvic viscera. Almost 75% of all parasympathetic nerve fibres are in the VAGUS nerves, which serve the entire thoracic and abdominal regions of the body. The predominant secretion of the nerve endings of the parasympathetic nervous system is acetylcholine, which acts on the various organs of the body to either excite or inhibit certain activities.

parathyroid glands four small endocrine glands – two associated with each lobe of the thyroid gland, and sometimes embedded in it. Its hormone plays an important role in maintaining the plasma calcium level.

paratyphoid a notifiable infection caused by *Salmonella*.

parent–infant relationship 'bonding', or the relationship which develops between the parents and their baby. Breastfeeding is considered to strengthen the bond between the mother and her baby.

parenteral outside the alimentary tract. Used to describe the introduction of a substance into the body by any route but the alimentary tract.

parenthood education a series of classes to help parents prepare for labour and parenthood.

paresis partial paralysis affecting muscular action but not sensation.

parietal related to or attached to the wall of a cavity. One of two thin flat bones forming the major part of the vault of the skull. *See also* FETAL SKULL.

parity 1. para; the condition of a woman with respect to her having borne viable infants. 2. equality; close correspondence or similarity.

Parlodel bromocriptine mesylate, a dopamine receptor agonist.

paronychia inflammation of the folds of skin surrounding the fingernail. A fairly common infection in newborn babies, almost always staphylococcal in origin.

parotid near the ear. *P. glands* the largest of the 3 main pairs of salivary glands, located on either side of the face, just below and in front of the ears.

parous having borne one or more viable offspring. *See also* NULLIPARA *and* PRIMIPAROUS.

paroxysm 1. a sudden recurrence or intensification of symptoms. 2. a spasm or seizure. adj. *paroxysmal.*

partial pressure *See* PO₂; Appendix 16.

partogram a graphical record of the progress of labour, particularly the dilatation of the cervix. Progress can be assessed from the visual patterns of cervical dilatation and descent of the presenting part in conjunction with the record of maternal and fetal well-being. When normal progress does not occur action such as augmentation with oxytocic drugs can be taken. *See* Appendix 5.

parturient being in labour; relating to childbirth.

parturition giving birth to a child.

pascal (Pa) the international (SI) unit of pressure, which corresponds to a force of 1 newton per square metre.

passive not active. *P. immunity see* IMMUNITY. *P. movements* manipulation by a physiotherapist without the help of the patient.

pasteurization heating of milk or other liquids to a temperature of 60°C for 30 minutes, killing pathogenic bacteria and considerably delaying other bacterial development.

Patau's syndrome trisomy 13 syndrome; a relatively rare chromosomal abnormality characterized by certain clinical features affecting the face, hands and feet and mental retardation.

patella the small, circular, sesamoid bone forming the knee-cap.

patent open. *P. ductus arteriosus* abnormal persistence of an open lumen in the ductus arteriosus, between the aorta and pulmonary artery, after birth. It places special burdens on the left ventricle of the heart and causes a diminished blood flow in the aorta. Closure of the patent ductus arteriosus can be produced in preterm infants by administration of an inhibitor of prostaglandin formation, such as indomethacin. Conversely, in neonates suffering from severe congenital heart defects in which an open ductus arteriosus could be beneficial, prostaglandins are given to keep the channel open.

paternity can now be proved by analysis of DNA in blood. The unsupported mother can apply for an affiliation order against the man she alleges to be the father of her child and, providing the court is satisfied about the paternity of the child, the putative father can be required to pay a fixed weekly sum for the maintenance of the child.

patho- a prefix denoting 'disease'.

pathogen any micro-organism or material which causes disease.

pathogenic causing disease.

pathological pertaining to the study of disease.

pathology the branch of medicine treating the essential nature of disease, especially the structural and functional changes in tissues and organs in the body.

Patients' Charter a charter which details standards of care which patients and clients can expect and have a right to receive when undergoing health care, in an attempt to improve the quality of services, both in the community and in hospitals. It includes issues such as hospital waiting times, the hospital environment, ambulance, dental, optical and pharmaceutical services. There is a special charter for maternity services to comply with the recommendations in the 'CHANGING CHILDBIRTH' REPORT.

Pawlick's Grip

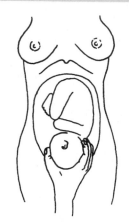

patulous distended or open. Used in reference to the external os in a multiparous woman and during pregnancy when the cervix is incompetent.

Paul–Bunnell test a method of testing for the presence of heterophil antibodies in the blood for the diagnosis of infectious mononucleosis.

Pawlik's grip a method of estimating the mobility and engagement or non-engagement of the presenting part by palpation of the lower pole of the uterus. It can cause discomfort if not performed gently and slowly, ensuring that the mother is well relaxed. It is particularly useful to feel under the apron of fat in a very obese mother.

pectineal pertaining to the os pubis.

pectoral 1. of or pertaining to the chest or breast. 2. relieving disorders of the respiratory tract, as an expectorant.

Caldwell and Moloy's Classification of the Brim of the Pelvis

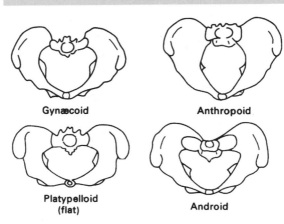

Gynaecoid

Anthropoid

Platypelloid (flat)

Android

---

pedicle the stem of a tumour.

pediculosis infestation with lice of the skin or hair.

Pediculus a louse.

pedigree a table, chart, diagram or list of an individual's ancestors, used in genetics in the analysis of Mendelian inheritance.

peduncle a large stalk or pedicle.

peer review the basic component of a QUALITY ASSURANCE programme in which the results of health and/or midwifery care given to a specific client population are evaluated according to defined criteria established by the peers of the professionals delivering the care.

pellagra a syndrome caused by a diet seriously deficient in niacin (or by failure to convert tryptophan to niacin). Most patients with pellagra also suffer from deficiencies of vitamin B$_2$ (riboflavin) and other essential vitamins and minerals. The disease also occurs in people suffering from alcoholism and drug addiction.

pelvic pertaining to the pelvis. *P. bone* hip bone, comprising the ilium, the ischium and pubis. *P. cellulitis see* PARAMETRITIS. *P. diameter* any diameter of the bony pelvis. *P. floor,* or *diaphragm,* consists of strong sheets of muscle fibres, the chief of which are the LEVATORES ANI, which form the principal support of the pelvic organs. *See also* PERINEUM. *P. girdle* the ossa innominata and sacrum. *P. inflammatory disease (PID)* infection involving the uterine tubes, ovaries and parametrium. Other

Pelvic Brim	Pelvic Outlet

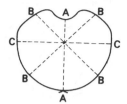

A–A, Anteroposterior diameter;
B–B, oblique diameters;
C–C, transverse diameter.

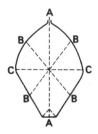

A–A, Anteroposterior diameter;
B–B, oblique diameters;
C–C, transverse diameter.

organs in the pelvis, especially the gut, may also be involved.

pelvimeter calipers for measuring the diameters of the pelvis, rarely used now.

pelvimetry measurement of the capacity and diameter of the pelvis, either internally or externally or both, with the hands, with a pelvimeter, or by radiography.

pelvis a bony girdle formed anteriorly and laterally by the innominate bones, and posteriorly by the sacrum and coccyx. It has a muscular floor, and contains the uterus, fallopian tubes, ovaries, urinary bladder and rectum. *False p.* the part lying above the brim (*see above*) bounded by the iliac fossae laterally, with the lumbar spine posteriorly and the abdominal wall anteriorly. Of little importance in obstetrics. *True p.* the part including and below the level of the brim. Of great obstetric importance, as it forms the bony canal through which the fetus must pass to be born normally. *Brim* or *inlet*, bounded by the sacral promontory and alae, upper part of the sacroiliac joints,

iliopectineal lines, and upper inner borders of the upper rami of the pubes and symphysis pubis. *Cavity*, bounded by the hollow of the sacrum, the sacrospinous ligaments, the ischial and pubic bones and the symphysis pubis. *Outlet*, bounded anatomically by the coccyx, the sacrotuberous ligaments, the ischial tuberosities and the pubic arch. An *obstetrical outlet* is bounded posteriorly by the lower aspect of the sacrum and laterally by the ischial spines, this being the lowest level at which the fetus has bone surrounding it within the birth canal. *Inclination of p.* the brim slopes at an angle of approximately 55° to the horizontal, and the bony outlet slopes at an angle of about 15°. *See also* CURVE OF CARUS. *Android p.* this has masculine characteristics, including a roughly triangular or heart-shaped brim and a narrow funnel shape, with an outlet which is narrower than in the gynaecoid pelvis.

Table of average measurements of pelvis: internal measurements			
	Anteroposterior (cm)	Right and left oblique diameters (cm)	Transverse (cm)
Brim	11	12	13
Cavity	12	12	12
Outlet	13	12	10–11

Diagonal conjugate 12–12.5 cm measured from the apex of the pubic arch to the sacral promontory.

Obstetric conjugate extends from the inner, upper border of the symphysis pubis – 11 cm.

True or anatomical conjugate measures slightly more than the obstetric conjugate as it extends from the sacral promontory to the centre of the upper surface of the symphysis pubis, but the extra space is not available for the passage of the fetus.

Anthropoid p. this has a brim which is long anteroposteriorly and narrow transversely. *Gynaecoid p.* this is the normal female pelvis. It is as nearly as possible round at the brim, cavity and outlet. It is roomy and shallow, and ideally shaped for the transmission of the fetus. *Platypelloid* or *flat p.* this has an oval brim, small anteroposteriorly and wide transversely. All these types of pelvis are normal, and only cause difficult labour if they are extreme or small. The pelvis may also be deformed as a result of rare inherited characteristics, disease or accident. Examples are: the *Naegele pelvis*, in which one sacral alae has failed to develop, producing asymmetry; the *Robert pelvis* (an extremely rare type) in which both sacral alae are undeveloped and the symphysis pubis is sometimes split; the *spondylolisthetic pelvis*, in which the 5th lumbar vertebra has slipped forwards on the sacrum, creating a false promontory; the *rachitic pelvis*, the brim of which is markedly flattened and kidney-shaped. *Assessment of the pelvis.* (a) Observation of the mother's general appearance; sometimes a rough guide. (b) Previous obstetric history may be very valuable. (c) Measurement of the pelvis.

The pelvis can be assessed more accurately by VAGINAL EXAMINATION. The ability of the fetal head to engage is a guide to the capacity of the pelvic brim in nulliparous women, but in multigravidae failure of the head to engage before labour is common due to laxity of the abdominal muscles. In cases of doubt, e.g. a head which fails to engage and cannot be made to do so, breech presentation or an obstetric history suggesting mechanical difficulty in labour, radiological pelvimetry is accurate and valuable.

pemphigus an acute or chronic skin disease, characterized by watery blisters. *P. neonatorum* bullous impetigo. It is an extremely infectious disease, and is usually due to infection with *Staphylococcus aureus*. The midwife should immediately report any blister. The child should be

191

strictly isolated until the cause of the condition has been found. *Syphilitic p.* may, rarely, occur in the neonate.

pendulous hanging down. *P. abdomen* a condition seen in multigravid women with extreme laxity of the abdominal muscles. The uterus falls forwards so much that the abdomen may hang below the symphysis pubis. Apart from the marked discomfort, this may cause malpresentation of the fetus.

penicillin an antibiotic substance obtained from cultures of the mould *Penicillium*.

penicillinase enzyme that inactivates penicillin, produced by many bacteria, particularly staphylococci.

penis the male organ of copulation.

pentazocine hydrochloride a synthetic narcotic analgesic developed as an attempt to produce a narcotic without abuse potential. It is used orally and by infusion for moderate to severe pain, although relief is variable. A proprietary brand is Fortral.

pepsin a proteolytic enzyme that is the principal digestive component of gastric juice. It acts as a catalyst in the chemical breakdown of protein to form a mixture of polypeptides. It also has a milk-clotting action similar to that of RENNIN and thereby facilitates the digestion of milk protein.

peptide the peptides form the constituent part of proteins; known as di-, tri-, tetra-, etc., peptides, depending on the number of amino acids in the molecule.

per through (Latin), e.g. in *per vaginam*: through the vagina.

percentile a term used in statistics to show how common some characteristic is. The line represents the percentage of the population who have this. The 90th percentile (or centile) for height means that 90% of the

population will be no taller than the figure. The 50th percentile is the median or average. The charts are widely used in midwifery to show the birth weight of babies at different gestations.

percussion tapping a surface with the fingers to determine, by the sound, the condition of the underlying organs.

perforation a hole or break in the containing walls or membranes of an organ or structure of the body. Perforation occurs when erosion, infection, or other factors create a weak spot in the organ and internal pressure causes a rupture.

performance indicators 'package' of routine statistics derived nationally and presented visually in ways which highlight the relative efficiency of health services in each health authority compared with other authorities.

peri- prefix meaning 'around'.

pericardium the smooth membranous sac enveloping the heart, consisting of an outer fibrous and an inner serous coat. Inflammation of this membrane is called *pericarditis*.

pericranium the external periosteum of the cranial bones.

perimetrium the peritoneum of the uterus.

perinatal around the time of birth. *P. period* the first week of life. *P. mortality rate* the number of stillbirths plus deaths of babies under 1 week old per 1000 total births in any 1 year.

perineal pertaining to the perineum. *P. lacerations* are classified as: (*a*) first degree, a tear of skin only, the muscle being intact; (*b*) second degree, a tear of skin and muscle which may be slight or severe, but which does not include the anal sphincter; (*c*) third degree or complete, where the tear extends through the whole of the perineal body, and through

Perineal Repair (Commonly Used Method)

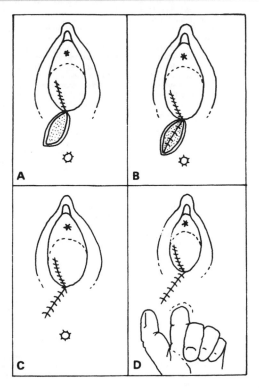

A, Vagina sutured with continuous catgut; B, muscle layer sutured with interrupted catgut; C, perineal skin sutured with interrupted catgut or silk; D, rectal examination to exclude rectal involvement.

the anal sphincter into the rectum. *P. repair* midwives who have received instruction and been assessed as competent may undertake the repair of the perineum. The perineum is closed in three layers using polyglycolic material or Dexon; the vagina is sutured, commencing just above the apex of the incision or tear, using interrupted sutures; deep and superficial muscle layers are sutured by starting in the centre of the incision to give good approximation; perineal skin is sutured. After removal of the tampon which was inserted to maintain a clear visual field, a gloved finger is passed into the rectum to ensure no sutures encroach into it. *See also* Appendix 3.

perineorrhaphy repair of the perineal body following injury sustained during childbearing.

perineum anatomically, the area extending from the pubic arch to the coccyx, with the underlying tissues. Obstetrically, the perineal body is the fibromuscular pyramid between the lower third of the vagina anteriorly and the anal canal posteriorly, and ischial tuberosities laterally. *See also* PELVIC FLOOR.

periosteum a specialized connective tissue covering all bones of the body, and possessing bone-forming potentialities. It also serves as a point of attachment for certain muscles.

peripheral relating to the periphery.

periphery the outer surface or circumference.

peristalsis a wave-like contraction which travels along the walls of a tubular organ, tending to press its contents onwards. It occurs in the muscle coat of the alimentary canal and in the fallopian tubes. Sometimes visible peristalsis occurs in PYLORIC STENOSIS.

peritoneum the serous membrane lining the abdominal cavity and forming a covering for the abdominal organs. *Parietal p.* that which lines the abdominal cavity. *Pelvic p.* that which covers the pelvic organs, in the female forming a pouch between the rectum and the uterus, the pouch of Douglas, and a shallow pouch between the uterus and the bladder, the uterovesical pouch. The peritoneum which hangs over the fallopian tubes is known as the broad ligament. *Visceral p.* the inner layer which closely covers the organs, and includes the mesenteries. adj. *peritoneal.*

peritonitis inflammation of the peritoneum, due to infection. *General p.* the whole of the abdominal cavity is affected. *Pelvic p.* the infection is restricted to the peritoneum of the pelvic cavity. It is an occasional complication of puerperal sepsis.

periventricular haemorrhage a serious complication occurring in preterm babies, especially those under 34 weeks' gestation. The haemorrhage can be graded from 0 to 3, with 3 being the most extensive.

periventricular leukomalacia cystic, ischaemic lesions occurring in the periventricular region. This condition is associated with periventricular haemorrhage and is diagnosed by ultrasound scanning. It is associated with a high incidence of spastic cerebral palsy.

permeable able to be penetrated. Applied to membrane which allows fluid to pass through, e.g. the walls of the capillaries (also semi-permeable).

pernicious highly destructive; fatal. *P. anaemia* a megaloblastic anaemia occurring in middle-aged people and caused by failure of the gastric secretion of intrinsic factor, and treated by the administration of vitamin B_{12}. Not to be confused with megaloblastic anaemia of pregnancy, which is due to lack of folic acid in the diet.

peroxide a compound of any element with more than the normal quantity of oxygen required to form an oxide. *P. of hydrogen* a compound of hydrogen and oxygen.

perphenazine (Fentazin) an oral antiemetic; should be avoided in the first trimester.

persistent mentoposterior a face presentation in which the sinciput has rotated forwards and the chin has been rotated backwards to the hollow of the sacrum. A rare cause of obstructed labour, when the thorax must present at the pelvic brim with the head.

persistent occipitoposterior a deflexed vertex presentation in which the sinciput has rotated forwards and the occiput has been rotated backwards to the hollow of the sacrum; this may cause delay in the second stage of labour. Spontaneous FACE-TO-PUBES delivery is possible.

personality that which constitutes, distinguishes, and characterizes a person as an entity over a period of time; the total reaction of a person to his environment. Many factors that determine personality are inherited; they are shaped and modified by the individual's environment. The early years of life influence personality development.

perspiration 1. sweating; the excretion of moisture through the pores of the skin. 2. sweat; the salty fluid, consisting largely of water, excreted by the sweat glands in the skin. In cystic fibrosis the sweat shows a raised level of sodium chloride.

pertussis whooping cough. A potentially serious infection of the respiratory tract, usually caused by the organism *Bordetella pertussis*. The incidence declined until the mid-1970s but has risen again in parallel with the fall in immunization rate. It is particularly serious in babies under 3 months and in children with asthma.

pessary an object inserted into the vagina. It may be a device to maintain anteversion of the uterus in early pregnancy, or a drug in a solvent base, e.g. antifungal or contraceptive. *Prostaglandin p.* a pessary containing prostaglandins, inserted into the posterior fornix of the vagina to facilitate cervical ripening and the onset of labour.

petechiae small spots caused by minute subcutaneous haemorrhages, seen in purpura and sometimes on the face of the normal newborn child, due to venous congestion during delivery. When seen over the whole body it is a feature of congenital RUBELLA, TOXOPLASMOSIS and CYTOMEGALOVIRUS infection.

pethidine hydrochloride an analgesic and antispasmodic drug, very effective in relieving pain in labour. Under the Misuse of Drugs Regulations, 1973, registered midwives working in the community are authorized to be in possession of pethidine. Because of depression of the fetal respiratory system and its adverse effect on neonatal behaviour, including breastfeeding, for the first few days of life, pethidine is now less popular for use in labour.

petit mal a relatively mild epileptic attack, contrasting with GRAND MAL, a major attack. In petit mal, the affected person loses consciousness only momentarily.

Pfannenstiel's incision a transverse abdominal incision just above the symphysis pubis.

pH the symbol used to express the hydrogen ion concentration or reaction of a fluid. In a scale ranging from 0 to 14, 7 is neutral, below 7 acid and above 7 alkaline. Blood, with a pH of 7.4, is slightly alkaline. It may be measured with an Astrup machine. The pH is used as a measure of whether the body is maintaining a normal ACID–BASE BALANCE. A favourable pH is essential to the functioning of enzymes and other biological systems.

phaeochromocytoma a rare growth usually a benign adrenal tumour, but occasionally found in other sites such as the bladder associated with an increased production of adrenaline and consequent hypertension. Typically the blood pressure has wide diurnal variations. The test considered most reliable to diagnose phaeochromocytoma is direct assay of adrenaline and noradrenaline in the plasma and urine. Another test involving measurement of vanillylmandelic acid (VMA) and of metanephrine and normetanephrine in urine may be carried out. The level of these substances in the urine in women with phaeochromocytoma is almost twice the upper limits of normal. Surgical removal of the tumour is necessary.

phage a virus which kills certain microorganisms. Viruses have differential susceptibility, which enables them to be distinguished into phage types.

phagocytes polymorphonuclear leucocytes and monocytes which engulf and digest bacteria and foreign particles.

phagocytosis the action of PHAGOCYTES.

phalanx any bone of a finger or toe. adj. *phalangeal*.

phallic pertaining to the penis.

phantom 1. an image or impression not evoked by actual stimuli. 2. a model of the body or of a specific part thereof. 3. a device for simulating the *in vivo* interaction of radiation with tissues. *P. pregnancy* pseudocyesis or false pregnancy.

pharmaceutical relating to drugs.

pharmacokinetics study of the metabolism and actions of drugs, especially absorption, duration of action, distribution within the body and method of excretion.

pharmacology the science of the nature and preparation of drugs.

pharmacopoeia an authoritative publication which gives the standard formulae and preparation of drugs as used in a given country. *British Pharmacopoeia (BP)*: that authorized for use in Great Britain.

pharmacy 1. the art of preparing, compounding and dispensing medicines. 2. a shop in which medicines are dispensed and sold.

pharynx the back of the mouth leading to the oesophagus and the larynx and communicating with the nose through the posterior nares, and the ears through the eustachian tubes.

Phenergan *See* PROMETHAZINE HYDROCHLORIDE.

phenindione oral anticoagulant similar to warfarin; should be avoided in pregnancy and breastfeeding.

phenobarbital a barbiturate drug which depresses the cerebral cortex. It is used in the treatment of epilepsy and eclampsia, but should be avoided in early pregnancy.

phenol a powerful and very poisonous antiseptic, which may also cause severe skin irritation in mild dilutions.

phenomenology an inductive descriptive approach to research developed from phenomenological philosophy, involving an understanding of the response of the whole human being;

it focuses on describing experiences as they are lived by a person, such as describing a person's pain as they perceive it.

phenothiazine a group of major tranquillizers, the phenothiazine derivatives.

phenotype 1. the outward, visible expression of the hereditary constitution of an organism. 2. an individual exhibiting a certain phenotype; a trait expressed in a phenotype.

phenoxymethylpenicillin oral antibiotic commonly used for mild streptococcal infections (penicillin V).

phenylalanine an essential amino acid, normally converted to tyrosine by an enzyme from the liver.

phenylketonuria the presence in the urine of phenylketones resulting from the incomplete breakdown of PHENYLALANINE to tyrosine. A high blood level of phenylalanine leads to mental retardation, fits and poor muscular coordination. Early diagnosis should be achieved by routine screening of infants' blood by the GUTHRIE TEST, for example, as urine tests are less accurate. A diet containing only a little phenylalanine must be given. The incidence is about 1 in 10 000. The inheritance is autosomal RECESSIVE. Persons with phenylketonuria are usually blue-eyed and blond, with defective pigmentation, the skin being excessively sensitive to light and tending to eczema.

phenylpyruvic acid abnormal constituent excreted in the urine of people with phenylketonuria.

phenytoin sodium (Epanutin) an anticonvulsant drug used to control epilepsy. It should be avoided in early pregnancy unless the potential benefits outweigh the risk of congenital abnormality.

phimosis constriction of the orifice of the prepuce so that it cannot be drawn back over the glans of the penis.

phlebitis inflammation of a vein. It is usually a vein of the leg, and a deep or superficial vein may be involved. Phlebitis in a deep vein can be a cause of THROMBOSIS and EMBOLISM.

phlebothrombosis clotting of blood in a vein, not associated with infection. The clot is loosely attached to the wall of the vein and there is considerable risk of separation of all or part of it, and, therefore, EMBOLISM. cf. THROMBOPHLEBITIS.

phlebotomist one who performs phlebotomy, i.e. obtaining samples of blood for testing.

phlebotomy venesection.

phlegmasia inflammation. *P. alba dolens* white leg. A condition, uncommon nowadays, of puerperal femoral THROMBOPHLEBITIS or PHLE-BOTHROMBOSIS, associated with venous obstruction and/or reflex arterial spasm. The leg is swollen and very painful. Treatment consists of elevating the leg without immobilization and giving antibiotics if the condition is caused by thrombophlebitis; in other cases anticoagulants may be given in addition.

phlegmatic of dull and sluggish temperament.

phobia any persistent abnormal dread or fear that appears to result from repressed inner conflicts of which the affected person is unaware. Used as a word ending designating abnormal or morbid fear of, or aversion to, the subject indicated by the stem to which it is affixed. A person with a phobia reacts uncontrollably and unreasonably to the situation of which he or she is afraid, e.g. acrophobia, fear of heights; claustrophobia, morbid fear of closed places.

phocomelia congenital absence of the proximal portion of a limb or limbs, the hands or feet being attached to the trunk by a small, irregularly shaped bone.

phospholipid any lipid that contains phosphorus, including those with a glycerol backbone (phosphoglycerides and plasmalogens) or a backbone of sphingosine or a related substance (sphingomyelins). They are the major lipids in cell membranes.

phosphorus a chemical element. Symbol P. It is an essential element in the diet. In the form of phosphates it is a major component of the mineral phase of bone and is involved in almost all metabolic processes. It also plays an important role in cell metabolism. It is obtained by the body from milk products, cereals, meat and fish, and its use by the body is controlled by vitamin D and calcium.

photophobia intolerance of light. One of the symptoms of meningitis.

photosensitivity abnormal degree of skin sensitivity to sunlight. During pregnancy, increased levels of melanocytic hormone can contribute to this. Also caused by certain drugs, e.g. chlorpromazine.

phototherapy treatment using fluorescent light, containing a high output of blue light, to reduce the amount of unconjugated bilirubin in the skin of a neonate. Complex changes occur and the non-toxic photodegradation products are excreted without the help of the enzyme system in the liver. Side-effects are skin rashes and loose green stools. The latter requires an extra fluid intake of about 30 mg/kg per 24 hours to compensate, and conventionally the eyes and gonads are covered in case the light may cause problems. Phototherapy also may be used prophylactically in preterm infants with bruising, and in babies affected by Rhesus incompatibility. It is used therapeutically with levels of bilirubin of 340 μmol/l at term, 210 μmol/l at 34 weeks, and about 150 μmol/l at 28 weeks.

phrenic pertaining to the diaphragm or to the mind. *P. nerve* a major branch of the cervical plexus. Nerve impulses from the inspiratory centre in the brain travel down the phrenic nerve, causing contraction of the diaphragm, and inspiration occurs.

phthisis pulmonary tuberculosis.

physiological third stage management of the third stage of labour in which the placenta separates from the uterine wall physiologically without the use of oxytocic drugs to expedite the process. Signs of separation and descent of the placenta are awaited: the uterus rises in the abdomen, feels small, hard and mobile, the cord lengthens and there is a small gush of blood from the vagina. The placenta may then be delivered with maternal effort, or if CONTROLLED CORD TRACTION is to be used, it is imperative that the midwife ascertains that separation of the placenta has occurred. *See also* ACTIVE MANAGEMENT OF LABOUR.

physiology the science of the function of living organisms.

physiotherapist practitioner of physiotherapy who uses massage, manipulation, remedial exercises, heat, light and electrical impulses to treat and rehabilitate. *Obstetric p.* one who specializes in treating pregnant women.

physique the body organization, development, and structure.

phytomenadione (Konakion) a preparation of vitamin K, effective in treating haemorrhage occurring during anticoagulant therapy, and due to vitamin K deficiency. Prophylactic vitamin K is given orally or intramuscularly to the newborn to prevent haemorrhagic disease.

phytotherapy treatment using plant substances such as herbal medicine and aromatherapy.

pia mater the innermost membrane enveloping the brain and spinal cord.

pica a craving to eat unnatural substances, sometimes occurring during pregnancy, possibly related to nutritional deficiencies.

pie chart a circular diagram divided into segments showing the proportional distribution of observations of particular events.

Pierre–Robin syndrome a congenital abnormality where there is MICROGNATHIA and a cleft palate. If it is not recognized at birth, severe respiratory obstruction may occur, as the tongue occludes the pharynx. The baby should be nursed prone, with the tongue pulled forwards if necessary to clear the airway.

pigment any dye or colouring agent. *Bile p.* BILIRUBIN and biliverdin. *Blood p.* haematin.

piles HAEMORRHOIDS.

pilonidal having a nest of hairs. *P. cyst* an implantation dermoid in the natal cleft. The cyst results from penetration of hairs in the natal cleft through the skin of the fold thus causing a sinus (pilonidal sinus) and epithelium cell implantation. Prone to recurrent infection. *P. depression* a depression in the midline near the coccyx, seen in the newborn child. It is of no significance. *P. sinus* a small sinus, opening near the coccyx. It is seen on routine examination of the newborn child soon after birth. It is a remnant of the neural canal and may become infected, necessitating excision.

pilot study small-scale version of a planned investigation or observation, used to test the design of the larger study.

Pinard's stethoscope a trumpet-shaped instrument which can be placed on the maternal abdomen over the fetal chest to hear the fetal heart sounds. Called also fetal or monoaural stethoscope.

pineal 1. shaped like a pine cone. 2. pertaining to the pineal body. *P. body, p. gland* a small conical structure attached by a stalk to the posterior wall of the third ventricle of the cerebrum, believed to be an endocrine gland.

pinna the projecting part of the ear lying outside the head.

Piriton See CHLORPHENAMINE (CHLORPHENIRAMINE) MALEATE.

Pitressin See VASOPRESSIN.

pituitary gland an endocrine gland lying in the pituitary fossa of the sphenoid bone. It has an anterior and a posterior lobe. The anterior lobe produces GONADOTROPHIC hormones, GROWTH HORMONE, lactogenic hormone (prolactin), ADRENOCORTICOTROPHIC HORMONE and thyrotrophic hormone. The posterior lobe secretes OXYTOCIN and antidiuretic hormone.

place of safety order court order whereby a child is arbitrarily removed from the care of its parents in the interests of the child's safety.

placebo a substance given to a patient as medicine or a procedure performed on a patient that has no intrinsic therapeutic value and relieves symptoms or helps the patient in some way only because the patient believes or expects that it will. Placebos are used in controlled clinical trials of new drugs. While some patients selected at random are given the new drug, others are given a placebo. Neither the patients nor those administering it know who is receiving the real drug, but the

Manual Removal of the Placenta

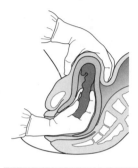

effects are closely monitored on all patients.

placenta the afterbirth. A flat organ measuring 17.5–20 cm in diameter and 2.5 cm in thickness tapering to 1.2 cm at the periphery. It weighs approximately one-sixth of the baby's birth weight at full term. The placenta is developed from the trophoblastic layers with a lining of mesoderm in which the blood vessels develop. It is formed by the 12th week of pregnancy, and is composed of large numbers of chorionic villi grouped together in cotyledons, and embedded in the decidua basalis of the uterus. The villi contain the fetal blood vessels (which ultimately join together to form the umbilical vessels), whilst they are separated by intervillous spaces through which the maternal blood circulates. The branches of the umbilical vessels can be seen on the fetal surface, radiating from the insertion of the cord which is usually placed centrally. This surface

is covered by the amnion, which can be stripped from it up to the insertion of the cord. The chorion is continuous with the edge of the placenta.

Functions of the placenta

Glycogen storage
Respiration
Excretion
Endocrine
Nutrition
Partial barrier

Abruptio placentae premature separation of a normally situated placenta. *Battledore p.* one in which the cord is attached to its margin and not the centre. *Bipartite p.* one having 2 lobes. *P. accreta* one abnormally adherent to the myometrium, with partial or complete absence of the decidua basalis. *P. circumvallata* one encircled with a dense, raised, white nodular ring, the attached membranes being doubled back over the edge of the placenta. *P. fenestrata* one having a gap or 'window' in its structure. *P. membranacea* one that is abnormally thin and spread over an unusually large area of the uterus. May occur as a PLACENTA PRAEVIA. *P. percreta* an abnormal insertion in which the chorionic villi have invaded the perimetrium; hysterectomy is usually required to control haemorrhage. *Succenturiate p.* one that has a separate or accessory lobe joined to the main placenta by blood vessels. If it is retained when the placenta is expelled it could cause serious postpartum haemorrhage.

placenta praevia an abnormally situated placenta in the lower segment of the uterus, either completely or partially covering the internal os. This leads to unavoidable haemorrhage towards the end of pregnancy

Placenta with Succenturiate Lobe

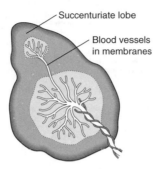

Succenturiate lobe

Blood vessels
in membranes

when the lower uterine segment stretches in preparation for labour. The bleeding is *painless* and often occurs when the mother is at rest; it recurs with increasing severity and requires hospital admission. The placenta occupies part or all of the lower uterine segment so that there will be a high presenting fetal part possibly with a malpresentation such as an oblique lie. Ultrasound scan will identify the exact position of the placenta. Occasionally a careful examination under anaesthetic is performed with all preparations having been made for immediate caesarean section in the event of tumultuous haemorrhage; usually the cautionary measure of an elective caesarean section will be performed where possible, unless the degree of placenta praevia is so minimal that controlled rupture of the membranes and induction of labour can be performed. Four grades are described; grade 1: the edge of the placenta encroaches into the lower uterine segment; grade 2: the whole placenta is in the lower segment; grade 3: the placenta reaches to the internal cervical os; grade 4: the entire placenta covers the central cervical os.

placental lactogen a hormone affecting growth and development of the breast in pregnancy. It also has a role in glucose metabolism in pregnancy. This hormone is similar to pituitary human GROWTH HORMONE, although it does not actually promote growth.

placentography radiological visualization of the placenta after injection of a contrast medium.

placentophagy the practice of consuming the placenta, usually in the belief that the large amount of hormones contained within it can assist in preventing postnatal depression.

plagiocephaly asymmetry of the head resulting from irregular closure of the sutures.

planned parenthood birth control.

plantar pertaining to the sole of the foot.

plasma a straw-coloured fluid which, with red and white blood cells, makes up the blood. Of the total volume of blood, 55% is made up of plasma. It is 92% water, in which are contained plasma proteins, inorganic salts, foods, gases, waste materials from the cells, and various hormones, secretions and enzymes. These substances are transported to or from the tissues of the body by the plasma. Plasma may be transfused to increase plasma proteins or in cases of shock.

plasmapheresis method of removing a portion of the plasma from the circulation. Venepuncture is performed, plasma is removed from the blood sample, and the red cells are returned to the circulation. Used in treatment of diseases caused by circulating antibodies in the plasma.

plasmin an enzyme, FIBRINOLYSIN, which dissolves the fibrin in a thrombus. It is present in blood as plasminogen before it is activated.

Plastibell a presterilized plastic device used for circumcision. The bell is slipped inside the foreskin and a string is tied around it. The foreskin becomes gangrenous and then drops off with the bell.

platelets thrombocytes. Blood platelets are disc-shaped, non-nucleated blood elements with a very fragile membrane; they tend to adhere to uneven or damaged surfaces. They are formed in the red bone marrow and average about 250×10^9 per litre of blood. The functions of platelets are related to coagulation and the clotting of blood. Because of their adhesion and aggregation capabilities platelets can occlude small breaks in blood vessels and prevent the escape of blood.

platypelloid flat. *See* PELVIS.

plethora an excess; in medicine, usually used to describe an excess of blood.

plethoric having the appearance of plethora, i.e. a florid colouring. Describes the condition usually seen in a baby with a large placental transfusion or in one of the twins with TWIN-TO-TWIN TRANSFUSION syndrome.

pleura the serous membrane lining the thorax and enveloping each lung, the 2 layers enclosing a potential space, the pleural cavity.

pleurisy inflammation of the pleura.

plexus a network of veins or nerves. *Brachial p.* the network of nerves of the neck and axilla. *Solar* or *coeliac p.* the network of nerves and ganglia at the back of the stomach, which supply the abdominal viscera.

pneumonia inflammation of the lung. It may be (*a*) *lobar p.* usually a pneumococcal infection of one or more lobes of the lung; (*b*) *bronchopneumonia* in which the bronchioles are affected. A number of bacteria may be responsible, including *Staphylococcus aureus*, streptococcus or *Haemophilis influenzae*; (*c*) *viral p.* the newborn child is predisposed to pneumonia by the RESPIRATORY DISTRESS SYNDROME.

pneumonitis inflammation of the lungs.

pneumothorax accumulation of air or gas in the pleural cavity, resulting in collapse of the lung on the affected side. The condition may occur spontaneously, as in the course of a pulmonary disease, or it may follow trauma to, and perforation of, the chest wall. It may be a complication of vigorous resuscitation, ventilation, CONTINUOUS INFLATING PRESSURE or follow MECONIUM ASPIRATION. pl. *pneumothoraces*.

Po₂ partial pressure of oxygen. In the blood of an adult it is about 100 mmHg, and of a baby rather lower, about 60–90 mmHg. In a preterm infant there is a danger of RETROLENTAL FIBROPLASIA if it exceeds 100 mmHg. *See also* Appendix 16.

podalic version the internal correction of a transverse lie by grasping a foot, thus converting it to a longitudinal lie and breech presentation.

polarity the gradient of the strength of uterine contractions between the fundus (the upper pole where the activity is the strongest) and the lower uterine segment and cervix (the lower pole where contractions are very weak or absent), which brings about dilatation of the cervix.

pole one extremity or end of an organ of the body, e.g. the uterus, or of the fetus.

policy a course or plan of action, in health care, a written plan of action for specific situations, either clinical or managerial.

poliomyelitis infantile paralysis. Inflammation of the anterior cells of the spinal cord. A virus infection which is a notifiable disease. It affects chiefly young people and can cause such injury to the grey matter that paralysis results. It can be prevented by vaccination.

poly- prefix meaning 'much' or 'many'.

polycystic containing numerous cysts. *P. kidneys* a congenital malformation in which the kidneys are enlarged because they contain many cysts. In mild cases the condition may remain undiagnosed, and a woman may have a normal pregnancy, although it predisposes her to urinary tract infection and hypertension. In other cases the baby's kidneys are enlarged at birth and survival is unlikely.

polycythaemia an excess of red blood cells. The newborn child is normally polycythaemic due to high levels of fetal haemoglobin.

polydactyly the existence of supernumerary fingers.

polygraph an apparatus for simultaneously recording several mechanical or electrical impulses, such as blood pressure, pulse, and respiration, and variations in electrical resistance of the skin.

polyhydramnios sometimes used synonymously with HYDRAMNIOS. A demonstrable excess of amniotic fluid. It is associated with maternal diabetes, congenital abnormalities especially of the central nervous system, uniovular twins and a rare tumour of the placenta (CHORIOANGIOMA).

polymorphonuclear possessing multilobed nuclei like most of the white blood cells.

polyneuritis multiple neuritis.

polypus a small pedunculated tumour arising from any mucous surface. *Cervical p.* in the cervical canal. *Fibroid p.* occurs in the uterus and contains fibrous myomatous tissue. *Placental p.* consists of remains of the placenta. pl. *polypi.*

polysaccharide a complex type of carbohydrate, e.g. starch.

polyuria an excessive increase in the secretion of urine, due to diuretics or to diabetes. In the first few days of the puerperium, polyuria is normal due to the autolysis which occurs as a part of the process of INVOLUTION.

pons 1. that part of the metencephalon lying between the medulla oblongata and the midbrain, ventral to the cerebellum. 2. any slip of tissue connecting 2 parts of an organ.

popliteal relating to the posterior part of the knee which is described as the *p. fossa* or *p. space.*

pore a minute circular opening on a surface, such as of sweat glands.

port-wine stain naevus flammeus.

portal vein the large vein which carries nutritive material from the digestive tract to the liver. Formed from the gastric, splenic and superior mesenteric veins.

portfolio collection of competency evidence assembled by the practitioner to demonstrate professional development. May include marked assessments, evidence of reflective practice, certificates of attendance at conferences or study days.

position attitude or posture. *Dorsal p.* lying flat on the back. *Genupectoral* or *knee–chest p.* resting on the knees and chest with arms crossed above the head. More probably, resting on knees and elbows. It is the traditional position to help relieve pressure on a cord which has prolapsed. However, if the foot of the bed can be elevated, and the woman put into Sims' position, the same effect is achieved with more comfort and less indignity. *Left lateral p.* on the left side with right knee drawn up towards the chin. *Lithotomy p.* lying on the back with thighs raised and knees supported and held widely apart. *Prone p.* lying face down. *Recumbent p.* lying down. *Sims' p.* similar to *left lateral,* but almost on the face, and semiprone with the right knee and thigh drawn up and resting on the bed in front of the left one. *Trendelenburg p.* lying on the back on a tilted plane (usually an operating table at an angle of 30° to the floor), with the head lowermost and the shoulders supported.

position of the fetus the relation of a particular part of the fetus, the DENOMINATOR to a particular part of the mother's pelvis. In the vertex presentation the denominator is the occiput. Eight positions may be described. If the occiput is directed

towards the symphysis pubis, the position is direct occipitoanterior; if to the left or right iliopectineal eminence, it is left or right occipitoanterior; if to the mid-point of the left or right iliopectineal line, left or right occipitolateral; if to the left or right sacroiliac joint, left or right occipitoposterior; and if towards the sacrum, direct occipitoposterior. In practice it has been found that the head commonly lies transversely with the occiput lateral, and thus a left occipitolateral and a right occipitolateral position are described. The breech positions are similar, but with the sacrum as the denominator. *See* Appendix 4.

positive end-expiratory pressure (PEEP) in mechanical ventilation, a positive airway pressure maintained until the end of expiration.

posseting regurgitation of a small amount of milk immediately after a feed.

post- prefix meaning 'after', e.g. postnatal clinic.

postcoital contraceptive oral contraceptive pills, used as an emergency measure, to be taken within 72 hours of unprotected sexual intercourse (Schering PC4). Inserting an intrauterine contraceptive device to prevent the embedding of a fertilized ovum may be used as an alternative method of postcoital contraception, up to 5 days after unprotected intercourse.

posterior placed at the back.

posthumous occurring after death. *P. birth* one occurring after the death of the father, or by caesarean section after the death of the mother.

postmaturity a state in which the pregnancy is prolonged after the expected date of delivery. Owing to the many variables it is difficult to estimate, but may exist when a pregnancy has lasted 41–42 weeks from the last menstrual period. There is a danger of hypoxia to the fetus once placental degeneration commences.

post mortem after death. *P. m. examination* autopsy.

postnatal after childbirth. *P. examination* physical and psychological examination of the mother undertaken frequently during the first 10 days of the puerperium to ensure that INVOLUTION is taking place, lactation is becoming established and the mother is adapting emotionally and psychologically to motherhood; also refers to the medical/midwifery examination at the end of the 6 week puerperium to ensure that her body has returned to the non-pregnant state without complications. *P. exercises* exercises which may be taught by the midwife or physiotherapist and which the mother should be strongly encouraged to practise several times daily during the puerperium and regularly for the rest of her life. They focus especially on strengthening the pelvic floor and abdominal muscles, but also include deep breathing and leg exercises in an attempt to prevent some of the complications of childbearing.

postnatal period a period not less than 10 and not more than 28 days after the end of labour, during which the continued attendance of a midwife on the mother and baby is mandatory. This is a rule of the Nursing and Midwifery Council.

postpartum after labour. *P. haemorrhage (PPH)* excessive bleeding from the genital tract at any time from the birth of the baby up to 6 weeks after delivery. *Primary PPH* occurs within the first 24 hours and usually refers to blood loss of more than 500 ml or any amount which is detrimental to the health of the mother; *secondary PPH*

occurs after the first 24 hours. *See* Appendix 6. *P. shock* collapse due to circulatory failure, occurring after delivery, which may be haemorrhagic or non-haemorrhagic. The main causes are ante- or postpartum haemorrhage, uterine inversion or rupture, acid aspiration syndrome, pulmonary or amniotic fluid embolism, hypotension or endotoxic shock as a result of septicaemia. Hypotension and tachycardia occur, the skin is cold, clammy and white and the mother suffers air hunger. The mother must be resuscitated urgently by maintaining an airway, administration of intravenous fluids to increase the blood volume, which is measured by the use of a central venous pressure line, administration of oxygen, a sedative and, in the cases of endotoxic shock, appropriate antibiotics.

post-traumatic stress disorder condition in which there is an immediate or delayed reaction to a seriously stressful event, commonly rape, drowning or disasters such as aeroplane accidents or natural disasters. May also occur following a highly stressful and traumatic birth experience such as the immediate need for a caesarean section or a forceful forceps delivery, or in some cases, where the mother feels she has suffered abuse as a result of the childbirth experience. Manifests as acute anxiety, insomnia, nightmares, 'flashbacks' and depression, loss of concentration, apathy, guilt and difficulties with sexual relationships. Support and counselling are needed. Where possible, all mothers should be debriefed after delivery, preferably by the midwife or doctor who conducted it.

posture the general attitude of body and limbs.

potassium a metallic element. Symbol K. Forms one of the electrolytes of the blood and tissue fluids and plays an essential role in maintenance of the acid–base and water balance in the body. A proper balance between sodium, calcium and potassium in the blood plasma is necessary for proper cardiac function.

potential existing as a possibility but not in fact. *P. diabetic* a person with normal glucose tolerance but with an increased risk of developing clinical DIABETES, e.g. a woman who has one or both parents as diabetics, or who has given birth to a live or stillborn baby weighing 4.5 kg (10 lb) or more at birth.

Potter's syndrome a congenital condition consisting of renal agenesis and pulmonary hypoplasia. The baby has low-set ears and furrows under the eyes (Potter's facies), and it is commonly associated with only 2 vessels in the umbilical cord. Absence of the kidneys is a rare and fatal condition.

pouch a pocket-like space or cavity. *P. of Douglas* the lowest fold of the peritoneum between the uterus and rectum. *Uterovesical p.* the fold of peritoneum between the uterus and bladder.

Poupart's ligament inguinal ligament. The tendinous lower border of the external oblique muscle of the abdominal wall, which passes from the anterior superior spine of the os ilium to the os pubis.

practitioner a person who practises a profession.

prandial pertaining to a meal.

pre- prefix meaning 'before', e.g. prenatal, premature.

precipitate 1. to cause settling in solid particles of a substance in solution. 2. a deposit of solid particles settled out of a solution. 3. occurring with undue rapidity, as *precipitate labour*. There is a danger to the mother of

severe perineal lacerations, and to the child of intracranial trauma as a result of the rapid passage through the birth canal.

preconception prior to conception. *P. care* health education and medical examination before conception in order that any problems can be detected and where possible treated, thus promoting optimum health at the time of conception and during the period of organogenesis in the first trimester of pregnancy. It is hoped that such care will reduce the incidence of congenital malformations and improve the mother's health and that of the fetus. Foresight is one of the organizations for the promotion of preconception care in the UK. Medical screening includes a detailed personal, medical, family and reproductive history, plus a lifestyle history such as diet, smoking, alcohol and drug intake and occupational hazards. A full medical examination including a gynaecological examination and cervical smear is performed. Investigations include full urinalysis and blood tests for rubella antibodies, haemoglobin, and haemoglobinopathies, syphilis and HIV antibodies. Hair and domestic water analysis may be carried out to test for toxic metals and semen analysis and stool tests for infestation may also be undertaken. Referral to an appropriate physician or for genetic counselling may follow.

precursor something that precedes. In biological processes, a substance from which another, usually more active or mature substance is formed. In clinical medicine, a sign or symptom that heralds another.

pre-diabetes a state which precedes diabetes mellitus, in which the disease is not yet clinically manifested.

In pregnancy the diabetes may become evident, or the woman may remain well but give birth to an unusually large child.

predisposition a latent susceptibility to disease which may be activated under certain conditions.

prednisone, prednisolone synthetic preparations with the same action as hormones from the adrenal cortex. These glucocorticoid drugs are used as anti-inflammatory and anti-allergic agents.

pre-eclampsia the precursor of ECLAMPSIA. Now commonly termed pregnancy-induced hypertension. A syndrome with three physical signs which occurs only in pregnancy, usually during the second half. The cause of the arteriolar spasm is still unknown, but it produces the following signs: (a) an elevated blood pressure – over 130/80 mmHg is often taken as the significant level, but a rise of 15–20 mmHg above the individual's previous diastolic level is more comprehensive; (b) generalized oedema; and (c) proteinuria; this is the most serious sign. The diagnosis is usually made when two out of the three signs are present. The disease resolves within 48–72 hours of delivery. In cases where the disease develops before term, unless very severe, the treatment is conservative, allowing the pregnancy to mature as near to 38 weeks as possible, thereby avoiding the risks associated with an immature baby.

Pregaday proprietary iron, preparation, specifically for the prevention and treatment of iron deficiency and megaloblastic anaemia in pregnancy.

pregnancy the condition of having a developing embryo or fetus within the body; the state from conception to delivery of the fetus. The normal duration is 280 days (40 weeks or 9 months and 7 days) counted from the first day of the last normal menstrual period. The interval from conception to birth – more nearly accurate but less easy to ascertain – averages 265 days. *Ectopic p.* extrauterine pregnancy. This occurs relatively frequently in the fallopian tube and very rarely in the ovary or the abdominal cavity. adj. *pregnant.*

pregnancy-induced hypertension asymptomatic rise in blood pressure during pregnancy which occurs in 5–20% of women, typically primigravidae, those with a multiple pregnancy, diabetes mellitus or essential hypertension. It is most common in the third trimester, but may develop into PRE-ECLAMPSIA if accompanied by oedema and proteinuria. Dangers include placental abruption, renal and cardiac failure, cerebral haemorrhage, placental insufficiency and intrauterine growth retardation.

pregnancy tests these detect the HUMAN CHORIONIC GONADOTROPHIN (HCG) produced by the embryo 8 days after the first missed period. Immunological laboratory tests, e.g. Gravindex or Pregnosticon, now give 98% accuracy.

pregnanediol a derivative of pregnane, formed by reduction of progesterone and found especially in urine of pregnant women.

pregnant with child; gravid; having a developing embryo or fetus within the uterus.

premature early.

premedication drugs given prior to a general anaesthetic, e.g. atropine, hyoscine or papaveretum. Opiates, however, are not used before caesarean section to avoid respiratory depression of the baby.

premenstrual preceding menstruation. *P. syndrome* condition affecting many women in the 7–10 days prior to menstruation as a result of fluctuating hormone levels, and characterized by a variety of symptoms such as irritability, aggression, anxiety, mood changes, headache, breast tenderness and oedema, cravings, particularly for sweet or salty foods, lack of coordination or concentration. The condition subsides once menstruation commences.

premonition a forewarning. *See* AURA.

prenatal occurring before birth.

preoperative preceding an operation.

prepuce foreskin; a loose fold of skin covering the glans penis.

pre-registration midwifery education education and training of women and men wishing to practise as midwives. In the UK they may undertake a 3 year diploma or degree course; those who are qualified nurses undertake a shortened programme of 18 months. Students undertaking the long course are supernumerary to NHS staffing establishments and receive a bursary.

prescription a formula written by a physician, directing the pharmacist to prepare a drug, or mixture of drugs. NHS prescriptions are free for expectant mothers and mothers who have a child under 12 months old.

presentation that part of the fetus which first enters the pelvis, occupying the lower pole of the uterus. Normally cephalic with the vertex presenting, sometimes the breech, and occasionally the face, brow or shoulder.

presenting part that part of the fetus which lies lowest in the birth canal; the first part felt on examination *per vaginam*. In a normal vertex presentation this is the occiput.

pressor tending to increase blood pressure.

pressure stress or strain, by compression, expansion, pull, thrust or shear.

Arterial p. the blood pressure in the arteries. Also *see* BLOOD PRESSURE.

preterm before term, i.e. before the 37th completed week of pregnancy. *P. infant* baby born before 37 weeks' gestation. The baby will be of low birth weight, but may also be SMALL FOR GESTATIONAL AGE. Gestational age is assessed using the DUBOWITZ SCORE. Preterm infants are prone to RESPIRATORY DISTRESS SYNDROME, feeding problems due to immature sucking, swallowing and coughing reflexes, hypothermia, jaundice and infection. There is also the risk of a poor maternal–infant relationship due to the baby's prolonged admission to the neonatal intensive care unit. *P. labour* labour which occurs before 37 weeks' gestation. It may occur spontaneously as a result of changing hormone levels, an overstretched uterus or weak cervix or due to infection; the obstetrician may attempt to arrest labour by the administration of tocolytic drugs such as ritodrine hydrochloride, until conditions are more favourable for the baby to be born. Occasionally, due to maternal illness or the poor condition of the fetus, labour is induced before term when it is considered that the health of the mother or baby would be better served by discontinuing the pregnancy. A very controlled delivery of the baby either by an experienced midwife or by the doctor, using obstetric forceps, is required to protect the delicate fetal head.

prevalence the total number of cases of a specific disease in existence in a given population at a certain time.

preventive serving to avert the occurrence of; prophylactic.

pre-viable before viability. A pre-viable infant is one born alive before the 24th week of pregnancy.

Price precipitation reaction (PPR) a serological test for syphilis.

primary first in order of time or importance. *P. postpartum haemorrhage see* POSTPARTUM HAEMORRHAGE.

primary care group (PCG) grouping of general practitioners and their services within a defined geographical area agreed with the health authority. Encompasses a community of approximately 100 000 people. Direct means for GPs, community nurses and other professionals to secure appropriate high quality care for local people. Responsible for commissioning services, promoting good health and combating health inequalities.

primary care trust (PCT) responsible for planning, securing local services, improving health of the local community and local integration of health and social care. There are 303 PCTs for England which receive 75% of the NHS budget.

primary health care medical, midwifery and nursing care provided in the community.

primary health care team the people who provide primary health care in the community. The team is made up of general practitioner, community midwife, community nurse and health visitor. It may also include a social worker. They may be based in a health centre or a general practice area.

primigravida a woman pregnant for the first time.

primipara a woman who has given birth to a viable child, whether alive or stillborn.

primiparous having borne one child.

probability (*P*) a statistical term meaning the likelihood of an association between variables being due to chance.

probe a blunt, malleable instrument for exploring sinus tracks, wounds, cavities or passages.

procaine a local anaesthetic; the hydrochloride salt is used in solution for infiltration.

procaine benzyl penicillin intramuscular antibiotic, commonly used in the treatment of syphilis and gonorrhoea.

process 1. a prominence or projection, as from a bone. 2. a series of operations or events leading to achievement of a specific result. *Midwifery or nursing p.* a systematic, problem-solving approach to the task of meeting the needs and healthcare problems of clients.

prochlorperazine a major tranquillizer and antiemetic, sometimes administered in labour with pethidine.

procidentia complete prolapse of the uterus so that the cervix protrudes through the vulva.

procreation the act of begetting young.

proctalgia pain in the rectum.

proctitis inflammation of the anus or rectum.

proctoscope an instrument for examination of the rectum.

prodromal preceding. Warning of approaching disease, e.g. visual disturbances occurring before ECLAMPSIA.

profession 1. an avowed, public declaration or statement of intention or purpose. 2. a calling or vocation requiring specialized knowledge, methods and skills, as well as preparation, in an institution of higher learning, in the scholarly, scientific and historical principles underlying such methods and skills. Members of a profession are committed to continuing study, to enlarging their body of knowledge, place service above personal gain, and are committed to providing practical services vital to human and social welfare. A profession functions autonomously and is committed to high standards of achievement and conduct.

professional profile a resumé of an individual practitioner's personal professional training programmes, courses subsequently attended and other relevant experiences, including learning acquired through reflection on and in practice. This is a mandatory requirement of the Nursing and Midwifery Council for all midwives, nurses and health visitors; supervisors of midwives or an officer from the NMC can request to examine the profile to ensure it is being maintained.

profibrinolysin plasminogen, the precursor of fibrinolysin.

profile 1. a simple outline, as of the side view of the head or face; by extension, a graph representing quantitatively a set of characteristics determined by tests. A record of achievements developed during a course of study or subsequently. 2. *See* PROFESSIONAL PROFILE.

progeny issue. Descendants.

progesterone the female sex hormone essential to normal life and to maintaining pregnancy. It is produced from the corpus luteum and also the placenta. During the menstrual cycle it is responsible for the secretory changes in the endometrium in preparation for the reception of a fertilized ovum, a slight rise in body temperature at the time of ovulation and premenstrual retention of water and electrolytes. In pregnancy it promotes the formation and maintenance of the decidua, the development of the glandular tissue of the breasts, the relaxation of plain muscle throughout the body and the retention of water and electrolytes in the body tissues.

progesterone-only contraceptive oral pills, taken daily with no pill-free interval, and prescribed when combined contraceptive pills, containing

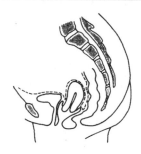

Uterovaginal Prolapse

oestrogen as well as progesterone, are contraindicated, e.g. during breastfeeding. There is a higher failure rate than with the combined pill; should be taken within the same 3-hour time limit every day.

progestogen any substance having progestational activity.

prognosis a forecast of the course and duration of a disease.

projectile vomiting *See* VOMITING.

prolactin a hormone from the anterior lobe of the pituitary gland that stimulates and sustains milk production in postpartum women.

prolapse the descent of an organ or structure. *P. of the umbilical cord* this is when, following rupture of the membranes, the cord lies in front of the presenting part. The fetus is in great danger of HYPOXIA or ANOXIA when the cord is compressed. Immediate delivery must follow the diagnosis. *P. of rectum* protrusion of the rectal mucosa and, occasionally, of the muscle, through the anal canal to the exterior. *P. of an arm* the fetal arm falls into or through the vagina. A serious complication of uncorrected shoulder presentation. *P. of the uterus* the uterus protrudes into the lower part of the vagina, as a result of the weakening of its supports. Prolapse, unqualified, refers to the descent of one or more of the pelvic structures due to weakness of the pelvic floor. The uterus, vaginal walls, bladder or rectum may be involved.

proliferation rapid multiplication of cells, as may occur in a malignant growth.

prolonged labour labour lasting more than 24 hours. This may be due to inadequate or incoordinate uterine action, cephalopelvic disproportion or a poorly fitting presenting part as in the case of malpresentation or malposition. The midwife is responsible for ensuring that the mother receives adequate pain relief and is as comfortable as possible, that progress is being made, albeit slowly, and that the conditions of mother and fetus are satisfactory. Risks to the fetus include hypoxia and trauma, especially excessive moulding of the fetal skull resulting in intracranial haemorrhage; for the mother there are risks of exhaustion and dehydration, uterine rupture, and physical trauma leading to long-term uterine, cervical or urinary tract problems.

prolonged pregnancy pregnancy lasting 42 weeks (294 days) or more from the first day of the last normal menstrual period. Many obstetricians do not, however, induce labour unless the condition of the mother or fetus warrant it. Daily investigations to monitor their conditions are undertaken.

promazine hydrochloride a tranquilizer; a phenothiazine derivative. Often given with pethidine in labour to combat nausea and vomiting, in doses of 25–50 mg intramuscularly.

promethazine hydrochloride (Phenergan) an antihistamine drug, often allied with pethidine in labour. Also used in the treatment of vomiting in pregnancy; a phenothiazine derivative.

promontory a projection. The *sacral p.* is an important landmark of the pelvis formed by the projection of the upper border of the first sacral vertebra.

pronation turning downwards. *P. of the hand* the palm is downward.

prone lying face downward.

pronucleus the haploid nucleus of a sex cell.

prophylactic pertaining to prophylaxis.

prophylaxis measures taken to prevent a disease; preventive treatment.

propranolol a β-adrenergic blocking agent used in the treatment of hypertension and some cardiac conditions.

propylthiouracil a thyroid inhibitor used in the treatment of thyrotoxicosis.

prostacyclin potent vasodilator and inhibitor of platelet aggregation. An intermediate in the metabolic pathway of arachidonic acid, formed from prostaglandin endoperoxides in the walls of arteries and veins.

prostaglandins a group of substances, first discovered in semen, now known to be present in menstrual blood, amniotic fluid and many other cells. They have an oxytocic effect, so are used to induce abortion before 10 weeks and to ripen the cervix and induce labour. A proprietary preparation of prostaglandin E_2 may be used for this purpose.

prostate a gland in the male which surrounds the neck of the bladder and the prostatic urethra. It contributes a secretion to the seminal fluid.

prosthesis the replacement of an absent part by an artificial substitute;

an artificial substitute for a missing part. adj. **prosthetic.**

Prostin E *See* PROSTAGLANDINS.

protamine sulphate an antidote to heparin overdosage.

protease proteolytic enzyme in the digestive juices which causes protein breakdown.

protein a material composed of carbon, hydrogen, nitrogen and oxygen. It is the essential constituent of body tissue. Animal sources are meat, fish, milk and eggs; vegetable sources are peas, beans and lentils. During digestion, proteins are broken down into 20 varieties of amino acid. Of these, 8 are essential including PHENYLALANINE and TYROSINE. These are then built up into new cells and used to repair others. Excess amino acids cannot be stored, but are broken down by the liver and excreted in the urine as urea. The proteins in blood plasma are divided into 4 major classes: specific protein carriers, that are involved in the transport of hormones and other substances; acute phase reactants, such as alpha$_1$-antitrypsin or fibrinogen, that are involved in inflammation or in clotting; complement components; and immunoglobulins. Albumin plays an important role in the maintenance of normal distribution of water by exerting osmotic pressure at the capillary membrane. This pressure prevents fluid of the plasma from leaking out of the capillaries and into the space between the tissue cells.

proteinuria any protein, usually albumin, found in the urine.

Proteus a Gram-negative bacteria usually found in faecal and other putrefying matter.

prothrombin a plasma protein synthesized in the liver. It is vital for the blood clotting mechanism as, in the presence of calcium, it forms thrombin when activated by thromboplastin released when tissues are damaged and platelets broken down. The thrombin, with fibrinogen, then forms insoluble fibrin. *P. time* the time, in seconds, required for a specimen of blood brought into contact with thromboplastin, to clot.

prothrombinase thromboplastin.

protocol an agreement between parties; in health care, a multidisciplinary planned course of suggested action in relation to specific situations.

proton a positively charged particle forming part of the nucleus of an atom.

protoplasm the essential chemical compound of which living cells are made.

provider self-governing trusts, directly managed units and private institutions which provide health care services for those wishing to purchase them. *See also* PURCHASER.

proximal in anatomy, nearest that point which is considered to be the centre of a system; the opposite of distal.

pruritus great irritation of the skin. It may affect the whole surface of the body, as in certain skin diseases and nervous disorders, or it may be limited in area. *P. vulvae* in pregnancy may be associated with glycosuria or with candidal (*Monilia*) VAGINITIS.

pseudo- prefix meaning 'false'.

pseudocyesis a false pregnancy. Subjective manifestation of the symptoms of pregnancy, in the absence of conception.

pseudohermaphroditism apparently having male and female characteristics. More precisely defined as INTERSEX.

pseudomenstruation a blood-stained vaginal discharge which may occur on about the third day of life in baby girls due to withdrawal of maternal oestrogens.

Pseudomonas a Gram-negative, aerobic bacteria, some species of which are pathogenic for plants and vertebrates.

psoas a muscle forming part of the posterior abdominal wall.

psoriasis chronic recurrent skin disease characterized by reddish marginated patches with profuse silvery scaling on extensor surfaces such as knees or elbows, but can be more widespread. Non-infectious. Cause unknown. Tends to occur in families.

psyche the mind, both conscious and unconscious.

psychiatrist a doctor who specializes in psychiatry.

psychiatry study of mental disorders and their treatment.

psychologist one who studies normal and abnormal mental processes, development and behaviour.

psychology the science of the mind and its functions.

psychomotor pertaining to motor effects of cerebral or psychic activity.

psychopath a person with an antisocial personality.

psychoprophylaxis a method of preparation for labour aimed at preventing pain and modifying the perception of painful sensations associated with normal uncomplicated childbirth. Preparation includes education about the process of labour and breathing patterns linked with disassociation and muscular control. This method usually requires intensive practice during the antenatal period.

psychosexual relating to the mental aspects of sexual activity.

psychosis a severe mental illness affecting the whole personality. Of organic or emotional origin. It is marked by derangement of the personality and loss of contact with reality, often with delusions, hallucinations, or illusions. adj. *psychotic*.

psychosomatic relating to the mind and the body. *P. disorders* those illnesses in which emotional factors have a profound influence.

psychotherapy any of a number of related techniques for treating mental illness by psychological methods. These techniques are similar in that they all rely mainly on establishing communication between the therapist and the patient as a means of understanding and modifying the patient's behaviour.

ptosis drooping of the upper eyelid from 3rd nerve paralysis. Dropping downwards of an organ or other structure.

ptyalin the ENZYME in saliva which starts digestion of starches.

ptyalism abnormally increased salivation. A rare complication of pregnancy.

puberty the age at which the reproductive organs become functionally active. Generally between the 10th and 14th years.

pubes the region over the pubic bones.

pubic pertaining to the pubes, e.g. *p. arch*, the bony arch formed by the junction of the *inferior pubic rami*, forming the anterior part of the pelvic outlet.

pubiotomy cutting through the pubic bone to enable birth to take place.

pubis the anterior portion of the hip bone; called also pubic bone.

public health the field of medicine that is concerned with safeguarding and improving the physical, mental and social well-being of the community as a whole. Environmental aspects are the responsibility of the district local authority, whereas communicable disease control is supervised by the Medical Officer for Environmental Health, from the District Health Authority. Central government formulates national policy and is responsible for international aspects.

pubococcygeus one part of the levator ani muscle extending from the symphysis pubis to the coccyx.

pubovesical pertaining to the pubis and bladder.

pudenda the external genitalia.

pudendal pertaining to the external genital organs. *P. block* a form of local analgesia induced by injecting a solution of 0.5 or 1% lidocaine (lignocaine) around the pudendal nerve.

pudendum external genitalia of a woman.

puerperal pertaining to the puerperium. *P. pyrexia* a rise of temperature in the puerperium. *P. psychosis* any psychosis appearing in the puerperium. *P. sepsis* infection of the genital tract following childbirth.

puerperium the period following childbirth during which the maternal uterus and other organs and structures are returning to the non-pregnant state. A period of 6–8 weeks.

pulmonary pertaining to or affecting the lungs. *P. circulation see* CIRCULATION. *P. embolism see* EMBOLISM. *P. haemorrhage* neonatal death can sometimes be caused by massive haemorrhage into both lungs. *P. infarction* is due to the occlusion of a small blood vessel in the lung by a clot, which causes death of the tissue supplied by that vessel. *P. tuberculosis see* TUBERCULOSIS.

pulsation a beating or throbbing.

pulse the local rhythmic expansion of an artery, which can be felt with the finger, corresponding to each contraction of the left ventricle of the heart. It may be felt in any artery sufficiently

near the surface of the body. The normal adult rate is about 72 per minute. In childhood it is more rapid, varying from 130 in infants to 80 in older children. *P. pressure* the difference between the diastolic and systolic blood pressures, as measured by the sphygmomanometer.

puncture to pierce. *Lumbar p.* to remove cerebrospinal fluid by puncture between the 3rd and 4th, or 4th and 5th lumbar vertebrae to relieve cerebral pressure, or to obtain cerebrospinal fluid for diagnostic purposes.

pupil the opening in the centre of the iris through which light enters the eye.

purchaser health authorities purchase healthcare services from PROVIDERS for the local population. They are responsible for identifying the total health needs of their resident population, planning how to meet these needs and then securing the best and most cost-effective services within the area.

purgative a drug which produces evacuation of the bowels.

purine heterocyclic compound that is the nucleus of the purine bases such as adenine and guanine, which occur in DNA and RNA.

purpura haemorrhagica a condition characterized by extravasation of blood in the skin and mucous membranes, causing purple spots and patches. It is sometimes associated with a deficiency of THROMBOCYTES (THROMBOCYTOPENIA).

purulent containing or resembling pus.

pus a thick, semi-liquid substance consisting of dead leucocytes and bacteria, debris of cells and tissue fluids. It results from inflammation caused by invading bacteria which have destroyed the phagocytes and set up local suppuration.

pustule a small, elevated, circumscribed, pus-containing lesion of the skin.

putative supposed, reputed. *P. father* the man believed to be the father of an illegitimate child.

pyaemia a condition resulting from invasion of the blood stream by bacteria. Blockage of small blood vessels occurs with resultant formation of abscesses, the development of which causes rigors and high fever.

pyelitis literally inflammation of the renal pelvis. Usually called PYELONEPHRITIS.

pyelography radiology of the renal pelvis after the injection of radio-opaque contrast medium. *Intravenous p.* (IVP) a water-soluble, iodine-containing contrast medium is injected intravenously and radiographs are exposed as the contrast medium is excreted by the kidneys, and passes down the ureters into the bladder.

pyelonephritis inflammation of the kidneys and ureters, usually caused by ESCHERICHIA COLI. The acute symptoms are severe lumbar pain, hyperpyrexia, often rigors, tachycardia, vomiting and general malaise; the chronic symptoms are backache, vomiting and anaemia, though this type is often symptomless. Either form may occur during pregnancy, usually between 18 and 24 weeks, owing to stasis of urine in the ureters, which have dilated and relaxed under the influence of progesterone, and of pressure from the pregnant uterus particularly on the right side. Multiplication of bacteria can then take place; asymptomatic bacteriuria often occurs at the start of pregnancy. All women should be screened for bacteriuria early in pregnancy and

treated at once if necessary. This urinary tract infection is not uncommon in newborn infants. There are no obvious signs but the condition may be suspected in any infant who is pale, not feeding well, losing weight and generally not thriving.

pyelonephrosis any disease of the kidney and its pelvis.

pyloric stenosis congenital hypertrophic pyloric stenosis occurs in 3 per 1000 births. In the affected baby the pyloric sphincter becomes thickened, strong and spastic. The stomach enlarges and becomes more powerful from forcing the gastric contents through the narrowed pylorus. Waves of peristalsis can be seen abdominally during feeding and the pylorus can be felt as a tumour. Persistent projectile vomiting occurs. These signs rarely occur before 3–4 weeks of age. An anti-spasmodic drug (e.g. atropine) may be given with feeds but RAMSTEDT'S OPERATION is often necessary for rapid and complete recovery.

pylorus the opening between the stomach and the duodenum.

pyo- prefix meaning 'pus'.

pyogenic producing pus.

pyometra the condition in which pus is present in the uterus.

pyosalpinx pus in the fallopian tube.

pyretic pertaining to fever.

pyrexia fever; a rise of body temperature above 37.2°C (99°F).

pyridoxine one of the forms of vitamin B$_6$, chiefly used in the prophylaxis and treatment of vitamin B$_6$ deficiency.

pyrogen a fever-producing substance, possibly of bacterial origin.

pyuria the presence of pus in the urine. The urine is generally cloudy and pus cells will be seen if the urine is examined microscopically.

Q

QRS complex a group of waves depicted on an electrocardiogram, consisting of 3 distinct waves created by the passage of cardiac electrical impulses through the ventricles; occurs at the beginning of each contraction of the ventricles. Normally the R wave is the most prominent of the three.

quadrant 1. one fourth of the circumference of a circle. 2. one of 4 corresponding parts, or quarters, as of the surface of the abdomen or of the field of vision.

quadruplets four children born at the same labour. Formerly very rare; more common since the use of fertility drugs.

qualitative research a systematic subjective approach to research used to describe life experiences and give them meaning, it may be conducted to describe and promote understanding of human experiences such as pain, caring, powerlessness and comfort.

quality assurance in the healthcare field, a pledge to the public by those within the various health disciplines such as midwifery that they will work towards the goal of an optimal achievable degree of excellence in the services rendered to every client. A quality assurance programme takes into account the need to define that which is to be measured. The development of criteria based on acceptable standards of care and norms of professional behaviour are formulated. The criteria are then used as the 'yardstick' against which actual practice and its results can be evaluated. Evaluation is conducted by a review committee. The ultimate goal is improvement of client care.

Quality Assurance agency organization which approves higher education institutions offering courses and awards. Monitors delivery of subjects in universities. Has established codes of practice and guidance for programme development, and a contract with the Department of Health to carry out subject review in England.

quantitative research a formal objective systematic approach to research in which numerical data are utilized to obtain information. It is used to describe variables, examine relationships among variables and to determine cause and effect interactions between variables. Some researchers believe this form of research provides a sounder knowledge base to nursing and midwifery practice than QUALITATIVE RESEARCH.

quarantine the period during which known infected persons, contacts and suspects are isolated to prevent the spread of infection.

'quickening' the first perceptible fetal movements, felt by the mother at approximately the 18th to 20th week in a nulliparous woman and recognized at the 16th to 18th week in the multigravida.

quintuplets five children born at the same labour.

quotient a number obtained by division. *Intelligence q. (IQ)* a numerical expression of intellectual capacity obtained by multiplying the mental age of the subject concerned, ascertained by testing, by 100 and dividing by his/her chronological age.

R

racemose grape-like. *R. cells* those arranged round a central duct. *R. glands* are compound and lobulated in structure, e.g. salivary glands, cells of the breasts, glands of the cervix.

rachi(o)- word element meaning 'spine'.

rachitic pelvis a flat pelvic brim similar to that of the platypelloid pelvis. This deformity of the pelvic brim is caused by rickets in early childhood.

radial relating to the radius. *R. artery* the artery at the wrist. *R. palsy* a palsy characterized by wrist drop; it can be seen soon after birth. It usually recovers spontaneously over a varying time.

radical dealing with the root or cause of a disease. *R. cure* one which cures by complete removal of the cause.

radioactive emitting electromagnetic waves, alpha (α), beta (β) or gamma (γ). A radioactive substance may do this naturally, as does radium, or the effect may be produced artificially by bombardment in an atomic pile, e.g. radioactive iodine (^{131}I).

radiograph a picture taken by X-rays.

radiographer a professional healthcare worker in a diagnostic X-ray department (diagnostic radiographer) or in a radiotherapy department (therapy radiographer).

radiography examination by means of Röntgen or X-rays. This may yield valuable information in pregnancy and labour.

radioimmunoassay (RIA) a sensitive assay method that can be used for the measurement of minute quantities of specific antibodies or any antigen such as a hormone or drug, against which specific antibodies can be raised. It is a standard method for clinical laboratory measurements of hormones and is also used for therapeutic drug monitoring, drug abuse screening, and other laboratory tests.

radioisotope a radioactive form of an element. A radioisotope consists of unstable atoms that undergo radioactive decay emitting alpha, beta or gamma radiation. Radioisotopes occur naturally, as in the cases of radium and uranium, or may be created artificially.

radio-opaque capable of obstructing the passage of X-rays.

radiotelemetry measurement based on data transmitted by radio waves from the subject to the recording apparatus. Continuous fetal heart monitoring may be carried out by radiotelemetry when the mother is ambulant in labour.

radiotherapy the treatment of disease by ionizing radiation such as X-rays, beta rays and gamma rays; it is mainly used in malignant disease. The source of radiation may be outside the body of the patient or it may be an isotope that has been implanted or instilled into abnormal tissue or a body cavity.

radium a metallic element. Symbol Ra. A metal which is naturally RADIOACTIVE.

Ramstedt's operation division of a hypertrophied pyloric sphincter to relieve PYLORIC STENOSIS.

ramus a branch, as of the pubic bone which has an upper and lower branch. pl. *rami*.

random blood sugar test blood glucose test undertaken when an expectant mother presents with unexplained glycosuria. If the random blood sugar test result is suspicious a glucose load or glucose tolerance test may be performed.

randomized controlled trial a research trial in which subjects to be studied are chosen at random from a suitable group of potential participants; it usually involves a control group and an experimental group. The purpose of random sampling is to increase the extent to which the sample is representative of the target population, although it is rarely possible to obtain a purely random sample for clinical studies because of informed consent requirements.

ranitidine an H_2 receptor antagonist which may be given to women in labour prior to general anaesthesia in order to inhibit the production of hydrochloric acid, thereby reducing the risk of Mendelson's syndrome.

rape sexual assault or abuse; criminal forcible sexual intercourse.

raphe a seam or ridge of tissue indicating the juncture of two equal parts, e.g. the median raphe of the perineal body, the anococcygeal raphe.

rash a temporary eruption on the skin. *Heat r.* miliaria. *Napkin r.* a cutaneous reaction in an infant, localized in areas ordinarily covered by the napkin. It is due to various primary irritants, such as ammonia in decomposed urine; improperly washed nappies and other contact factors may also be responsible. *Nettle r.* urticaria.

raspberry leaf tea a herbal preparation which many women like to take during pregnancy to tone the uterus and prepare the reproductive organs for labour. Raspberry leaf facilitates cervical ripening and enhances contraction efficiency; it may also help to relieve contraction pain. The mother should only take raspberry leaf tea (or tablets) in the third trimester, gradually increasing from 1 cup (or tablet) daily to three by term. The tea can be sipped during labour, and may help involution in the puerperium.

raspberry mark congenital haemangioma.

Rastelli's operation surgical procedure used in the treatment of transposition of the great vessels. The circulation of blood through the heart is diverted to effect adequate oxygenation.

rate the speed or frequency with which an event or circumstance occurs per unit of time, population, or other standard of comparison. *Basal metabolic r. (BMR)* an expression of the rate at which oxygen is utilized in a fasting subject at complete rest as a percentage of a value established as normal for such a subject. *Birth r.* the number of live births in a population in a specified period of time (crude birth rate), for the female population (refined birth rate), or for the female population of childbearing age (true birth rate), usually expressed per year per 1000 of the estimated mid-year population. *Death r.* the number of deaths per stated number of persons (1000 or 10 000, or 100 000) in a certain region in a certain time (crude death rate). The death rate calculated with allowances made for age and sex distribution in the population is termed the standardized death rate. Called also mortality rate. *Glomerular filtration r.* an expression of the quantity of glomerular filtrate formed each minute in the nephrons of both kidneys, calculated by measuring the clearance of specific substances, e.g. insulin or creatinine.

ratio an expression of the quantity of one substance or entity in relation to that of another; the relationship between 2 quantities expressed as the quotient of one divided by the other. *Lecithin–sphingomyelin r.* the ratio of lecithin to sphingomyelin in amniotic fluid.

reabsorption the act or process of absorbing again, as in the absorption by the kidneys of substances (glucose, proteins, sodium, etc.) already secreted into the renal tubules.

reaction counteraction; a response to the application of a stimulus. Evidence of acidity or alkalinity. The pH of a solution.

reagent a substance employed to produce a chemical reaction so as to detect, measure, produce, etc., other substances.

real-time scanner an ULTRASOUND scanner which gives a moving visual display.

receptor 1. a molecule on the surface or within a cell that recognizes and binds with specific molecules, producing some effect in the cell; e.g. the cell-surface receptors of immunocompetent cells that recognize antigens, complement components, or lymphokines, or those of neurons and target organs that recognize neurotransmitters or hormones. 2. a sensory nerve ending that responds to various stimuli.

recession receding or drawing back. *Rib r.* or *sternal r.* is commonly seen in the RESPIRATORY DISTRESS SYNDROME of neonates.

recessive tending to recede. In genetics the opposite of dominant – capable of expression only when borne

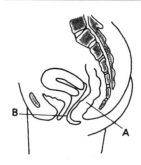

Rectocele

A, Rectum; B, posterior vaginal wall.

by both sides of a set of homologous chromosomes, i.e. HOMOZYGOUS and not HETEROZYGOUS.

recipient one who receives, as a blood transfusion, or a tissue or organ graft. *Universal r.* a person thought to be able to receive blood of any 'type' without agglutination of the donor cells.

recombinant 1. a new cell or individual that results from genetic recombination. 2. pertaining or relating to such cells or individuals. *R. DNA technology* the process of taking a gene from one organism and inserting it into the DNA of another; called also gene splicing.

rectal relating to the rectum. *R. examination* digital examination of the rectum or adjacent structures, e.g. during labour, of the cervix uteri and presenting part.

rectocele hernia of the rectum, caused by overstretching of the vaginal wall at childbirth. Treated by posterior colporrhaphy.

rectovaginal pertaining to rectum and vagina. *R. fistula see* FISTULA.

rectovesical pertaining to or communicating with the rectum and bladder.

rectum the lower 15 cm (6 in) of the large intestine extending from the pelvic colon to the anal canal.

recumbent lying down.

recurrent occurring again.

reduction the correction of a fracture, dislocation or hernia.

referred pain that which occurs at a distance from the place of origin, and which is related to the distribution of sensory nerves.

reflection in midwifery, a process of conscious, systematic thinking about one's actions; review, analysis and synthesis of situations that have occurred, usually after an event. Active process by which the practitioner learns from experience, with a view to improving future practice.

reflex reflected or thrown back. *R. action* an involuntary movement resulting from a stimulus, e.g. the knee jerk, or the withdrawal of a limb from a pinprick. Certain reflexes are present in the mature newborn child, e.g. the sucking, swallowing and MORO REFLEXES. *Conditioned r.* one that is not natural but acquired by regular association of a physiological event with an unrelated outside event, e.g. the draught, milk ejection or milk flow reflex that causes the myoepithelial cells in the breast to contract at the sight or sound of the hungry baby, so mobilizing the milk into the lacteal sinuses where it is immediately available to the baby.

reflex zone therapy a system of complementary therapy, similar to reflexology, in which it is believed the body is divided into ten longitudinal and three transverse zones, with corresponding divisions in the feet. Reflex zone therapy can be used to identify areas of disorder or disease in the body and a sophisticated grip technique is used to massage the feet and so treat the problem. The therapy can also be performed on the hands, which correspond closely to the feet, the tongue, the face and the back.

reflexology a system of complementary therapy in which the feet represent a map of the rest of the body, so that by working on the feet, using a sophisticated massage technique, other areas of the body can be influenced and treated. It is particularly beneficial for stress-related conditions such as hypertension, and for mechanical problems such as constipation. In midwifery it has successfully been used to treat urinary retention, and to stimulate the pituitary gland as in labour or for lactation.

register an epidemiological term meaning an index on file of all cases with a particular disease or condition in a defined population.

registered midwife a midwife registered to practise in the country in which s/he resides. A midwife's name may be on the Register of Midwives but s/he must also be eligible to practise by complying with the mandatory requirements of the Midwives' Rules. *See* Appendix 15.

registrar of births, marriages and deaths the official recorder of births, marriages and deaths. In England and Wales, the office comes under the Office for National Statistics, which also regulates and records civil marriages, conducts demographic research and analyses demographic material. Local registry offices are available in most towns. Births should be registered within 6 weeks in England (21 days in Scotland).

regulatory bodies organizations responsible for defining and monitoring preparation and practice of a specific professional group, e.g. Nursing and Midwifery Council, General Medical Council, Health Professions Council.

regurgitation backward flow, e.g. of food from the mouth from the stomach. Sometimes occurs in newborn babies, when it is associated with weakness of the cardia of the stomach. *Aortic r.* backward flow of blood into the left ventricle when the aortic valve is incompetent. *Mitral r. see* MITRAL. *Gastro-oesophageal r. see* HEARTBURN.

rehabilitation re-education.

Reiter's protein complement fixation (RPCF) a serological test used to aid the diagnosis of syphilis.

relapse the return of a disease, following an apparent recovery.

relaxant causing relaxation; an agent that causes relaxation. *Muscle r.* an agent that either acts at the neuromuscular junction, causing muscle paralysis, and used in anaesthesia, or relieves muscle spasticity and tension by acting on muscle itself, or more commonly on the central nervous system.

relaxation a lessening of tension, as may be observed when muscles slacken after they have contracted. It is important that the mother in labour should rest and relax her muscles between the contractions of labour. Classes may be given to the pregnant woman to prepare her for this. *See also* PSYCHOPROPHYLAXIS.

relaxin a hormone which is thought to cause general 'softening' of the pelvic tissues and joints in the preg-nant woman, thereby providing some increase in pelvic capacity. A cause of lumbar lordosis.

releasing factor a substance produced in the hypothalamus which causes the anterior pituitary gland to release hormones.

reliability a research technique concerned with the degree of consistency, dependability, accuracy and comparability of a test or investigation.

renal concerning or affecting the kidney. *R. calculus* stone in the kidney. *R. disease in pregnancy* a rare but serious problem. There may be a history of nephritis in childhood, and proteinuria is present from early pregnancy. Prolonged hospital admission may be necessary, to reduce the risks of miscarriage, pre-eclampsia, placental abruption and further renal impairment. The fetus is at risk of intrauterine growth retardation and death *in utero*. Women already undergoing dialysis do not have a good prognosis for a successful outcome to their pregnancies, although those who have had a renal transplant have a better prognosis of achieving a live healthy baby. *R. failure* failure of the renal function, which gives rise to uraemia. *R. threshold* the level of substances in the blood beyond which they are excreted in the urine. Normally the renal threshold for glucose is 10 mmol/l (180 mg/100 ml) and if the blood sugar rises above this level glycosuria results.

renin an enzyme synthesized, stored and secreted by the kidneys; it plays a role in regulation of blood pressure by catalysing the conversion of angiotensinogen to angiotensin I. This, in turn, is converted to angiotensin II which is a powerful vasoconstrictor and also stimulates aldosterone secretion. Aldosterone results in retention of salt and water by the kidneys.

rennin the milk-curdling enzyme found in gastric juice of human infants. Rennin catalyses the conversion of casein from a soluble to insoluble form.

reproduction 1. the process by which a living entity or organism produces a new individual of the same kind. 2. the creation of a similar object or situation; duplication; replication.

reproductive organs, female the ovaries, which produce the ova, or eggs; the uterine tubes; the uterus; the vagina, or birth canal; and the vulva, comprising the external genitalia. The breasts are the secondary sexual characteristics, enclosing the mammary glands. *R. o., male* the external genitalia (the penis, testes and scrotum), accessory glands that secrete special fluids, and the ducts through which these organs and glands are connected to each other and through which the spermatozoa are ejaculated during coitus.

Rescue Remedy one of the Bach Flower remedies, based on homoeopathic principles, and available from health food stores in liquid form, which is particularly effective in reducing stress, panic, anxiety and hysteria. Useful for women who have a fear of needles for venepuncture and injections, for the transition stage of labour and at any other time when the mother is especially anxious or nervous, e.g. before surgical intervention. Four drops of the remedy are given neat on the tongue or can be added to a small glass of water or applied to the temples or wrists; it is preserved in brandy so some women may object to the (minimal) alcohol content.

research an attempt to increase available knowledge by the discovery of new information through systematic scientific enquiry.

resection removal of a part.

residential care (for children) care provided by the local authority social services department, or voluntary organizations registered with the social services department for children up to the age of 18 years. Residential nurseries are provided for the under 5-year-olds, and community homes and hostels for children in care up to the age of 18 years. Boarding out with foster parents is arranged whenever possible.

residual remaining. *R. urine* urine remaining in the bladder after micturition.

resistance the power to overcome. The natural power of the body to withstand and recover from infection or disease. The ability of bacteria to become insensitive to antibiotics, e.g. some staphylococci are resistant to penicillin.

respiration breathing; the exchange of oxygen and carbon dioxide between the atmosphere and the body cells, including inspiration and expiration, diffusion of oxygen from the pulmonary alveoli to the blood and of carbon dioxide from the blood to the alveoli, and the transport of oxygen to and carbon dioxide from the body cells. *Inspiration* is accomplished by contraction of the external intercostal muscles (which raise the ribs and sternum), and of the diaphragm which descends. In *expiration* the internal intercostal muscles contract, the ribs return to their normal position and the diaphragm relaxes. The normal rate of respiration varies. In neonates it is about 40–50 per minute at rest, and in adults 16. *Artificial r.* the production of respiratory movements by other than natural means.

respiratory distress syndrome (RDS)
a condition occurring mainly in preterm babies due to lack of SUR-FACTANT. It also affects mature babies of diabetic mothers and those born by caesarean section. The onset of respiratory difficulty occurs within 4 hours of birth and the condition gradually worsens.

restitution restoration, putting right. A corrective movement of the fetal head after it is born in the antero-posterior diameter, to right it in relation to the shoulders.

resuscitation restoration from a state of collapse. *Neonatal r.* may be necessary if the baby fails to breathe after birth. In order for respiration to be established the lungs must normally be developed, the respiratory centre functioning adequately and the air passages clear. Preterm infants may be difficult to resuscitate without mechanical ventilation as there is immaturity of the lungs, respiratory centre and respiratory muscles. Medullary depression which causes neonatal asphyxia and the need for resuscitation may be due to maternal drugs used in labour which depress the respiratory centre of the fetus; this can be reversed by the administration of an antagonist; hypoxia from fetal distress; intracranial damage during delivery, particularly as a result of excessive or abnormal moulding. For management *see* Appendix 7.

retained placenta a placenta which fails to be evacuated from the vagina after the normal length of time has elapsed following delivery of the baby. The placenta may be morbidly adherent to the decidua due to placenta accreta, increta or percreta, in which case a manual removal under anaesthetic, or occasionally hysterectomy, is required. More commonly

the placenta is partially separated with resulting haemorrhage from the decidual sinuses, so that the mother should be treated for shock and haemorrhage. This is often due to poor uterine action following birth of the baby so that the uterus fails to contract sufficiently to cause placental separation. Manual stimulation per abdomen or the administration of oxytocic drugs should encourage the uterus to contract more effectively so that the placenta separates and can be delivered. If separation does not occur, MANUAL REMOVAL of the placenta and membranes under general anaesthetic will be necessary. *See also* POSTPARTUM HAEMORRHAGE, Appendix 6.

retardation delay; hindrance; delayed development. *Mental r.* subnormal general intellectual development, associated with impairment either of learning and social adjustment or of maturation, or of both.

retching an involuntary, spasmodic, but ineffectual effort to vomit.

retention holding back. *R. of urine* inability to pass urine from the bladder, which may rarely be due to obstruction or, more commonly in obstetrics, of nervous origin. During labour, as the fetus occupies a large part of the pelvis, there is considerable stretching of the urethra and trigone, which disturbs micturition. In the puerperium both these areas take time to recover. There may be diminished sensation in the bladder and perineal discomfort, coupled with anxiety and lack of privacy, and retention of urine may occur. The woman should be encouraged to empty her bladder within a very few hours of delivery, using various measures. Catheterization should be avoided if possible, as chronic urinary tract infection can occur as a result, leading to renal failure in severe cases.

reticular resembling a net.

reticuloendothelial system a network of tissues and cells found throughout the body, especially in the blood, general connective tissue, spleen, liver, lungs, bone marrow and lymph nodes. The very large reticuloendothelial cells are concerned with blood cell formation and destruction, storage of fatty materials, and metabolism of iron and pigment, and they play a role in inflammation and immunity. Some of the cells are motile, that is, capable of spontaneous motion and phagocytic, i.e. they can ingest and destroy unwanted foreign material. The reticuloendothelial cells of the spleen possess the ability to dispose of disintegrated erythrocytes. The reticuloendothelial cells located in the blood cavities of the liver are called Kupffer cells. These cells together with the cells of the general connective tissue and bone marrow, are capable of transforming into bile pigment the haemoglobin released by disintegrated erythrocytes.

retina the inner lining of the eyeball formed of nerve cells and fibres, and from which the optic nerve leaves the eyeball and passes to the visual area of the cerebral cortex. The impression of the image is focused upon it.

retinopathy a general term denoting pathological conditions of the retina; they may occur in conjunction with certain systemic disorders, such as hypertension, severe pre-eclampsia or eclampsia, and diabetes. *R. of prematurity* is caused by vasoconstriction of retinal capillaries due to the presence of very high concentrations of oxygen in these blood vessels. This produces the development of an overgrowth of blood vessels in the retina. The vascular proliferation and exudation of blood and serum detaches the retina, and produces scarring and inevitable blindness. Careful monitoring of the newborn and of oxygen tension level is essential because no totally safe dosage of oxygen that will prevent the retinal changes has been found.

retraction drawing back. The process of permanent and progressive shortening of the muscle of the uterus which accompanies contractions during labour (*a*) to dilate the cervix, (*b*) to expel the fetus and (*c*) to separate the placenta and to control bleeding. Over-retraction of the uterus in obstructed labour may cause a *r. ring* to become apparent. *See* BANDL'S RING.

retractor a surgical instrument for drawing apart the edges of a wound to make the deeper structures more accessible.

retro- prefix meaning, 'behind' or 'backward', e.g. retroversion of the uterus.

retroflexion a bend backwards; applied to the uterus when the corpus is bent backwards at an acute angle, the cervix being in its normal position.

retrograde going backwards. *R. pyelography* X-ray of the kidneys and ureters following the injection of a radio-opaque substance into the renal pelvis via the urethra.

retrolental behind the crystalline lens. *R. fibroplasia* see RETINOPATHY OF PREMATURITY.

retroplacental behind the placenta *R. clot* clot of blood behind the placenta.

retrospection morbid dwelling on memories. Looking back.

retroversion a turning back; applied to the uterus when the whole organ is tilted backwards. cf. RETROFLEXION.

Retroversion of Uterus

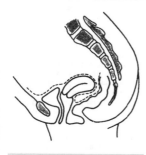

retroverted gravid uterus a pregnant uterus that is tilted backwards. This is a common occurrence, and the uterus almost always becomes spontaneously corrected to an anteverted position. Occasionally the retroversion persists, and a state of INCARCERATION of the retroverted gravid uterus develops, with retention of urine.

retrovirus a large group of RNA viruses, including human T-cell leukaemia viruses, lentiviruses, and the causative virus of AIDS, HIV (human immunodeficiency virus).

Rhesus factor an antigen, the presence or absence of which determines the Rhesus type of human blood as positive or negative. There are three pairs of Rhesus antigens Cc, Dd and Ee. The D antigen is responsible for Rhesus immunity in the majority of cases. A capital letter indicates that the person is Rhesus positive to the factors C, D or E, and a small letter indicates that a person is Rhesus negative to factors c, d or e. About 83% of Caucasians are Rhesus positive and 99–100% of other races.

rheumatism a term used to describe muscular and joint pains, often called fibrositis. *Acute r.* rheumatic fever. An acute fever associated with streptococcal infection and related to chorea and acute tonsillitis. It causes acute rheumatic ENDOCARDITIS, myocarditis and pericarditis and, as sequelae, MITRAL STENOSIS and aortic incompetence may occur. When mild they can be asymptomatic until pregnancy increases the load on the heart. Any pregnant woman who has had rheumatic fever when a child must have careful assessment of her cardiac condition.

rhinitis inflammation of the mucous membrane of the nose. *Staphylococcal r.* sometimes occurs in the newborn child.

rhomboid of Michaelis a diamond-shaped area at the base of the spine marked by dimpling of the skin. Beneath its superior angle is the spinous process of the 5th lumbar vertebra, and under the lateral angles the posterior superior iliac spines are palpable. Inferiorly is the beginning of the gluteal cleft.

rhythm a measured movement; the recurrence of an action or function at regular intervals. adj. *rhythmic, rhythmical. R. method of family planning* the natural methods of family planning which include calculating the so-called 'safe' period during which the woman is least likely to conceive, taking the temperature daily and observing the mucoid discharge from the vagina, i.e. the Billings' method.

rib any one of the paired bones, 12 on either side, extending from the thoracic vertebrae toward the median line on the ventral aspect of the trunk, forming the major part of the thoracic skeleton. Called also costal.

riboflavin vitamin B₂, necessary for certain enzymes that catalyse many oxidation–reduction reactions. Found in liver, kidney, heart, brewer's yeast, milk, eggs, greens and enriched cereals.

ribonucleic acid (RNA) the nucleic acid of a cell which translates the 'code' of DEOXYRIBONUCLEIC ACID (DNA) into action.

ribosome a minute granule seen with an electron microscope in the cytoplasm of a cell. Ribosomes are concerned with protein synthesis.

rickets rachitis. A disease of deficient calcification of bone. It results from lack of vitamin D, necessary for the proper absorption of calcium and phosphorus. It leads to characteristic bony deformity of skull, ribs, legs and pelvis. It is preventable, by the administration of vitamin D and by exposure to sunlight or ultraviolet light, and is nowadays uncommon.

rigor a sudden shivering attack in which the temperature usually rises rapidly, remains high for a short time and, following a phase of sweating, declines. It may occur in severe pyelonephritis in pregnancy, of in puerperal SEPTICAEMIA. *R. mortis* the stiffening of the body, occurring soon after death owing to coagulation of the muscle protoplasm.

risk management use of a structured approach to care to reduce identifiable risks before problems arise in order to protect the interests and increase the satisfaction of patients and clients and reduce the number of complaints and consequent costs of litigation. Agreed standards of care based upon current research findings are written into clinical guidelines; regular systematic reviews of clinical notes are undertaken to assess for completeness; case discussion for a

are initiated and case conferences are held in the event of any adverse outcomes to treatment; and continuous training programmes are developed. Health and safety risks are also considered.

ritodrine hydrochloride a β₂-adrenergic receptor stimulant used to decrease uterine activity and prolong gestation in the management of preterm labour. (Yutopar)

Ritter's disease exfoliative dermatitis. A rare and severe form of PEMPHIGUS NEONATORUM.

rockerbottomfeet a feature of certain chromosomal disorders such as Edwards' syndrome (trisomy 18) and Patau's syndrome (trisomy 13) when the infant has prominent heels.

Rogitine phentolamine, an adrenolytic used to test for the presence of phaechromocytoma.

role a pattern of behaviour developed in response to the demands or expectations of others; the pattern of responses to the persons with whom an individual interacts in a particular situation.

Röntgen rays X-RAYS.

rooming-in the baby remains by the mother's bedside when she is in hospital, rather than being cared for in a nursery. This enables the mother to get to know her baby and strengthens the bond between them as she learns to handle and care for him.

rooting reflex a reflex which can be elicited in the newborn by stroking the cheek or side of the mouth and in response the baby will turn to the side stimulated and open his mouth ready to suckle.

rotation the turning of a body on its long axis. In midwifery, the turning of the fetal head (or presenting part) for proper orientation to the pelvic axis. It should occur naturally, but if it does not it must be accomplished manually or instrumentally by the obstetrician.

rotator a muscle which causes rotation of any part.

rotavirus a virus which, under the microscope, looks like a wheel. It is considered one of the commonest causes of acute infantile diarrhoea. Respiratory signs often precede the diarrhoea and vomiting.

Rothera's test a test for the presence of acetone in urine.

roughage indigestible vegetable fibre. Cellulose. It gives bulk to the diet and stimulates peristalsis. Found in bran, cereals, fruit and vegetable fibres.

round ligaments extend from the cornua of the uterus to the labia majora.

Royal College of Midwives (RCM) founded in 1881 as the professional body concerned with the education and standards of professional practice of midwives. It is the only professional organization solely for midwives. The RCM is now concerned primarily with standards of professional practice, statutory and other post-basic education for midwives and negotiation of conditions of service and salaries. Headquarters: *see* Appendix 13.

Royal College of Nursing–Midwifery Society a division of the Royal College of Nursing devoted to the needs of its members who are midwives; often these midwives hold dual registration and continue to practise as nurses as a part of their work.

rubella German measles. A mild infective disease causing a faint macular rash on the body and enlargement of the posterior cervical lymph nodes. It is spread by droplets from an infected person 7 days before the rash appears but is of low infectivity. Rubella is uncommon in pregnancy,

but the virus crosses the placenta to the fetus and causes abortion, stillbirth or congenital rubella. The incidence of congenital malformations such as cardiac, ear and eye defects, varies according to the period of gestation at which the disease occurs. If in the first month the incidence is 50–60% with multiple defects, and this slowly falls until, in the case of infection in the 16th week, it is about 5%. From this time until the 31st week the fetus may suffer growth retardation and be born with thrombocytopenic purpura. Later in life it may be mentally retarded, physically retarded or deaf. The baby itself may be a source of infection for up to 2 years. When a woman is exposed to rubella during the first 4 months of pregnancy, serum should be taken to test for immunity to rubella. If this shows immunity and no infection, reassurance can be given to continue the pregnancy. The second serum should be taken 4 weeks later, if the first showed no immunity. Only if this shows evidence of infection should termination be considered. Rubella vaccination is given, in conjunction with immunization against mumps and measles (MMR) when an infant is approximately 1 year old. Rubella vaccination alone is repeated for all schoolgirls between the ages of 11 and 14 years.

Rubin test a test for patency of the uterine tubes, made by transuterine inflation with carbon dioxide gas. Called also tubal insufflation.

rugae ridges or creases, e.g. of the mucosa of the stomach, and the squamous epithelium of the vagina.

Rules for Midwives the compliance with the NMC Midwives Rules is the responsibility of any midwife practising in the United Kingdom whether employed within or without the National Health Service or self-employed. Failure to do so is likely to result in allegation of professional misconduct. *See* Appendix 15.

rupture 1. tearing or bursting of a part, as in rupture of an aneurysm, of the membranes during labour or of a tubal pregnancy. *R. of the uterus* may follow obstructed labour, or may occur during pregnancy or labour following previous caesarean section. In obstructed labour Bandl's retraction ring can be seen as a ridge running obliquely across the abdomen and marks the junction between the grossly thickened upper uterine segment and the danger-ously thinned and over-stretched lower segment. If there is a uterine scar from a previous caesarean section or hysterostomy, DEHISCENCE may occur insidiously towards term or uterine rupture may occur as a result of the powerful contractions during labour. Shock and blood loss must be treated before attempting to suture the rupture; occasionally hysterectomy may be required.

Ryle's tube a thin rubber tube with a weighted end, introduced via the nose into the stomach. It may be used for the withdrawal of gastric contents or for the administration of fluids.

S

Sabine vaccine an oral vaccine against poliomyelitis consisting of three types of live, attenuated polioviruses. It may be given in a capsule, on a lump of sugar, or by medicine dropper.

sac a pouch-like cavity.

saccharide one of a series of carbohydrates, including the sugars; they are divided into monosaccharides, disaccharides, trisaccharides, and polysaccharides according to the number of saccharide groups composing them.

sacculation of the uterus a rare complication of incarceration of the retroverted gravid uterus, in which the fundus remains under the sacral promontory and the anterior wall grows to accommodate the fetus.

sacral relating to the sacrum. *S. promontory* the upper anterior border of the body of the prominent first sacral vertebra.

sacro- concerning the sacrum. *Sacroanterior* and *sacroposterior* the positions that may be encountered in a breech presentation, the sacrum being the denominator.

sacrococcygeal concerning the sacrum and the coccyx. *S. joint* a slightly movable joint of the pelvis, between the sacrum and the coccyx.

sacrocotyloid concerning the sacrum and the acetabulum. *S. diameter* the measurement between the sacral promontory and the nearest point of the iliopectineal eminence on either side of the pelvis. It measures 9.5 cm (3.75 in).

sacroiliac concerning the sacrum and the ilium. *S. joint* or *s. synchondrosis* the slightly movable joint between the sacrum and the ilium.

sacrum a wedge-shaped bone composed of 5 united vertebrae, situated between the lowest lumbar vertebra and the coccyx. It forms the posterior wall of the pelvis.

Safe Motherhood Initiative a campaign initiated in 1987 by the World Health Organization to reduce maternal mortality and morbidity throughout the world by the implementation of simple, appropriate, cost-effective strategies to enable mothers to have access to high quality, affordable care during pregnancy and childbirth and associated events such as fetal loss. The campaign aims to improve the health, nutrition and general well-being of girls and women of reproductive age before conception and into parenthood, and to reduce the long-term sequelae of childbirth which often result in lifelong disabilities. *See* Appendix 13.

Saf-T-Coil an intrauterine contraceptive device.

sagittal arrow-shaped. *S. section* an anteroposterior midline section. *S. suture* the junction of the parietal bones. A *sagittal* or *third fontanelle* may be noted in the sagittal suture. This condition is sometimes, though not always, associated with DOWN'S SYNDROME.

salbutamol a beta-sympathomimetic drug used to try to suppress premature labour. Contraindicated in pre-eclampsia and antepartum haemorrhage.

salicylate any salt or ester of salicylic acid. Aspirin is a salicylate which is used for its analgesic, anti-pyretic and anti-inflammatory effect. The mechanism of most of the effects of aspirin and other salicylates is inhibition of prostaglandin synthesis, thus blocking pyretic and inflammatory processes that are mediated by prostaglandin.

saline containing a salt or salts. *Physiological s.* formerly called *normal s.* a solution of 0.9% sodium chloride. It is isotonic with blood and may be given intravenously as a temporary means of replacing fluid in shock and haemorrhage, but it is rapidly excreted.

saliva the secretion of the salivary glands, which is poured into the mouth when food is taken. It moistens and dissolves certain substances, and begins carbohydrate digestion by its enzyme ptyalin, the salivary amylase.

salivation the normal flow of saliva. When this is excessive it is referred to as PTYALISM.

Salk vaccine a preparation of killed polioviruses of three types given in a series of intramuscular injections to immunize against poliomyelitis.

Salmonella a genus of bacteria responsible for GASTROENTERITIS.

salpingectomy excision of one or both of the fallopian tubes.

salpingitis inflammation of a fallopian tube.

salpingogram radiological outline of the interior of the fallopian tubes, usually to determine whether they are patent or have some other disorder.

salpingography radiography of the fallopian tubes after intrauterine injection of a radio-opaque medium.

salpingo-oöphorectomy removal of a fallopian tube and ovary.

salpingotomy surgical incision of a uterine tube.

salpinx a tube, notably the fallopian tube.

salt 1. sodium chloride, common salt, used in solution as a cleansing agent or for infusion into the blood to replace fluid. 2. any compound of an acid with an alkali or base. *S. depletion* loss of salt from the body due to sweating, persistent vomiting or diarrhoea.

sample a selected group of a population.

sanguineous pertaining to or containing blood.

saphenous the name given to two superficial veins, the long and the short, which carry blood up the leg from the foot.

sarcoma a highly malignant tumour developed from connective tissue cells and their stroma. *Kaposi's s.* a multifocal, metastasizing, malignant reticulosis principally involving the skin, although visceral lesions may be present. It usually starts on the toes or feet as reddish-blue or brownish soft nodules and tumours. It is viral in origin and is frequently seen in AIDS.

saturated solution a liquid containing the largest amount of a solid which can be dissolved in it without forming a precipitate.

scalp the layer of tissue covering the cranial bones.

scan an image produced using a moving detector or a sweeping beam of radiation, as in scintiscanning, B-mode ULTRASONOGRAPHY, scanography, or COMPUTED TOMOGRAPHY.

scanner scintiscanner; called also computed tomography (CT) scanner.

scapula the large flat triangular bone forming the shoulder blade.

Schilling test test used to confirm diagnosis of pernicious anaemia by estimating absorption of ingested radioactive vitamin B_{12}.

schizophrenia a psychosis of unknown cause, but showing hereditary links. The person feels him/herself influenced by external forces and suffers delusions and hallucinations. Pregnancy tends to aggravate the condition.

school health service the provision of medical and dental inspection and treatment in schools maintained by local education authorities.

Schultze expulsion of the placenta at the end of the third stage of labour the placenta is expelled inverted, the fetal surface appearing first at the vulva. This is commoner than the MATTHEWS DUNCAN EXPULSION; there is less associated bleeding and the placenta was probably lying at a higher level in the uterus.

sciatic relating to the sciatic nerve which runs down the back of the thigh.

sciatica severe pain in the back of the leg, running along the course of the sciatic nerve. In pregnancy this can be very debilitating and is due to undue pressure of the heavy uterus on the nearby nerves and ligaments. Bedrest may be necessary; transcutaneous electrical nerve stimulation or acupuncture may relieve the problem. It should resolve following delivery.

sclera the tough, white outer coat of the eyeball, covering approximately the posterior five-sixths of its surface, continuous anteriorly with the cornea and posteriorly with the external sheath of the optic nerve. adj. *scleral*.

sclerema an uncommon disease sometimes seen in newborn babies. It is characterized by hardening of the skin and subcutaneous fat and occurs in HYPOTHERMIA.

sclerosis the hardening of any part from an overgrowth of fibrous and connective tissue, often due to chronic inflammation.

scoliosis abnormal curvature of the spine, most commonly applied to a lateral deviation. *See also* LORDOSIS *and* KYPHOSIS.

scopolamine HYOSCINE.

screening 1. examination of a large number of individuals to disclose certain characteristics, or an unrecognized disease, as phenylketonuria or hypothyroidism in the neonate. 2. fluoroscopy.

Scriver test a biological test used for diagnosing a whole range of inborn errors of metabolism, including phenylketonuria. If the phenylalanine level is found to be above 725 µmol/l treatment for phenylketonuria is necessary.

scrotum the pouch of skin and soft tissues containing the testicles.

scurvy a disease due to a deficiency in vitamin C. It is characterized by weakness, anaemia, haemorrhage from mucous membranes, purpuric rash, swelling and pain in joints, and ulceration in the mouth. It rapidly improves with a proper diet containing adequate vitamin C.

sebaceous fatty or pertaining to the sebum. *S. glands* are found in the skin, communicating with the hair follicles and secreting sebum.

sebum the fatty secretion of the sebaceous glands.

second degree perineal lacerations *See* PERINEAL LACERATIONS.

second stage of labour the stage of expulsion, lasting from full dilatation of the cervix uteri to complete birth of the child.

secondary second in order of time or importance. *S. postpartum haemorrhage* haemorrhage from the genital tract which occurs after the first

24 hours following delivery and up to 6 weeks after the birth of the baby; classified as any amount of excessive bleeding which adversely affects the health of the mother. The usual causes are retained products of conception and/or sepsis. Evacuation of the retained products, intravenous or oral oxytocics and antibiotics are the normal treatments. *See also* POSTPARTUM HAEMORRHAGE.

secretin a hormone secreted by the mucosa of the duodenum and jejunum when acid chyme enters the intestine; carried by the blood, it stimulates the secretion of pancreatic juice and, to a lesser extent, bile and intestinal secretion.

secretion a substance produced by a gland.

sedative a drug which allays excitement and calms a patient, often helping her to sleep, but not relieving pain.

sedimentation formation of sediment. *S. rate, see* ERYTHROCYTE SEDIMENTATION RATE.

segment a section or part. *Upper uterine s.* the upper three-quarters of the uterus, the part which contracts and retracts during labour. *Lower uterine s.* including the cervix, the lowermost quarter of the uterus, which becomes stretched and dilated in the first stage of labour.

segmentation the division of the fertilized ovum into 2 cells, then 4, 8, 16, etc., as it traverses the fallopian tube.

seizure a convulsion or attack of epilepsy.

self-actualization a level of psychological development in which innate potential is realized to the full.

self-governing trust hospitals or other establishments or facilities which assume responsibility for their own ownership and management by 'opting out' of direct NHS control. Trust status is approved by the

Secretary of State and each trust has a Board of executive and non-executive directors and a Chairman who is approved by the Secretary of State.

Sellick's manoeuvre the application of backward pressure on the cricoid cartilage in the throat in order to occlude the oesophagus and prevent regurgitation of stomach contents into the pharynx with consequent risk of aspiration into the lungs. The pressure is not released until an endotracheal tube has been inserted and the respiratory tract sealed off.

semen the male secretion of seminal fluid from the prostate gland, and spermatozoa from the testis, produced following ejaculation.

semi-permeable property of a membrane, permitting the passage of some molecules and hindering that of others.

semi-prone position in which the person is lying face down with knees turned to one side.

senna a laxative derived from the cassia plant. A standardized proprietary preparation, Senokot, can be used in pregnancy, but may be too purgative for some women.

sense a faculty by which the conditions or properties of things are perceived, e.g. hunger, thirst and pain; a sense of equilibrium or well-being and other senses are also distinguished. The five major senses comprise vision, hearing, smell, taste and touch.

sensitive reacting to a stimulus.

sensitization 1. the initial exposure of an individual to a specific antigen, resulting in an immune response. 2. the coating of cells with antibody as a preparatory step in eliciting an immune reaction. 3. the preparation of a tissue or organ by one hormone so that it will respond functionally to the action of another.

sensitized rendered sensitive.

sensory pertaining to sensation. *S. nerve* a peripheral nerve that conducts impulses from a sense organ to the spinal cord or brain; called also afferent nerve.

sepsis infection of the body by pathogenic bacteria. *Puerperal s.* that occurring in the genital tract during the PUERPERIUM.

septic relating to sepsis.

septicaemia the presence and multiplication in the blood of pathogenic bacteria. The signs are a rapid rise of temperature, which is later intermittent, rigors, sweating, and all signs of acute fever. Puerperal sepsis occasionally takes the form of septicaemia. *See also* ENDOTOXIC SHOCK.

septum a division or partition, e.g. that between the right and left ventricles of the heart. One form of congenital heart malformation is characterized by a defect in the interventricular septum.

septuplet one of seven offspring produced at one birth.

sequela a morbid condition following a disease and resulting from it. pl. *sequelae.*

serology the study of antigen–antibody reactions *in vitro.* adj. *serological.*

serotonin amine present in blood platelets, intestine and central nervous system, acts as a vasoconstrictor. Derived from the amino acid tryptophan and inactivated by monoamine oxidase.

serrated with saw-like edge, e.g. the bones of fetal skull.

serum clear straw-coloured fluid which is left after blood has clotted. The clear residue of blood, from which the corpuscles and fibrin have been removed. Serum from the blood of a convalescent patient (or animal) may be used to protect another person, from the same disease, e.g. in diphtheria or tetanus.

service provider clinical institutions which provide placement experiences for student midwives and nurses, staff to support students and evidence of good practice from clinical audit.

sex 1. the fundamental distinction, found in most species of animals and plants, based on the type of gametes produced by the individual or the category to which the individual fits on the basis of that criteria. Ova, or macrogametes, are produced by the female, and spermatozoa, or microgametes, are produced by the male. The union of these distinctive germ cells results in the production of a new individual in sexual reproduction. 2. to determine the sex of an organism.

sex-linked genes carried on the sex chromosome, usually the X or female chromosome.

sextuplet one of six offspring produced at the same birth.

sexual intercourse the process of coitus. *S. i. in pregnancy* libido in pregnancy may be either reduced or increased, depending on a variety of factors. Intercourse is not contraindicated although some couples may require information and suggestions about changing their positions or alternative means of sharing intimacy. *Resumption of s. i.* following delivery may be delayed due to perineal or vaginal trauma, although women should be advised that it is wise to attempt coitus within 6 weeks of delivery and before they attend for their postnatal examination, as occasionally, difficulties with penetration may highlight inadequate wound healing or other pathological problems resulting from the delivery.

sexually transmitted diseases (STD) an infectious disease that is usually transmitted by means of sexual intercourse, either by heterosexual or homosexual individuals, or by intimate contact with the genitals, mouth and rectum. STDs include syphilis, GONORRHOEA, HUMAN IMMUNO-DEFICIENCY VIRUS (HIV) infection, HERPES GENITALIS, NON-SPECIFIC URETHRITIS, TRICHOMONIASIS, PEDICULOSIS pubis, scabies, genital or venereal WARTS, HEPATITIS B infection and AIDS.

shaken baby syndrome presence of unexplained fractures in the long bones, together with evidence of subdural haematoma, in a baby, as a result of child abuse; caused by violent shaking which produces a whiplash effect, and rotational movement of the head, resulting in vomiting, convulsions, irritability, coma and death.

shared care antenatal care shared between a midwife and an obstetrician or a general practitioner.

sheath a tubular case or envelope. A sheath, also known as a condom, can be worn over the erect penis during intercourse to trap the seminal fluid, thereby reducing the incidence of pregnancy. The use of a spermicidal preparation with sheaths increases their reliability up to about 97%. Sheaths are advocated as a means of preventing transmission of sexually transmitted diseases and HUMAN IMMUNO-DEFICIENCY VIRUS (HIV) from one partner to another.

Sheehan's syndrome hypopituitarism. This uncommonly occurs following severe and prolonged shock after ABRUPTIO PLACENTAE and POSTPARTUM HAEMORRHAGE, where there is necrosis of the anterior pituitary, giving rise to AMENORRHOEA, genital atrophy and premature senility.

shiatsu a form of alternative medicine based on principles similar to acupuncture in which it is believed that the body has a series of energy lines called meridians running through it from top to toe. When the body, mind and spirit are in optimum health the energy along the meridians will be in equilibrium; when there is stress in the physical, emotional or spiritual body, shiatsu can be used to re-establish energy equilibrium. The system involves the use of pressure from the practitioner's fingers, hands, elbows, heels or feet applied to specific points on the body. It is a useful therapy for pregnant and childbearing women, particularly for conditions such as nausea and vomiting, pain in labour and for colic and fractiousness in babies.

shingles HERPES ZOSTER.

Shirodkar operation an operation to prevent abortion resulting from cervical incompetence. The internal os is closed by means of a nylon suture which is removed shortly before term, or earlier if labour should begin. Now commonly known as cervical cerclage.

shock collapse due to acute peripheral circulatory failure, resulting usually from severe trauma or haemorrhage. The main causes of shock are ante- or more commonly postpartum haemorrhage, uterine rupture or inversion, acid aspiration syndrome, pulmonary or amniotic fluid embolism, severe hypotension or endotoxic shock as a result of septicaemia. Hypotension and tachycardia occur, the central venous pressure fluctuates and the woman may appear cold, clammy, white and searching for air. Urgent resuscitation is required before the condition becomes irreversible. The airway must be maintained; oxygen should be administered if dyspnoea is present. Intravenous fluids to combat dehydration and plasma substitutes are given, the amount dependent on the central venous pressure reading. The foot of the bed can be raised if the baby has been delivered and the mother may be positioned on her left side to prevent inferior vena cava pressure. A sedative may be given; the mother should be kept as quiet as possible and overheating must be avoided. Endotoxic shock occurs when there is a serious infection by Gram-negative organisms, especially *Escherichia coli* and *Clostridium welchii*. There is widespread dilatation of the arterioles so that the venous return is diminished and shock occurs. The signs are similar to hypovolaemic shock but rigors may also occur. The infection must be treated urgently with the appropriate antibiotics.

shoulder dystocia a rare complication occurring after delivery of the fetal head, in which the shoulders fail to rotate, descend and deliver, usually as a result of a large baby or a contracted pelvic outlet. The midwife should turn the mother into the left lateral position or ask her to squat in an attempt to enlarge the outlet and then deliver the baby. Alternatively the McRobert's manoeuvre is performed, in which the woman lies on her back and assumes an exaggerated knee–chest position with the thighs abducted, in order to enlarge the pelvic outlet. External or internal rotation of the shoulders may be necessary; occasionally symphysiotomy is performed or in extreme cases the baby's shoulders are fractured in order to deliver a live baby and prevent serious complications in the mother. Alternatively the Zavanelli manoeuvre, i.e. cephalic replacement

followed by caesarean section, is performed.

shoulder presentation the state which develops when labour begins with the fetus lying obliquely and this lie is not corrected. The shoulder is driven down into the maternal pelvis, and labour becomes obstructed. This may occur during the second stage of a twin labour, after the birth of the first child. On examination the uterus appears broad and the fundal height is less than expected for the gestation. On examination *per vaginam*, if the presenting part is not too high, the fetal ribs (which are quite distinctive) are palpated; an arm may prolapse into the vagina. Caesarean section is necessary, or in parts of the world where this is not possible, internal podalic version and breech extraction would be carried out if the fetus was alive, or possibly a destructive operation if the baby was dead, although the risk to the mother of a ruptured uterus is extremely high.

'show' a term used to denote the blood-stained discharge at the onset of labour which comes from the cervical canal plug, the operculum.

shunt 1. to turn to one side; to divert; to bypass. 2. a passage or anastomosis between two natural channels, especially blood vessels, either by natural means or operation.

SI units the units of measurement generally accepted for all scientific and technical uses. Together they make up the International System of Units. The abbreviation SI, from the French Système International d'Unités, is used in all languages. *See* Appendix 9.

Siamese twins identical (monozygotic) twins joined together at birth. The connection may be slight or extensive. It involves skin and usually muscles or cartilage of a limited region, such as the head, chest or hip. The twins may share a single organ, such as an intestine, or parts of the spine. Where possible the twins are separated by surgery soon after birth.

sibling one of two or more children having the same parents.

sickle cell disease a severe type of anaemia found in the West African and West Indian races. It is hereditary and results in abnormal sickling of haemoglobin beta chains when oxygen tension falls. This leads to interruption of local blood flow and increased haemolysis of erythrocytes, and in severe cases causes sickle cell crises, particularly precipitated by infection. Women with sickle cell disease can become very ill during pregnancy and death may occur from rupture of the spleen or pulmonary embolism; the fetus is likely to have growth retarded in 50% of cases. Women found antenatally to have a sickle cell trait should be advised that their partner should be tested and counselling offered about the potential effects on the fetus.

sign objective evidence or manifestation of a change in the physiology or pathology of the body. Signs of pregnancy would be abdominal growth and palpation of fetal parts, whereas the subjective experience of nausea is a SYMPTOM.

silver nitrate $AgNO_3$. A crystalline salt. Used in solid form as a caustic for reducing excessive granulation tissue.

Silverman–Anderson score a system for evaluation of breathing performance of preterm infants. It consists of five items: 1. chest retraction as compared with abdominal retraction during inspiration; 2. retraction of the lower intercostal muscles;

3. xiphoid retraction; 4. flaring of the nares with inspiration; and 5. expiratory grunt. Each of the five is graded 0, 1 or 2. A sum of these factors yields the score. Adequate ventilation is indicated by a 0, severe respiratory distress is indicated by a score of 10.

Simmonds' disease underactivity of the whole PITUITARY GLAND (HYPOPITUITARISM), so affecting the total endocrine system. It may follow SHEEHAN'S SYNDROME.

Sims' position similar to left lateral position but almost on the face, semiprone with the right knee and thigh drawn up and resting on the bed in front of the left leg.

Sims' speculum See Appendix 3.

sinciput the brow. That part of the skull between the coronal suture and the orbital ridges.

Singer's test a blood test to distinguish fetal from maternal blood.

sinoatrial node a collection of specialized muscle fibres in the wall of the right atrium where the rhythm of cardiac contraction is usually established; also called pacemaker of the heart.

sinus a cavity. A general anatomical term for all cavities in the cranial bones or the dilated channels for venous blood also found in the cranium. See INTRACRANIAL MEMBRANES.

skeleton the bone structure of the body, which supports and protects the organs and soft tissues.

Skene's ducts the largest of the female urethral glands, which open within the urethral orifice; they are regarded as homologous with the prostate.

skull the bony structure of the head enclosing and protecting the brain. The fetal skull is considered in three parts, the vault, the base and the face. The bones of the base and face are firmly united and, therefore, incompressible. The vault is made up of two frontal bones, two parietal bones, two temporal bones and one occipital bone. At birth the vault is not fully ossified and thus there are membranous spaces between the bones called sutures. Where three or more sutures meet the membranous space is called a fontanelle. During labour there is considerable pressure on the fetal skull and moulding takes place whereby the bones overlap the sutures. *See also* FETAL SKULL.

slough a mass of dead tissue either in or which separates from the adjacent tissue.

small for gestational age baby a baby who is smaller or lighter than expected for its gestational age. The definition varies: some authorities include those below the 10th PERCENTILE and some below the 5th percentile. *In utero* there is a higher than normal risk of hypoxia leading to birth asphyxia, so the midwife should ensure that where possible a paediatrician is present at delivery to resuscitate the infant. Meconium-stained liquor during the first stage of labour may alert the midwife to this risk; if the fetus inhales the contaminated liquor respiratory distress may develop due to congestion in the bronchioles and pneumonitis. This can be prevented by intubating the baby before the first inspiration which avoids the liquor being sucked further down the pharynx and trachea. Babies who are small for gestational age are also prone to hypoglycaemia as the liver has been depleted of glycogen stores *in utero*; apnoeic attacks and brain damage may occur as a result of the hypoglycaemia. Regular estimations of blood glucose levels are necessary and frequent feeding to prevent the problem. Hypothermia, infection

and subsequent poor growth are also features of these babies.

smear a specimen of superficial cells, e.g. from the vagina or cervix, which, when examined microscopically, gives information about the level of hormones or early malignant disease.

smegma secretion of sebaceous glands of clitoris and prepuce.

smoking in pregnancy smoking is harmful in pregnancy because carbon monoxide reduces oxygen transport and nicotine causes vasoconstriction of arterioles. The result is a diminished supply of food and oxygen to the fetus. Fetal growth and development may therefore be retarded. The babies of smokers will also be continually exposed to cigarette smoke in their early years, which predisposes them to asthma and other allergenic and respiratory conditions.

snuffles the noisy breathing and nasal catarrh noted in infants with congenital SYPHILIS.

social class a classification, by the Registrar General, of persons by their occupation from I to V: I, professionals; II, intermediate; III, skilled workers; IV, semi-skilled; V, unskilled.

social services services provided by the community to meet certain individual needs. It excludes those provided for profit.

social services department a department of the local authority, set up in 1971 following the Local Authority Social Services Act 1970. Its purpose is to coordinate the social services. It has a responsibility to children and young persons, the elderly, the mentally and physically handicapped, the socially inadequate, and the unsupported parent. It has the power to delegate some areas to voluntary organizations. It may also act as an adoption agency.

social worker a specially trained and qualified person to assess social need and provide the necessary resources.

sociology the scientific study of relationships and phenomena.

sodium symbol Na. A metallic element widely distributed in nature, and forming an important constituent of animal tissues. Sodium is the major cation, i.e. positively charged ion, of the extracellular fluid (ECF) and thus determines the osmolality of the ECF. The serum sodium level is normally about 140 mEq/l. If the sodium level and osmolality fall, osmoreceptors in the hypothalamus are stimulated and cause the release of an antidiuretic hormone (ADH) from the posterior lobe of the pituitary gland. ADH increases the absorption of water in the collecting ducts in the kidneys so that water is conserved while sodium and other electrolytes are excreted in the urine. If the sodium level and osmolality rises, neurons in the thirst centre in the hypothalamus are stimulated and the thirsty person drinks enough fluid to restore the osmolality of the ECF to the normal level. A decrease in serum sodium concentration below normal levels can occur in a variety of conditions associated with fluid volume deficit such as diarrhoea and vomiting, acute or chronic renal failure and in diuretic therapy. An increase in serum sodium concentration above normal levels (HYPERNATRAEMIA) occurs when insensible water loss is not replaced by drinking, and in the newborn when artificial feeds are made up incorrectly with too high a concentration of milk powder. *S. bicarbonate* is used to reverse metabolic ACIDAEMIA following hypoxia to the tissues. It is used in varying strengths, 8.4 or 5%, the more concentrated used where fluid levels are critical, as in the neonate. *S. citrate* a substance added to donor blood to prevent clotting.

soft chancre a venereal ulcer, not due to syphilis. The infecting organism is *Haemophilus ducreyi* (Ducrey's bacillus).

soft palate the fleshy structure at the back of the mouth which, together with the hard palate, forms the roof of the mouth. From the middle of the free border of the soft palate hangs the uvula. In swallowing the soft palate is drawn upward against the back of the pharynx, and prevents food and fluids from entering the nasal passage while they pass through the throat.

solar plexus network of sympathetic nerve ganglia in the abdomen; nerve supply to abdominal organs below the diaphragm.

solute a substance dissolved in a solution.

solvent a liquid which dissolves, or has the power to dissolve.

somatic relating to the body as opposed to the mind.

somatome 1. an appliance for cutting the body of a fetus. 2. a somite.

somatotrophin growth hormone. adj. *somatotrophic.*

somite one of the paired segments along the neural tube of the vertebrate embryo, formed by transverse subdivision of the thickened mesodeum next to the mid-plane, that develop into the vertebral column and muscles of the body.

sonar a term for ULTRASOUND in medical diagnosis.

sonogram a record or display obtained by ultrasonic scanning.

sonography ultrasonography. adj. *sonographic.*

soporific causing sleep.

sordes brown crusts which form on the teeth and lips of unconscious

239

patients, or those suffering from acute or prolonged fevers. The result of neglecting mouth hygiene.

sore buttocks a non-specific term generally referring to perianal excoriation which is commonly associated with frequent loose stools. It is more likely to occur in babies who are artificially fed. Other causes include infrequent changing of the napkin, poor hygiene, loose frequent stools, incorrect laundering of napkins, diet (extra sugar) and infection such as candidiasis. Treatment includes good hygiene, exposure of the buttocks to the air and investigations of feeding, laundering napkins and for infection. *See* NAPKIN RASH.

souffle a soft blowing sound heard on auscultation of the abdomen in pregnancy. *Uterine s.* is due to the blood passing through the uterine arteries of the mother, particularly over the placental site. It is synchronous with the maternal pulse.

soya milk used as a milk substitute for babies who cannot tolerate constituents of breast or cows' milk such as lactose. There are now soya-based milk substitutes prepared specifically for infant formulae. They contain only vegetable fats.

Spalding's sign gross overlapping of the fetal cranial bones, seen on abdominal radiograph. It indicates that intrauterine death has occurred several days previously.

spasm a sudden involuntary muscle contraction.

spastic pertaining to spasm. The term is used to describe special types of increased tone in muscles which results from brain or spinal cord injury. It is also used as a term for CEREBRAL PALSY.

specific gravity the weight of a substance compared with that of an equal volume of another substance,

Spalding's Sign

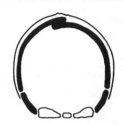

e.g. the specific gravity of water is taken to be 1000. That of other substances such as urine (1010–1020) or blood (1055) may thus be compared.

specular reflection reflecting as from a surface. A term used in ULTRASOUND to describe an interface which gives a strong reflection or echo, e.g. the fetal skull.

speculum an instrument used to open up a cavity, normally not visible, to enable a hidden structure to be inspected. pl. *specula. See* Appendix 3.

Spencer Wells a variety of artery forceps. *See* Appendix 3.

sperm the male reproductive cell; spermatozoon. *S. count* method of determining the concentration of spermatozoa in a semen sample. *S. donation* seminal fluid provided by donors for the fertilization of women whose partners are sterile.

spermatic pertaining to the spermatozoa or to semen. *S. cord* the structure extending from the abdominal inguinal ring to the testis, comprising the pampiniform plexus, nerves, ductus deferens, testicular artery and other vessels.

spermatogenesis the development of mature spermatozoa from spermatogonia.

spermatozoa (pl.) the male generative cells which form the essential part of semen. The normal count of cells is 50 million per ml. sing. *spermatozoon*.

spermicide an agent that destroys spermatozoa. Often used as a cream or paste applied to vaginal or cervical caps, as vagitories or as foam.

sphenoid wedge-shaped. *S. bone* forms part of the base of the skull.

spherocyte a small, globular completely haemoglobinated erythrocyte without the usual central pallor; characteristically found in hereditary spherocytosis but also in acquired haemolytic anaemia.

spherocytosis the presence of spherocytes in the blood.

sphincter a ring shaped muscle, contraction of which closes a natural orifice.

sphingomyelin a complex molecule of protein and fatty acid which is used as a standard to measure the ratio of LECITHIN in the liquor.

sphygmomanometer an instrument used to measure arterial blood pressure.

spigot small peg or bung to close the opening of a tube.

spina bifida a condition in which the arches at the back of the spine are incomplete. Sometimes there is only a bony gap (*spina bifida occulta*) but sometimes the spinal cord is exposed. When there is a sac over the spinal cord it is called a MENINGOCELE or, if nerves are exposed or involved in the sac, a MENINGOMYELOCELE.

spinal relating to the spine. *S. cord see* CORD. *S. anaesthesia* a technique in which the dura is pierced and local anaesthetic is injected directly into the cerebrospinal fluid. It is usually a single dose, fast-acting and reliable form of analgesia using smaller doses of anaesthetic than epidural analgesia. However there is a limited time in which pain relief is effective, and risks of dramatic hypotension, nausea and vomiting, post-spinal headache, and a serious risk of infection unless sterility is scrupulously maintained.

spine 1. the vertebral column. 2. a sharp process of bone.

spinnbarkeit thread of mucus secreted by cervix uteri. Used to determine ovulation as this usually coincides with the time at which the mucus can be drawn out on a glass slide to its maximum length.

spirit an alcoholic solution of a volatile substance, or an alcohol itself.

Spirochaeta a group of microorganisms with a flexible, spiral filament, e.g. *Treponema pallidum*, the cause of SYPHILIS.

spirograph an apparatus for measuring and recording respiratory movements.

spirometer an instrument for measuring air taken into and expelled from the lungs.

splanchnic pertaining to viscera. *S. nerves* three nerves from the thoracic sympathetic ganglia distributed to the viscera.

spleen a very vascular lymphoid organ, situated in the left hypochondrium under the border of the stomach. The framework of the organ consists of fibrous trabeculae with pulp in the spaces. The functions are (*a*) formation of erythrocytes in fetal life only; (*b*) production of lymphocytes throughout life; (*c*) control of red cell breakdown and excretion of the resulting products; and (*d*) formation of ANTIBODIES.

splenomegaly enlargement of the spleen.

splint a piece of wood or metal used to support, and possibly to immobilize, an injured limb.

spondylolisthesis a forward displacement of the 5th lumbar vertebra on the first sacral segment. This narrows the true conjugate by the formation of a false promontory, and is a rare cause of DYSTOCIA.

spondylosis ankylosis of a vertebral joint; also, a general term for degenerative changes in the spine.

spontaneous occurring naturally with no external aid. *S. evolution, see* EVOLUTION. *S. version* the change of the fetus from one lie to another with no obstetrical interference.

sporadic scattered or discontinuous. Applied to isolated cases of a disease which occurs in scattered and scattered places.

spore the reproductive element of certain plants, fungi and bacteria. Tetanus bacilli are spore-bearing, and the spores are resistant to high temperatures and strong antiseptics, and thus difficult to kill, as they can remain dormant for years.

spurious labour false labour. *See* LABOUR.

squamous scaly or plate-like. *S. bone* the thin part of the temporal bone which articulates with the parietal bone. *S. epithelium* thin-celled skin, e.g. the lining of the vagina.

squatting a position with the hips and knees flexed, the buttocks resting on the heels; partial or a full squatting position may be adopted by the parturient at delivery in order to facilitate delivery, both by the effects of gravity and by a slight enlarging of the pelvic outlet.

standard deviation (σ) a measure of the dispersion of a random variable: the square root of the average squared deviation from the mean. For data that have a normal distribution about 68% of the data points fall within one standard deviation from

the mean and about 95% fall within two standard deviations.

Staphylococcus a genus of pyogenic bacteria which, under the microscope, appear grouped together in small masses like bunches of grapes. Staphylococci cause skin infections, including PEMPHIGUS NEONATORUM, MASTITIS and, sometimes, PUERPERAL SEPSIS. *S. aureus* or *S. pyogenes* is coagulase-positive, can cause severe infections and, in hospital, may be resistant to antibiotic drugs. *S. albus* is a skin COMMENSAL but may also cause urinary tract infection.

stasis stagnation or stoppage. *Intestinal s.* sluggish movement of the muscles of the bowel wall, causing constipation. *S. of urine*, which occurs in pregnancy, predisposes to urinary tract infection. *See* PYELONEPHRITIS.

stat *statim* (immediately).

station the location of the presenting part of the fetus in the birth canal, designated as −5 to −1 according to the number of centimetres the part is above an imaginary plane passing through the ischial spines, 0 when at the plane, and +1 to +5 according to the number of centimetres the part is below the plane.

statistical significance in research, a conclusion that the results achieved have little probability of occurring by chance. If the result is below 1 in 20 or the 0.05 probability level, something other than chance produced the result.

statistics 1. numerical facts pertaining to a particular subject or body of objects. 2. the science dealing with the collection, tabulation and analysis of numerical facts.

status condition, state. *S. epilepticus* rapid succession of epileptic spasms without intervals of consciousness; brain damage may result.

statutory bodies the statutory control of the practice of midwives is the responsibility of the NURSING AND MIDWIFERY COUNCIL, established in 2002. *See* Appendix 15.

Stein–Leventhal syndrome a condition in which either AMENORRHOEA or OLIGOMENORRHOEA occurs, associated with hirsutism and infertility. Enlarged cystic ovaries are often found, from which excessive male hormones may be produced.

Stemetil *See* PROCHLORPERAZINE.

stenosis narrowing or contraction of a channel or opening. *Aortic s.* narrowing of the aortic valve of the heart due to scar tissue resulting from inflammation. *Mitral s.* of the mitral orifice from the same cause. *Pyloric s.* due generally to congenital hypertrophy.

stercobilin a bile pigment derivative formed by air oxidation of stercobilinogen; it is a brown–orange–red pigmentation contributing to the colour of faeces and urine.

sterile 1. barren; incapable of producing young. 2. free from microorganisms.

sterilize 1. to make sterile by operation, e.g. ligation of the fallopian tubes. 2. to render sterile dressings, instruments, etc.

sterilizer an apparatus in which objects can be sterilized.

sternum a plate of bone forming the middle of the anterior wall of the thorax and articulating with the clavicles and the cartilages of the first seven ribs. At 36 weeks' gestation the uterine fundus normally reaches the xiphoid process at the lower end of the body of the sternum.

steroids substances of a particular chemical structure of carbon and hydrogen and including sex hormones, adrenocortical hormones, cholesterol and bile acids.

stethoscope an instrument used to auscultate sounds within the body, e.g. of heart, lungs. *Binaural s.* branches into two flexible tubes, one for each ear of the examiner. *Fetal or monaural s.* a metal trumpet-shaped instrument which can be placed on the abdomen over the fetal shoulders to hear the heart sounds. Sometimes called Pinard's stethoscope.

stilboestrol *See* DIETHYLSTILBESTROL.

stilette a wire for keeping clear the lumen of hollow structures such as needles. A fine probe.

stillbirth a baby which has issued forth from its mother after the 24th week of pregnancy and has not, at any time after being completely expelled from its mother, breathed or shown any sign of life. adj. *stillborn*. The statutory duties of the midwife in a case of stillbirth are: 1. notification of stillbirth. 2. certification of stillbirth. 3. registration of stillbirth. 4. notification to the supervisor of midwives.

stillbirth certificate a certificate issued by a registered medical practitioner or a registered midwife who was present at the birth, or examined the body. It is a statutory duty to give it to the qualified informant (usually the father or mother) so that the registration of birth can be made and a Certificate of Burial or Cremation be issued to them. The midwife normally only completes the certificate if no arrangements for maternity care have been made with a medical practitioner. In cases where there has been an inquest, the coroner will issue the order for burial.

stomach the dilated portion of the alimentary canal between the oesophagus and the duodenum, just below the diaphragm. Its wall consists of four coats: serous, muscular, submucous and mucous. The gastric juice contains the enzymes PEPSIN and RENNIN, and HYDROCHLORIC ACID.

stomatitis inflammation of the lining of the mouth.

stool a motion or discharge from the bowel. The stool of the newborn child is at first meconium, then gradually changes to brown, then to a soft bright yellow stool.

strabismus deviation of the eye that the patient cannot overcome; the visual axes assume a position relative to each other different from that required by the physiological conditions; called also squint.

straight sinus venous sinus in the fetal skull at the junction of the falx cerebri and the tentorium cerebelli, a point which may rupture and cause intracranial haemorrhage if excessive or abnormal moulding of the fetal head occurs during delivery.

strawberry mark congenital haemangioma.

Streptococcus a genus of bacteria occurring in a chain-like formation. Streptococci may be haemolytic or non-haemolytic, and aerobic or anaerobic. The beta-haemolytic streptococcus of Lancefield group A (*Streptococcus pyogenes*) is the cause of scarlet fever, severe tonsillitis and can cause severe PUERPERAL SEPSIS. Puerperal sepsis may also be caused by anaerobic streptococci.

streptokinase an enzyme produced by streptococci that catalyses the conversion of plasminogen to plasmin. Streptokinase, when administered as a thrombolytic, requires careful usage to avoid haemorrhage. It is also capable of producing severe antigenic reactions upon readministration.

stress undue strain exerted upon mind or body. Strain liable to cause impairment of mental or physical function. The body's reaction to

emergency stress is set off by the adrenal medulla which pours adrenaline into the blood stream. This causes a rise in heart rate, blood pressure and blood glucose, and dilatation of the blood vessels in the muscles to give them immediate use of this energy. In cases of continuing stress the glands continue to produce a steady supply of hormones that apparently increase the body's resistance. Psychological situations can have the same effect. The diseases most often associated with a stressful environment are coronary artery disease and 'heart attack', high blood pressure and cancer.

striae gravidarum the marks due to skin stretching, which are seen on the abdomen, and to some extent on the breasts and thighs, during and after pregnancy. They occur first as reddish marks, and later fade to a silvery white colour.

sub- prefix meaning 'under' or 'below'.

subacute moderately acute. Applied to a disease that progresses moderately rapidly, but does not become acute.

subarachnoid below the arachnoid. *S. space* the space between the arachnoid and the pia mater, in which the cerebrospinal fluid circulates. *S. haemorrhage* haemorrhage into this space.

subclavian beneath the clavicle. *S. artery* the main artery to the arm.

subcutaneous beneath the skin, e.g. subcutaneous injection.

subdural under the dura mater. *S. haemorrhage* bleeding under the dura mater. One form of intracranial haemorrhage seen in the neonate, often as the result of a traumatic delivery. A subdural tap is sometimes used to withdraw blood to relieve the pressure.

subfertility a state of less than normal fertility.

subinvolution incomplete or delayed return of the uterus to its non-pregnant size during the puerperium, usually due to retained products of conception and infection.

subluxation partial dislocation.

submucous beneath the mucous membrane.

subnormal below normal.

subtotal hysterectomy *See* HYSTEREC-TOMY.

succenturiate additional or accessory. *S. placenta, see* PLACENTA.

sudden infant death syndrome (SIDS) the sudden and unexpected death of an apparently healthy infant, typically occurring between the ages of 3 weeks and 5 months, and not explained by careful post-mortem studies. They are often found dead in the cot, hence the popular name 'cot deaths'. Sometimes the baby has had a slight cold, but more often there have been no symptoms. It is more common in babies born before term and less common in breastfed babies. The incidence is about 6 per 1000 live births. The prone position, tobacco smoke and overheating have been found to increase the risk of cot death, so should be avoided.

sugar a class of carbohydrates which includes monosaccharides such as glucose, fructose and galactose, and disaccharides such as sucrose (cane sugar) and lactose (the sugar in milk). The sugar in the blood is glucose.

sulcus a groove or furrow, as between the cotyledons of a placenta.

sulphonamides a group of chemo-therapeutic drugs much used in the treatment of bacterial infections. They are given orally and are often effective in the treatment of infections with streptococci, gonococci, *E. coli* and other bacteria, although some of these organisms are now resistant.

super- prefix meaning 'over' or 'above'.

superfecundation the fertilization of two ova from the same ovulation by spermatozoa from two different individuals.

superfetation fertilization of an ovum occurring during the course of pregnancy.

superior 1. higher than, above. 2. better than. 3. one in charge of others. *S. longitudinal sinus* upper venous sinus between the layers of the falx cerebri which separates the two hemispheres of the brain.

supervisor of midwives a practising midwife, appointed by the LOCAL SUPERVISING AUTHORITY in accordance with Rule 44 of the Nurses, Mid-wives and Health Visitors (Midwives Amendment) Rules Approval Order 1986 to exercise supervision over midwives in its area. The supervisor must have a minimum of 3 years' experience as a midwife of which at least 1 year must have been in the 2 years immediately prior to appointment or s/he must be eligible to practise and undertake any fur-ther experience required by the NMC. Within 12 months of appoint-ment the supervisor must undertake a course of instruction and refresher courses at intervals of not more than 3 years. Supervisors are responsible for receipt and monitoring of noti-fication of intention to practise forms from all midwives working in the area and submitting them to the local supervising authority (LSA); moni-toring standards of midwifery prac-tice and providing professional, clinical and educational support and guidance; issuing supply orders for controlled drugs, witnessing the destruction of controlled drugs where appropriate and ensuring that midwives are competent to administer medicines; monitoring and, if necessary, storing written records from all midwives in the area; investigating allegations of malpractice, negligence or misconduct; referral of midwives to the Health Committee of the NMC and notifying the LSA of midwives liable to be a source of infection.

supination turning upwards. *S. of hand* the palm is upward. cf. PRONATION.

supine lying on the back. *S. hypotensive syndrome* hypotension occurring from pressure of the gravid uterus on the inferior vena cava, thus reducing the venous return and the cardiac output. It may happen when a woman in late pregnancy lies in the dorsal position, and can be aggravated by EPIDURAL ANALGESIA. It has the effect of reducing the blood pressure, sometimes making the woman feel faint, and ultimately will affect placental perfusion, and thus the flow of oxygen to the fetus.

supplement something added to supply a deficiency.

supplementary of the nature of a supplement. *S. feed* a feed given to an infant instead of or in addition to a breast feed. cf. COMPLEMENTARY.

supply of controlled drugs midwives working in the community obtain supplies of controlled drugs such as pethidine by applying to the supervisor of midwives who issues a supply order form. The midwife then goes to the approved pharmacist who issues the new stock, with the midwife and pharmacist entering the details in the midwife's personal register and drug book. All controlled drugs supplied to the midwife must be kept in a fixed locked cupboard which is only accessible to her/him.

supply order form the official authorization, provided by the supervisor of midwives, to a practising midwife to enable her/him to obtain a supply of PETHIDINE.

suppository a solid cone-shaped medicated compound to be introduced into the rectum, either to cause a bowel action (e.g. glycerine or bisacodyl suppositories) or to administer drugs, particularly analgesics (e.g. Anusol suppository for painful haemorrhoids). Medicated suppositories may also be introduced into the vagina or urethra.

suppression complete cessation of a secretion. Lactation is suppressed in cases where breastfeeding is not desired or contraindicated. It may be achieved naturally, i.e. by not removing the milk, or with the use of drugs such as bromocriptine which inhibits the release of prolactin from the pituitary gland.

suppuration the formation or discharge of pus.

supra- prefix meaning 'above'.

suprapubic above the pubic bones.

suprarenal above the kidney. *S. glands* two small triangular endocrine glands, one above each kidney. They secrete ADRENALINE and NORADRENALINE from the medulla and a number of hormones from the cortex.

surfactant a LECITHIN found in the lungs, which helps the alveoli to remain open. Babies who suffer from the RESPIRATORY DISTRESS SYNDROME do not have enough of this substance. This may be predicted by estimating the LECITHIN/SPHINGOMYELIN RATIO before delivery.

surrender of controlled drugs unwanted controlled drugs may be surrendered by the midwife to an 'authorized' person such as the pharmacist from whom the drugs were originally obtained, or to a medical officer but not to the supervisor of midwives. See also DESTRUCTION OF CONTROLLED DRUGS.

surrogate a substitute. *S. mother* a woman who carries a child for another with the intention that the child be handed over after birth.

survey a systematic collection of information, not forming part of a scientific epidemiological study.

suture 1. a stitch or series of stitches used to close a wound. 2. the fibrous joint where the opposed bony surfaces are very closely united by thin connective tissue, permitting movement only in the neonate. For details, see FETAL SKULL.

symmetrical cortical necrosis a rare complication of severe concealed ABRUPTIO PLACENTAE where there is destruction of large areas of the cortex of both kidneys due to internal spasm of the renal cortical arteries. Impaired renal function or death from renal failure may follow. See also TUBULAR NECROSIS.

sympathetic exhibiting sympathy.

sympathetic nervous system that part of the autonomic system which, when stimulated, prepares the body for emergency or flight. The pulse rate increases, the blood pressure rises, the pupils are dilated, while peristalsis is slowed.

symphysiotomy division of the symphysis pubis, a method of facilitating delivery in cases of disproportion, used: (*a*) where caesarean section is not practicable; (*b*) to avoid delivering a woman too many times by caesarean section; and (*c*) in regions where the midwifery services are inadequate, to avoid leaving a woman with a scar in her uterus.

symphysis a joint where the bone surfaces are joined by fibrocartilage and movement is very slight. *S. pubis* the fibrocartilaginous junction of the two

pubic bones. *S. pubis diastasis* slight separation of the fibrocartilaginous junction from the two pubic bones, caused in pregnancy by the hormones progesterone and relaxin. Causes discomfort and pain in the region and difficulty in walking. Physiotherapy, osteopathy or chiropractic may help to reduce the pain.

symptom any evidence of a disease or condition observed by the woman herself. Thus AMENORRHOEA and certain breast changes are symptoms of pregnancy. See also SIGN.

syn- prefix meaning 'together'.

synapse the junction between the processes of two neurons or between a neuron and an effector organ, where neural impulses are transmitted by chemical means. The impulse causes the release of a neurotransmitter, e.g. acetylcholine or noradrenaline, from the presynaptic membrane of the axon terminal.

synclitism the state when the fetal head enters the pelvic brim with both parietal eminences at the same level. See ASYNCLITISM.

syncope fainting. Loss of consciousness, due to diminished cerebral blood flow.

syncytium, syncytiotrophoblast the outlet layer of the TROPHOBLAST which does not have cell boundaries but scattered nuclei in the protoplasm. This layer persists throughout pregnancy covering the CHORIONIC VILLI, unlike the CYTOTROPHOBLAST cells.

syndactyly webbed fingers or toes.

syndrome a group of symptoms and signs typical of a distinctive disease, and of that disease only.

synthesis the joining together of substances, either naturally or artificially. Substances thus built up artificially, e.g. diethylstilbestrol, are termed synthetic.

synthetic chemical, an artificially formed compound.

Syntocinon *See* OXYTOCIN.

Syntometrine an oxytocic drug containing 0.5 mg ergometrine and 5 units of Syntocinon in 1 ml which is commonly administered to the mother intramuscularly with the birth of the anterior shoulder of the fetus to manage the third stage of labour actively. Causes rapid and sustained uterine contraction and separation of the placenta from the uterine wall.

syphilis a contagious venereal disease, caused by *Treponema pallidum*. It may be *congenital* or *acquired*. The acquired type is manifested in four stages: *Primary* incubation, 2–6 weeks, when the specific primary chancre appears, usually on the vulva, followed by enlargement of the regional lymph glands. The sore is painless and heals quickly, hence this phase could easily be overlooked. *Secondary*, this develops a few weeks later with rashes, *condylomata* around the anus and vulva, and general enlargement of the lymph glands. This stage is highly infectious. It varies considerably, and in a number of cases the symptoms do not appear, or are very slight; the patient, however, is not cured, but has *latent* syphilis. *Tertiary* may appear years later. Characterized by gummatous tumours in various tissues. *Quaternary* lesions are: tabes dorsalis, general paralysis of the insane, etc. *Treponema* can cross the placenta and cause abortion or stillbirth, or the baby may be born with *congenital syphilis*. Signs are: a brownish-red rash on the buttocks, sores about the mouth and rhinitis with discharge from the nose (SNUFFLES). Later the 'saddle' nose, HUTCHINSON'S TEETH, deafness or impaired vision may occur. Screening of all pregnant women for syphilis is vital, as prompt treatment can prevent congenital syphilis. The Wassermann reaction (WR) and Kahn tests may give positive results which then need testing more specifically with *Treponema pallidum* haemaglutination (TPHA) test, *Treponema* immobilization test (TPI) and Venereal Disease Research Laboratory (VDRL) test. All tests, except the VDRL, may give false positives with YAWS, malaria and glandular fever. Treatment with large doses of penicillin is effective. The mother can be cured and the child will be healthy, but it is wise to treat her in any further pregnancies, as congenital syphilis may occur unexpectedly.

syringocele a cavity containing herniation of the spinal cord through the bony defect in spina bifida.

syringomyelocele hernial protrusion of the spinal cord through the bony defect in a spina bifida, the mass containing a cavity connected with the central canal of the spinal cord.

Système International d'Unités (SI units) the international system for measurement in science, industry and general use. It was agreed in 1960, and it is now illegal in the United Kingdom to prescribe or dispense drugs in any other units.

systemic pertaining to or affecting the body as a whole.

systole the contraction of the heart. cf. DIASTOLE. *Ventricular s.* the contraction of the ventricles, by which the blood is pumped into the aorta and pulmonary arteries.

systolic pertaining to systole. *S. murmur* an abnormal sound produced during systole, in heart affections. *S. pressure*, *see* BLOOD PRESSURE. *S. sound* the dull sound of the heart in ventricular systole, caused by its movement against the chest wall.

T

T cell a lymphocyte which is derived from the thymus and is responsible for cell-mediated immunity.

TAB a vaccine which gives some protection against typhoid fever, paratyphoid A and paratyphoid B. *TABT* protects against tetanus in addition.

taboo any of the negative traditions and behaviours generally regarded as harmful to social welfare and sometimes health.

tachycardia abnormally rapid action of the heart and pulse rate.

tachypnoea abnormally rapid respirations, as sometimes seen in the newborn child in RESPIRATORY DISTRESS SYNDROME.

tactile pertaining to touch.

tai chi Chinese system of movement, breathing and concentration, originally a martial art, but now used to promote and maintain general health and well-being. A very gentle form of exercise, eminently suitable for pregnant women.

taking up of cervix the effacement of the cervical canal early in labour. *See* DILATATION.

talipes clubfoot. A congenital deformity in which the foot has developed at an abnormal angle to the leg. The cause is not fully understood. In some cases, notably in women with OLIGOHYDRAMNIOS, the child has been cramped *in utero* and is born with mild positional talipes. Most commonly an equinovarus or a calcaneovalgus combination is seen. The condition should be noted when the baby is first examined and a paediatrician should be informed. In mild cases, the physiotherapist, starting on the day of birth, can quickly correct the deformity, but if it is more severe, stretching, massage, or splinting or even operative treatment may be needed.

talipomanus clubhand.

talus ankle bone; the highest of the tarsal bones.

tamoxifen a non-steroidal oral anti-oestrogen used in the palliative treatment of breast cancer in postmenopausal women and to stimulate ovulation in infertility.

tampon a gauze plug with a long tape. Commonly introduced into the vagina during repair of episiotomy or perineal laceration.

tapotement a manual technique used in massage, involving gentle tapping with the fingers to stimulate the circulation.

tarsus 1. the seven bones – talus, calcaneus, navicular, medial, intermediate and lateral cuneiform, and cuboid – composing the articulation between the foot and leg; the ankle or instep. 2. the cartilaginous plate forming the framework of either (upper or lower) eyelid.

taurine a crystallized acid from the bile; found also in small quantities in lung and muscle tissue. Taurine is present in high quantities in breast milk and is necessary for the conjugation of bile acids in the first week of life until glycine takes over the

Talipes

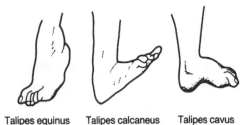

Talipes equinus Talipes calcaneus Talipes cavus

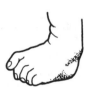

Talipes varus Talipes equinovarus Talipes calcaneovarus

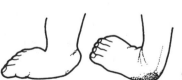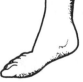

Talipes valgus Talipes calcaneovalgus Talipes equinovalgus

function and for the development of the nervous system.

Taussig–Bing syndrome transposition of the great vessels of the heart and a ventricular septal defect straddled by a large pulmonary artery.

taxonomy the orderly classification of organisms into appropriate categories (taxa) with application of suitable and correct names.

Tay–Sachs disease the infantile form of amaurotic familial idiocy, inherited as an autosomal recessive trait and affecting chiefly Ashkenazic Jews. It is a progressive disorder marked by a degeneration of brain tissue and the maculas (with the formation of a cherry red spot on both retinas) and by dementia, blindness and death. Antenatal diagnosis can be made at 14 weeks of pregnancy. An absence of the enzyme hexosaminidase A indicates conclusively that the fetus has Tay–Sachs disease. Carriers of the trait have a lower level of the enzyme in their blood.

tea tree oil an aromatherapy essential oil obtained from an Australian tree. It is highly effective as an anti-infective agent, being antibacterial, antifungal, antiviral and antimicrobial. It has been found to be useful for vaginal and other forms of candidiasis and is available in a proprietary pessary; also for herpes lesions; work is ongoing to evaluate its use for people with HIV infections.

team midwifery a system of midwifery management in which midwives are divided into teams to care for identified groups of women. The aim is to improve communication and thus continuity of care by reducing the number of midwives whom an individual mother sees during her pregnancy, labour and the puerperium. Unlike CASELOAD MIDWIFERY, however, it does not necessarily

improve continuity of care as a mother may be cared for by different midwives from the same team, some of whom work in the antenatal clinic, others are in the delivery suite, and others are based in the postnatal wards or in the community.

teat 1. nipple of the breast. 2. manufactured nipple used on infants' feeding bottles.

teething eruption of the teeth through the gums. The average baby cuts his/her first tooth between the 6th and 9th months. The full set of 20 baby teeth erupt gradually over a period of up to about 30 months; usually two teeth, one on each side of the jaw, appear at a time.

telemeter to transmit readings of an instrument by radio waves.

telemetry the record of fetal heart beats and uterine contractions by remote control, so that the mother is able to walk about during labour.

temazepam a hypnotic drug. Should be avoided in the first trimester.

temperature that degree of heat of a substance or body as measured by a thermometer. *Normal t.* of the human body 36–37°C (97–98.4°F). It varies slightly during the day, and in women it is higher during the second half of the menstrual cycle. It indicates the balance between heat production and heat loss. A thermometer inserted under the tongue or into the rectum will register slightly higher than when placed in the axilla or groin. *See* PYREXIA *and* FEVER.

temporal pertaining to the side of the head. *T. bone* an irregular bone of the skull, the squamous part of which forms part of the vault.

tendon a cord or band of strong white fibrous tissue that connects a muscle to a bone. When the muscle contracts, it pulls the tendon, which moves the bone.

tension 1. the act of stretching or the state of being stretched. 2. the pressure or concentration of a gas. *See* P_{O_2} *and* Appendix 16. *Premenstrual t.* symptoms occurring as a result of hormonal changes, in the 5–7 days before a menstrual period. Includes abdominal distension, headaches, emotional lability, poor coordination, fluid retention and others.

tentorium cerebelli a septum of dura mater, separating the cerebral hemispheres from the cerebellum. *See* INTRACRANIAL MEMBRANES.

tepid slightly warm; 32–37°C

teras a malformed fetus or infant. adj. *teratic.*

teratogen an agent or influence that causes physical defects in the developing embryo. adj. *teratogenic.*

teratoma a congenital tumour containing teeth, hair and cells of other tissues not normally found in the place where it is situated.

term the end of pregnancy. It is normally calculated as 280 days or 40 weeks from the first day of the last normal menstrual period, but is considered to be any time after the 37th week of pregnancy.

termination of pregnancy (TOP) an abortion which is induced, legally or illegally.

tertiary third *T. syphilis. See* SYPHILIS.

test 1. an examination or trial. 2. a significant chemical reaction. 3. a reagent. *Agglutination t.* one whose results depend on agglutination of bacteria or other cells; used in diagnosing certain infectious diseases and rheumatoid arthritis, the crossmatching of blood and in pregnancy tests. In the latter tests no agglutination indicates a positive pregnancy test, whereas when agglutination occurs the result is negative. *Complement-fixation t's* tests that utilize antigen–antibody reaction

and result in haemolysis to determine the presence of various organisms in the blood. *Concentration t.* a test of renal function based on the woman's ability to concentrate urine. *Creatinine clearance t.* a test for renal function based on the rate at which ingested creatinine is filtered through the renal glomeruli. *Early pregnancy t.* a do-it-yourself immunological test for pregnancy, performed as early as 9 days after menstruation was expected. *Glucose tolerance t.* a metabolic test of carbohydrate tolerance used to diagnose diabetes mellitus. *Glycosylated haemoglobin t.* measurement of the percentage of haemoglobin A_1 (HbA$_1$) molecules which helps to assess diabetic control. HbA$_1$ is a type of adult haemoglobin where one part of the beta chain has been combined with glucose, and increases in diabetes, especially when the blood glucose control is poor. *Histamine t.* following a rapid intravenous injection of histamine phosphate, the blood pressure normally falls, but in women with phaeochromocytoma, after the fall, there is a marked rise in blood pressure. *Pregnancy t's* laboratory procedures for early determination of pregnancy. *Sickling t.* a method to demonstrate haemoglobin S and the sickling phenomenon in erythrocytes, performed by reducing the oxygen concentration to which the red cells are exposed. *Treponema pallidum haemagglutination (TPHA) t., Treponema pallidum immobilization (TPI) t.* serological tests related directly to the causative organism, used in the diagnosis of syphilis. *VDRL t.* a slide flocculation test for syphilis designed by the Venereal Disease Research Laboratory, USA.

testicles, testes the two glands in the scrotum which produce spermatozoa and male sex hormones. *Undescended t.* when the organ remains in the pelvis or inguinal canal.

testosterone the hormone produced by the testes which stimulates the development of male characteristics.

tetanic relating to tetanus. *T. spasms* occur in strychnine poisoning.

tetanus a disease due to the *Clostridium tetani*, an anaerobe found in cultivated soil and manure, and therefore likely to infect accidental wounds. In persons thus exposed to the infection, tetanus antitoxin will confer passive immunity.

tetany a condition resulting from calcium deficiency, alkalaemia or impaired function of the parathyroid glands. The chief sign is tonic contraction of the muscles of the hands and feet (carpopedal spasm) with hypersensitivity of other muscles. It is sometimes seen in newborn babies who have been artificially fed. They have low calcium concentrations in the blood. *See also* HYPOCALCAEMIA.

tetracycline an antibiotic substance that is effective against many different micro-organisms. Tetracyclines should be used only with caution during pregnancy as they may cause yellow discoloration and subsequent premature degeneration of the child's first teeth.

tetradactyly the presence of four digits of the hand or foot.

tetralogy a group or series of four. *Fallot's t.* a congenital defect of the heart that combines four structural anomalies: pulmonary stenosis; ventricular septal defect; dextroposition of the aorta, in which the aortic opening overrides the septum and receives blood from both the right and left ventricles; and right ventricular hypertrophy. Surgical correction is required whenever possible.

thalamus that part of the brain at the base of the cerebrum. Most sensory impulses pass from the body to the thalamus and are transmitted to the cortex and forebrain.

thalassaemia Cooley's anaemia. It is most common in people of Mediterranean origin. Abnormal erythrocytes cause severe anaemia and folic acid is required as the bone marrow is very active in replacing the short-lived red blood cells.

thalidomide a sedative and hypnotic drug which, when used in early pregnancy, caused serious development deformities, mainly of one or more limbs.

theophylline a respiratory stimulant given to reduce the incidence of apnoeic attacks in the small preterm infant. It has no known long-term side-effects.

therapeutic abortion an abortion legally induced. It is performed when either the fetus is known to be so malformed that mortality or gross morbidity is certain, or in cases where the mother's physical or mental health is in jeopardy if the pregnancy continues.

therapy treatment. *Chemotherapy* treatment with chemical drugs.

thermometer an instrument for measuring temperature. *Clinical t.* a special type used to measure and record the body temperature.

thiamine vitamin B_1; a component of the B complex group of vitamins, found in various foodstuffs and present in the free state in blood plasma and cerebrospinal fluid. Deficiency results in neurological symptoms, cardiovascular dysfunction, oedema, and reduced intestinal motility.

thiazole any of a group of benzo thiadiazinesulphonamide derivatives, typified by chlorothiazide, that act as diuretics by inhibiting the reabsorption of sodium in the proximal renal tubule and stimulating chloride excretion, with resultant increase in excretion of water.

thiopental a barbiturate, given intravenously to induce general anaesthesia.

third degree perineal laceration a complete tear extending through the whole of the perineal body, through the anal sphincter and into the rectum.

third stage of labour the period from the birth of the child to complete expulsion of the placenta and membranes. It involves separation and expulsion of the placenta and membranes and the control of haemorrhage. The midwife may manage the third stage *physiologically* which may take any time from 5 minutes to 2 hours to complete, but which averages 20–30 minutes. *Active* management involves the administration of an oxytocic drug to expedite placental separation and to control haemorrhage. It may also involve the active delivery of the placenta and membranes by the use of CONTROLLED CORD TRACTION; active management of the third stage usually takes 5–10 minutes.

thoracic relating to the thorax. *T. duct* the large lymphatic vessel situated in the thorax along the spine. It opens into the left subclavian vein.

thorax the chest; cavity containing the heart, lungs, bronchi and oesophagus. It is bounded by the diaphragm below, the sternum in front and the dorsal vertebrae behind, and is enclosed by the ribs as a protective framework.

threatened abortion vaginal bleeding, usually slight, which may be accompanied by abdominal pain. There is no dilatation of the cervix, and often

the condition settles, the woman progressing to term. If the bleeding and pain are combined with cervical dilatation, the abortion becomes INEVITABLE. *See also* ABORTION.

threshold the level that must be reached for an effect to be produced, as the degree of intensity of stimulus which just produces a sensation.

thrill a tremor or vibration elicited by tapping the wall of a cavity containing fluid, e.g. a pregnant uterus with POLYHYDRAMNIOS.

thrombectomy surgical removal of a clot from a blood vessel.

thrombin a substance formed in the blood by the action of thromboplastin on PROTHROMBIN in the presence of calcium. The thrombin then converts the plasma protein fibrinogen into fibrin which, with the cells, forms a clot.

thrombocyte a blood platelet.

thrombocythaemia an increase in the number of circulating blood platelets.

thrombocytopenia an uncommon condition of deficiency of PLATELETS, sometimes seen in the newborn child especially of a mother with purpura, and characterized by purpuric haemorrhages. It usually resolves spontaneously. It also occurs in congenital RUBELLA.

thromboembolism obstruction of a blood vessel with thrombotic material carried by the blood from the site of origin to plug another vessel. Together with thrombosis, remains the major cause of maternal death in Britain.

thrombokinase activated clotting factor X.

thrombolysis dissolution of a thrombus.

thrombophlebitis inflammation of a vein, with clot formation. The clot tends to be adherent to the wall of the vein, and rarely separates, so that the danger of EMBOLISM is small. *Femoral t.* may occur following labour as an extension of pelvic infection. cf. PHLEBOTHROMBOSIS.

thromboplastin a substance liberated by injured tissue and platelets. *See* THROMBIN *and* PROTHROMBIN.

thrombosis the formation of a thrombus. *Coronary t.* formation of a clot in a coronary vessel, by which the heart muscle is deprived of blood according to the size of the vessel blocked. If the thrombus detaches itself from the wall and is carried along by the blood stream, the clot is called an embolus. The condition is known as EMBOLISM.

thrombus a stationary blood clot produced by coagulation of the blood, usually in a vein, and often the result of PHLEBITIS.

thrush a condition in which whitish spots form on the mucous membrane of the mouth, due to the fungus *Candida albicans*. In babies it may be transferred from the vulva of a woman with candidal (monilial) vaginitis during vaginal delivery. If untreated the infection will spread to other parts of the infant's neonatal tract. An erythematous napkin rash with small, white-headed pustules is usually due to *Candida albicans*. In artificially fed infants it may spread quickly, as it is killed only by autoclaving and not by other methods of sterilization. The treatment is to give antibiotics and fungicidal drugs such as nystatin. A herbal preparation, TEA TREE OIL, has also been found to be effective.

thymus a gland situated between the lungs and above the heart. It grows until puberty and then gradually involutes. The cortex contains many small T lymphocytes which play a part in the immunological reactions of the body.

thyroid gland an endocrine gland situated in the neck in front of the trachea. Its secretions, thyroxine and triiodothyronine, control metabolism. Overactivity causes thyrotoxicosis, and underactivity myxoedema. Infants whose thyroid secretions are defective are cretins.

thyrotoxic marked by toxic (excessive) activity of the thyroid.

thyrotrophin a hormone secreted by the anterior lobe of the anterior pituitary gland that stimulates the thyroid gland. Also called thyroid-stimulating hormone (TSH).

thyroxine a hormone of the thyroid gland that contains iodine and is a derivative of the amino acid TYROSINE. Thyroxine affects the metabolic rate (oxygen consumption); growth and development; metabolism of carbohydrates, fats, proteins, electrolytes and water; vitamin requirements; reproduction; and resistance to infection. Thyroxine can be extracted from animals or produced synthetically and is prescribed for HYPOTHYROIDISM and for some types of GOITRE.

tidal volume the amount of gas passing into and out of the lungs in each respiratory cycle.

tissue a mass of cells or fibres uniting to perform a particular function in the body. *Connective t.* there are many types: adipose (fatty), areolar (elastic supporting), bone, blood and cartilage. *Brown adipose t., brown fat t.* a thermogenic type of adipose tissue containing a dark pigment, and arising during embryonic life in specific areas such as between the shoulder blades, behind the sternum, in the neck and around the kidneys and suprarenal glands. It is utilized by the newborn for the production of heat, as required. *Epithelial t.* covers all inner and outer body surfaces. Some varieties are ciliated (e.g. the lining of the fallopian tubes), some columnar (e.g. the lining of the cervical canal) and some squamous (e.g. the lining of the vagina). *Erectile t.* spongy tissue that expands and becomes hard when filled with blood. *Granulation t.* material formed in repair of wounds and soft tissue, consisting of connective tissue cells and ingrowing young capillaries; it ultimately forms fibrous tissue; a scar; *muscular t.* the three types are striated (skeletal or voluntary), unstriated (plain or involuntary) and cardiac (striated but involuntary). *Nervous t.* this consists of nerve cells and their processes. *Subcutaneous t.* the layer of loose connective tissue directly under the skin.

tissue fluid the fluid in the tissue spaces between the cells, sometimes called extracellular fluid. A demonstrable excess constitutes OEDEMA.

titre the amount of a substance, e.g. an antibody, in the blood. It is estimated by finding the amount of it needed to correspond with a known amount of another substance.

toco-, toko- word element meaning 'childbirth', 'labour'.

tocograph an instrument for measuring the pattern and pressure of uterine contraction.

tocolytic drugs drugs used to arrest threatened preterm labour; ritodrine hydrochloride (Yutopar); salbutamol (Ventolin).

tocopherol vitamin E, present in wheatgerm, green leaves and milk.

tomography any method that produces images of single tissue planes. *Computed t.* (CT) a radiological imaging modality that uses computer processing of X-ray photons detected by a detector bank after passing through the patient. The image generated is a representation of tissue densities within a 'slice', 1–10 mm thick, through the patient's body. Called also computerized axial tomography (CAT). *Ultrasonic t.* the ultrasonographic visualization of a cross-section of a predetermined plane of the body; *see* B-mode ULTRASONOGRAPHY.

tone the normal degree of tension, e.g. in a muscle.

tongue tie shortening of the frenulum, a band of tissue which anchors the tongue to the floor of the mouth. It does not usually interfere with feeding.

tonic contraction of the uterus this may be *general*, where the uterus is in a state of powerful continuous contraction, leading to anoxia of the fetus, or *local*, a ring of tonic contraction called a *constriction ring*. It forms most commonly round the fetal neck, so preventing progress in labour. Deep anaesthesia is usually required to give relaxation, although inhaling amyl nitrite may sometimes help.

tonus muscle tone.

'topping up' epidural anaesthesia midwives are permitted by the NMC to top up epidurals provided they have been instructed and assessed in the technique, the drug and the dose are checked with another person, and the anaesthetist, who retains overall responsibility for the woman's care, has given written instructions regarding the dose of bupivacaine, and has detailed the mother's position, frequency of blood pressure recordings and the steps to be taken in the event of side-effects. The anaesthetist must administer the test dose and the first full dose of analgesia. Following administration of the first or a top-up dose, the midwife should record the mother's blood pressure every 5 minutes for 30 minutes and usually every 15 minutes thereafter. The mother should not be positioned flat on her back to avoid supine hypotension.

torsion twisting. May occur in the pedicle of a cyst which produces venous congestion in the cyst and consequent gangrene – a possible complication of ovarian cyst.

torticollis a contracted state of the cervical muscles, producing torsion of the neck. The deformity may be congenital, hysterical, or due to pressure on the accessory nerve, inflammation of the glands of the neck, or to muscle spasm.

tourniquet an instrument applied to a limb to arrest bleeding or to make a vein more prominent.

toxaemia poisoning of the blood by the absorption of toxins, once thought to be responsible for PRE-ECLAMPSIA.

toxic poisonous, relating to a poison.

toxin a poison, particularly that produced by pathogenic bacteria. Bacterial toxins do not produce symptoms until after a variable period of incubation while the microbes multiply sufficiently to overwhelm the leucocytes and other types of antibodies. Toxins cause antitoxins to form in the body, thus providing a means of establishing immunity to certain diseases.

toxoid toxin which has been rendered non-toxic but which retains its protective qualities. APT (alum-precipitated toxoid), used in diphtheria immunization, is such a preparation.

Toxoplasma a genus of protozoa which acts as parasites. They cause TOXOPLASMOSIS.

toxoplasmosis infection with *Toxoplasma*, causing a glandular-fever-like syndrome. When it occurs during pregnancy the fetus may become infected and as a result have hydrocephalus, intracranial calcification, splenomegaly, anaemia, jaundice and retinal damage.

trachea the windpipe; a cartilaginous tube lined with ciliated epithelium, extending from the lower part of the larynx to the bronchi.

tracheo-oesophageal fistula a congenital defect in which there is an opening between the trachea and the lower oesophagus. *See also* OESOPHAGEAL ATRESIA.

tracheostomy creation of an opening into the trachea through the neck, with insertion of an indwelling tube, undertaken in an emergency to restore the airway in acute obstruction, or to improve the airway and aspirate secretions.

traditional birth attendant women, usually mothers themselves, who traditionally help other women to deliver their babies. They are found in areas of the developing countries where midwifery or obstetric help may not be available. They are unqualified although there are moves to provide basic training to ensure that they adhere to safe standards of care. Sometimes called indigenous midwife, hilot, dunken, dai.

trait a characteristic behaviour pattern. *Sickle cell t.* a tendency for red cells to sickle, without accompanying anaemia, found when an individual is HETEROZYGOUS for the condition.

tranquillizers drugs which allay anxiety and calm the patient. Valuable for women who begin labour in great fear and anxiety. Chlorpromazine and promethazine are examples.

transcervical ligaments *See* CARDINAL LIGAMENTS.

transcutaneous blood gas monitors the application of a probe to the baby's skin which is heated to a temperature of 44°C and enables measurements of P_{O_2} and P_{CO_2} to be made. Accuracy depends on the quality of the peripheral circulation; thus transcutaneous blood gas monitoring is usually used in conjunction with intermittent arterial sampling.

transcutaneous electrical nerve stimulation (TENS) a procedure in which mild electrical stimulation is applied by electrodes in contact with the skin over a painful area. TENS stimulates the large myelinated nerve fibres and relieves pain in line with the GATE CONTROL THEORY. It also causes the release of endogenous opiates or endorphins in the cerebrospinal fluid, and this reduces the perception of pain. When used for pain relief in labour, four electrodes are placed parallel and close to the spine between T10 and T11 and in the sacral area between S2 and S4. Pain relief is controlled by the mother who is able to increase the degree of stimulation during a contraction, and is able to be ambulant if she wishes. The NMC has approved the use of TENS by midwives on their own responsibility, provided they have been instructed in its use.

transducer a device which transforms one form of energy into another. The one used in ULTRASOUND contains ceramic crystal moulded into a disc. This transforms vibrations from electrical charges into waves of ultrasound of a certain frequency.

transferase an enzyme that catalyses the transfer, from one molecule to another, of a chemical group that does not exist in free state during the transfer.

transferrin a serum globulin that binds and transports iron.

transfusion the direct administration into the blood stream of blood or other solutions to increase the blood

Positions of TENS Electrodes for Pain Relief in Labour

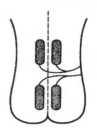

volume. *Exchange t.* repeated small withdrawals and replacement of blood to alter the constituents but not the blood volume, e.g. in haemolytic disease of the newborn it is used to decrease the amount of bilirubin. Sometimes called replacement transfusion. *Feto-maternal t.* from fetus to mother via the placenta. Also called transplacental transfusion (TPT).

transillumination the passage of a strong light through a body structure, to permit inspection by an observer on the opposite side.

translocation in GENETICS, the shifting of part of one CHROMOSOME on to another.

transmigration wandering. *External t.* the passage of an ovum from its ovary to the fallopian tube on the opposite side.

transplacental through the placenta.

transport movement of materials in biological systems, particularly into and out of cells and across epithelial layers. *Active t.* movement of materials across cell membranes and epithelial layers resulting directly from expenditure of metabolic energy.

transposition a cross-placement. *T. of the great vessels* the pulmonary artery arises from the left ventricle instead of the right, so that poorly oxygenated blood leaves the right ventricle by the aorta. Life can only be maintained if there is a patent ductus or if an atrioseptal shunt is created.

transudate any fluid which passes through a membrane, e.g. the vaginal fluid. In contrast to an exudate, it has a high fluid content and low protein and cellular content.

transvaginal through the vagina.

transverse arrest occurs when the fetal head is deflexed and is arrested above the level of the ischial spines with the sagittal suture in the transverse diameter of the pelvis. A cause of cephalopelvic disproportion and OBSTRUCTED LABOUR. *See* DEEP TRANSVERSE ARREST.

transverse lie a condition in which the longitudinal axis of the child lies across that of the mother's uterus. If it is not corrected before, or very shortly after the onset of labour, it can result in a SHOULDER PRESENTATION and obstructed labour. The commonest cause is lax abdominal and uterine muscles, often as a result of repeated pregnancies. It may also occur when the fetus is unable to settle into a cephalic presentation, as in the case of multiple pregnancy, placenta praevia or a contracted pelvic outlet. On abdominal inspection the uterus is typically broad and asymmetrical with the fundus low for the period of amenorrhoea. On palpation the fetal head is usually felt in the flank or the iliac fossa. If a persistent transverse or unstable lie is found after 30 weeks' gestation the midwife should refer the mother to the obstetrician who may perform external cephalic version each time the presentation is abnormal thereafter. The mother may be admitted to hospital for observation and a controlled membrane rupture/induction of labour towards term if this is appropriate. In serious cases caesarean section will be performed electively.

transverse sinuses venous sinuses in the tentorium cerebelli by which blood is drained from the head.

transvestite a person, usually a male, who experiences a habitual and strongly persistent desire to dress as a member of the opposite sex.

trauma injury.

traumatic caused by injury. *T. haemorrhage* bleeding from the vagina which commences immediately the baby is delivered and which continues despite good uterine contractions. It may be due to lacerations in the cervix, vagina or perineal body and can be treated by applying direct pressure to the bleeding point with artery or sponge-holding forceps or by digital pressure until the lacerations can be sutured.

travail labour, childbirth.

travel in pregnancy women may request advice regarding travel during pregnancy. Midwives can offer information which prompts the mother to take steps to make herself as comfortable as possible when travelling, such as postural and back-care advice, frequent stops for the lavatory and avoiding unnecessary travel in late pregnancy. Women who find the wearing of seatbelts in the car too uncomfortable should obtain a medical certificate allowing them to refrain from using them. Most airlines require a doctor's letter or medical certificate from a woman wishing to fly during late pregnancy, stating that she is fit to do so, although many refuse to accept pregnant passengers who are near term.

treatment mode of dealing with a patient or a disease. *Active t.* that in which specific medical or surgical intervention occurs. *Conservative t.* that which employs natural means, e.g. rest, fluid replacement rather than active or radical treatment. *Palliative t.* that which relieves distressing symptoms but not the disease. *Prophylactic t.* that aiming to prevent disease or pathology.

Trendelenburg position *See* POSITION.

Treponema pallidum the SPIROCHAETE causing syphilis.

trial labour this is conducted to see if normal vaginal delivery is possible despite the fact that the head is not engaged, owing to a slight degree of cephalopelvic disproportion. It should only be carried out in a well-equipped hospital. If good contractions occur, the head may flex more and descend with moulding through the pelvic brim, the joints of which relax a little in the process. A normal delivery should then result from the successful trial. Should the observer performing the vaginal examinations note a lack of progress in the descent of the head and in dilatation of the cervix, in spite of good contractions, or any sign of fetal or maternal distress, the trial labour should be ended quickly by caesarean section.

trial of scar a controlled, often induced labour in order to observe the condition and progress of a mother who has a uterine scar from a previous caesarean section or other uterine surgery. The increased risk of scar dehiscence, particularly in a multigravid woman, requires a carefully monitored labour in a consultant unit so that operative delivery can be effected if this occurs.

trichomoniasis, *Trichomonas vaginalis* one of the commonest sexually transmitted diseases caused by *Tri-*

chomonas vaginalis, an oval flagellate protozoon. The infection causes a thin and watery, or yellow-green and frothy vaginal discharge, vulval pruritus and inflammation. The usual treatment is metronidazole 200 mg daily for 10 days. The partner should be treated at the same time to avoid reinfection.

triglyceride a compound consisting of three molecules of fatty acids bound with one molecule of glycerol; a neutral fat that is the usual storage form of lipids in animals.

trigone a triangular area. *T. of the bladder* the triangular non-elastic area forming the base of the bladder, between the ureteric openings and the urethral orifice. It is embedded in the anterior vaginal wall, and so, when this is distended during labour, its functions may be disturbed.

trimester a period of 3 months.

trimethoprim oral or intravenous antibiotic used for urinary and respiratory tract infections. Contraindicated in pregnancy and neonates.

tripartite placenta a placenta divided into three lobes, each with a cord leaving it which join to form one cord a short distance from the lobes.

triple test blood screening test conducted at 16–18 weeks' gestation to assess the risks to the mother of having a baby with Down's syndrome or open neural tube defects. The three substances examined are alphafetoprotein, unconjugated oestriol and human chorionic gonadotrophin. Also called the BART'S TEST.

triple vaccine a combined dose of diphtheria, tetanus and pertussis immunization.

triplets three children carried in the uterus at once and born at one labour. Incidence formerly about 1 in 6400 births; now, as a result of treatment of infertility, more common.

trisomy an additional chromosome with one particular pair. *Trisomy 21* has the extra chromosome with the 21st pair and occurs in DOWN'S SYNDROME. *Trisomy 18* (EDWARDS' SYNDROME); *trisomy 13* (PATAU'S SYNDROME).

trocar a sharply pointed surgical instrument within a metal cannula used for aspiration or the removal of fluids from body cavities.

trochanter one of two prominences below the neck of the femur. *Greater t.* that on the outer side. *Lesser t.* the one on the inner side.

trophoblast the outer covering of the blastocyst, from which the placenta and chorion develop.

trophoblastic tissue SYNCYTIOTROPHO-BLAST and CYTOTROPHOBLAST.

true conjugate *See* CONJUGATE.

trypsin a powerful pancreatic enzyme which continues protein digestion to form amino acids.

tubal insufflation a test to assess patency of the fallopian tubes made by transuterine inflation with carbon dioxide gas.

tubal ligation ligation of the uterine tubes, a method of sterilization. Laparoscopic sterilization using diathermy, or the application of potentially removable clips to the uterine tubes are alternative methods commonly undertaken.

tubal mole a mass of blood clot retained in the fallopian tube after a tubal pregnancy.

tubal pregnancy a pregnancy embedded in the lining of the fallopian tube.

tube feeding administration of liquid (and for adults semi-solid foods) through a nasogastric, gastrostomy, or enterostomy tube. A common method of feeding for the preterm infant who easily tires when suckling and has immature swallowing and gag reflexes.

tuberculosis a specific infection caused by *Mycobacterium tuberculosis*. Occurs commonly in the lung, but any part of the body may be affected. During pregnancy care is shared between the obstetrician and chest physician, usually on an out-patient basis unless she has positive sputum, when hospital admission and isolation are necessary, and she will be cared for by staff who are immune to the infection. Treatment is usually with streptomycin, isoniazid, para-aminosalicyclic acid or ethambutol; rifampicin is contraindicated in the first trimester. Labour should be made as easy as possible to avoid respiratory exhaustion, by offering epidural anaesthesia, forceps delivery and intravenous ergometrine as the baby's anterior shoulder is delivered to limit blood loss. In the few mothers who have positive sputum lactation is suppressed and the baby is segregated from the mother until she is Mantoux test positive. The baby is given bacille Calmette–Guérin (BCG) vaccination as soon as possible after birth and may need to be cared for by a healthy relative or foster parents until the mother is better. The baby's name is entered on the 'at risk' register.

tuberosity an expanded portion of bone, or protuberance, *ischial tuberosities* between which is measured the transverse diameter of the pelvic outlet.

tubular necrosis (acute) 1. when protein is deposited in the collecting and distal convoluted renal tubules, as with an incompatible blood transfusion or septic abortion, the epithelium is damaged and urine dammed back, thus preventing further activity of the GLOMERULUS. It may clear in 7–14 days. 2. if the proximal convoluted tubule becomes ischaemic or bacterial toxins are released, the epithelium may necrose with death of the tubule. The kidney may recover its function in 10–30 days if there is only partial necrosis.

tubule a microscopic tube forming one part of the nephron.

tumescence swelling or enlargement of a part; penile erection.

tumour a growth or swelling.

tunica a coat. *T. albuginea* a dense layer of connective tissue below the germinal epithelium of the ovary.

tunnel a passageway through a solid body with open ends. *Carpal t.* the osseofibrous tunnel for the median nerve and the flexor tendons. Carpal tunnel syndrome occurs when the median nerve becomes compressed and results in pain and tingling paraesthesia in the fingers and hand, sometimes extending to the elbow. It is a fairly common disorder of pregnancy due to oedema causing compression of the median nerve.

Tuohy needle cannula and needle used for siting a catheter into the epidural space; usually either 16 or 18 gauge.

Turner's syndrome a congenital defect in which the person has 45 instead of 46 chromosomes. Only one sex chromosome (X) is present, described as XO, so the individual appears female with a normal vagina, uterus and fallopian tubes but, as the ovaries do not function, AMENORRHOEA and sterility occur. Webbing of the neck may also be evident and coarctation of the aorta may be present. Intelligence is usually normal.

twins two infants developing in the uterus together from one or two ova. *Binovular, dizygotic* or *fraternal t.* those developed from two separate ova fertilized by two spermatozoa. There are two complete pregnancies in the uterus, i.e. two fetuses, two placentae, two chorions, two amnions.

The infants may be of the same or different sexes, and as like or unlike each other as any two members of a family. *Uniovular, monozygotic* or *identical t.* Twins developed from the fertilization of a single ovum. The embryonic cell mass has divided into two identical halves, each of which has developed into a fetus. Thus there are two fetuses and two amniotic membranes, but only one placenta and one chorion. The babies are of the same sex, and alike in all characteristics. Rarely, incomplete division of the embryonic cell mass gives rise to conjoined, or Siamese, twins.

twin-to-twin transfusion transfer of blood from one fetus to its twin, resulting in the former being anaemic and the latter becoming plethoric.

tympanic of or pertaining to the tympanum. *T. membrane* a thin, semitransparent membrane that stretches across the ear canal separating the tympanum (middle ear) from the external meatus (outer ear); called also eardrum.

typing a method of measuring the degree of organ, solid tissue or blood compatibility between two individuals in which specific histocompatibility antigens, e.g. those present on leucocytes or erythrocytes, are detected by means of suitable isoimmune antisera.

tyramine enzyme present in cheese, game, yeast extracts, wine, beer, broad bean pods, with similar effect on the body to adrenaline. Foods containing tyramine should be avoided by women taking monoamine oxidase inhibitor drugs.

tyrosine a naturally occurring amino acid present in most proteins; it is a product of phenylalanine metabolism and a precursor of melanin, catecholamines, and thyroid hormones.

U

ulcer a lesion of the free surface of the skin or mucous membrane, caused by trauma, infection, pressure or nerve injury.

ultrasonic beyond the audible range; relating to sound waves having a frequency of more than 20 000 cycles per second.

ultrasonogram an echo picture obtained from using ULTRASOUND.

ultrasonography a radiological technique, originally developed in the 1960s, in which deep structures of the body are visualized by recording the reflections (echoes) of ultrasonic waves directed into the tissues. In diagnostic ultrasonography, the ultrasonic waves are produced by electrically stimulating a crystal called a transducer. As the beam strikes an interface or boundary between tissues of varying density some of the sound waves are reflected back to the transducer as echoes. The echoes are then converted into electrical impulses that are displayed as a television image, presenting a visual display of the tissues under examination. *A-mode u.* a display for measuring size and thickness accurately, particularly important in cephalometry. It uses impulses from the quartz crystal in the transducer and after amplication they are displayed on a cathode ray screen as vertical peaks from a horizontal line; the distances between the vertical lines are measured. *B-mode u.* builds up a picture of the deep tissues, each of which gives an echo according to its density and depth. It is possible to build up a valuable 2-dimensional sectional view by moving the transducer at right angles to the organs below it. GREY-SCALE DISPLAY shows more definition. *Real-time scanning* uses B-mode ultrasonography to view a moving image, for example to view fetal movements or beating of the fetal heart. Ultrasonography is used widely in obstetrics to confirm the presence and gestation of pregnancy, locate the placenta, estimate fetal size, weight and maturity, identify fetal abnormalities and to examine the uterine contents in cases of complete or incomplete abortion, ectopic or multiple pregnancy or hydatidiform mole. Liquor volume can be estimated and fetal ascites in cases of Rhesus incompatibility can be detected; fetal and uteroplacental blood flow can be measured. Fetal movements, including sucking, swallowing, breathing and eye movements, and filling and emptying of the fetal stomach and bladder can be observed. Ultrasonography is also used during invasive procedures such as amniocentesis and chorionic villus biopsy to avoid damage to the fetus and placenta.

ultrasound sound at frequencies above the upper limit of normal hearing, i.e. greater than about 20 000 Hz (cycles per second); used in medicine in the technique of ULTRASONOGRAPHY.

umbilical relating to the umbilicus. *U. catheterization* insertion of a

Prolapse of the Umbilical Cord

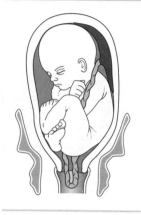

catheter into the umbilical vein or artery of the neonate, for the administration of drugs or fluids, continuous monitoring of blood gases, for exchange transfusion or obtaining blood samples for tests. *U. hernia* a protrusion of intestine through the umbilicus, usually slight but occasionally severe. *See* EXOMPHALOS.

umbilical cord the cord which connects the fetus and the placenta. It is usually 50–60 cm (20–24 in) long, has a spiral twist and consists of two umbilical arteries carrying deoxygenated blood and one umbilical vein carrying oxygenated blood, surrounded by Wharton's jelly and covered by amnion. Soon after birth the umbilical cord is clamped and cut. A stump of about 2.5 cm is left attached to the baby's umbilicus and this dies and separates naturally by a process of dry, aseptic necrosis

within 5–7 days. *Presentation of the u. c.* the cord lies below the presenting part, the membranes being intact. *Prolapse of the u. c.* the cord lies in advance of the presenting part, the membranes being ruptured. There is grave danger of pressure on the vessels of the cord and consequent fetal anoxia. The cause is a high or an ill-fitting presenting part, which allows a loop of cord to slip past. The principles in the treatment of this emergency are: (*a*) to lessen the pressure on the cord by any possible means, and permit the fetal oxygen supply to be maintained, and (*b*) to deliver the woman as quickly as possible.

umbilicus the navel; the scar in the abdomen marking the point at which the umbilical cord was attached.

unconscious 1. insensible; incapable of responding to sensory stimuli. 2. that part of the mental activity which includes primitive or repressed wishes, concealed from consciousness by the psychological censor.

uni- a prefix meaning 'one'.

unicellular consisting of one cell.

unilateral on one side only.

uniovular from one ovum. *See* MONOZYGOTIC.

universal donor *See* ABO BLOOD GROUPS.

universal recipient *See* ABO BLOOD GROUPS.

unstable lie when the lie of the fetus changes from one examination to another after 36 weeks' gestation. If the mother commences labour with the fetus in an abnormal lie, especially a compound lie, complications may arise which threaten the life of both the mother and the fetus, unless caesarean section can be undertaken. The mother may therefore be admitted before term for observation and external version of the fetus with a controlled membrane rupture and induction of labour.

unsupported mother a mother without a partner to support her; a one-parent family. The mother may be unmarried, separated, divorced or widowed.

urachal pertaining to the urachus. *U. cyst* congenital abnormality in which a small cyst persists along the course of the urachus. *U. fistula* one that forms when the urachus fails to close; urine may leak from the umbilicus.

urachus a fibrous band uniting the apex of the bladder to the umbilicus. It is a remnant of a canal present in the fetus.

uraemia the condition of renal failure in which the blood urea is very high. It is characterized by headache, vertigo, vomiting and convulsions, coma may ensue. It may complicate nephritis, concealed ABRUPTIO PLACENTAE or ECLAMPSIA.

urea the end product of protein metabolism, which is excreted in the urine. *Blood u.* the amount of urea present in the blood; normally 2.5–5.8 mmol/l (15–35 mg/100 ml) but in pregnancy usually 2.3–5.0 mmol/l (14–30 mg/100 ml).

ureter one of the two fibromuscular tubes which convey urine from the kidney to the bladder. They become dilated during pregnancy as PROGESTERONE relaxes the smooth muscle, leading to stasis of urine and multiplication of micro-organisms. *See* PYELONEPHRITIS.

ureteric relating to the ureter. *U. catheter* a fine catheter for insertion via the ureter into the pelvis of the kidney, either for drainage or for retrograde PYELOGRAPHY.

ureterovesical pertaining to a ureter and the vagina.

ureterovesical fistula an abnormal passage between a ureter and the vagina; a rare complication of prolonged or obstructed labour when the tissue of the ureter becomes devitalized due to prolonged pressure by the fetal head.

urethra the canal through which the urine is discharged from the bladder. The male urethra is 20–22.5 cm long, the female urethra 3.7 cm.

urethral relating to the urethra.

urethritis inflammation of the urethra. *Non-specific u.* a sexually transmitted disease, occurring in the male, the cause of which has not yet been identified.

urethrocele prolapse of female urethral wall, which may result from intrapartum pelvic floor damage.

uric pertaining to the urine. *U. acid* the end product of purine metabolism or oxidation in the body. It is present in the blood in a concentration of about 0.13–0.42 mmol/l and is excreted in the urine in amounts of slightly less than 1 g per day.

urinalysis analysis of the urine as an aid in the diagnosis of disease. In pregnancy the urine is regularly tested for the presence of protein, glucose and ketones. Blood and pus may also be detected in cases of infection. *U. tract infection* women are prone to urinary tract infection in pregnancy due to the stasis of urine which can occur in sections of the ureters kinked by the relaxation caused by progesterone. It commonly occurs between the 20th and 28th week of pregnancy, with the most common infecting organism being *Escherichia coli*. The woman is feverish and has frequency of micturition, dysuria, loin pain and nausea and vomiting. Hyperpyrexia with rigors and severe pain occur in severe cases and may precipitate the onset of preterm labour. Treatment includes the administration of antibiotics, analgesics, copious fluids.

Chronic PYELONEPHRITIS or renal failure are long-term complications.

urinary relating to urine.

urination micturition.

urine the fluid secreted by the kidneys, and excreted from the urinary bladder in micturition. The reaction is normally about pH 6. It consists of water (96%) in which are dissolved waste products of metabolism such as UREA and CREATININE, and other substances including sodium chloride and phosphates, but not normally glucose.

urinometer a glass instrument having a graduated stem weighted with a mercury bulb, used for measuring the specific gravity of urine.

urodynamics dynamics of the propulsion and flow of urine in the urinary tract.

urticaria a vascular reaction of the skin marked by transient appearance of slightly elevated patches which are redder or paler than the surrounding skin and often accompanied by severe itching; called also nettle rash. The cause may be certain foods, infection, or emotional stress.

uterine pertaining to the uterus. *U. souffle see* SOUFFLE. *U. tubes* FALLOPIAN TUBES.

uteroplacental pertaining to the uterus and placenta.

uterosacral pertaining to the uterus and sacrum. *U. ligaments* two ligaments which pass backward from the cervix to the sacrum, encircling the rectum. These ligaments help to maintain the uterus in a position of anteversion.

uterosalpingography radiography of the uterus and uterine tubes; hysterosalpingography.

uterotomy hysterotomy; incision of the uterus.

uterovesical referring to the uterus and bladder. *U. pouch* the fold of peritoneum between these two organs.

Uterus and Appendages

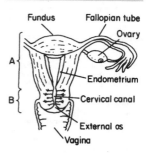

A, Body of uterus; B, cervix.

uterus the womb; a pear-shaped, hollow, muscular organ situated in the pelvic cavity between the bladder and the rectum, and supported by the parametrium. It is about 7.5 cm long, 5 cm at the widest part, and may be divided into two parts, the corpus, or body, which in the adult virgin uterus is the upper two-thirds, and the cervix, or neck, the lower third. The uppermost part, between the cornua, is termed the fundus, and the constriction between the corpus and cervix is described as the isthmus. The cavity of the body of the uterus is a triangular slit, communicating at the cornua with the fallopian tubes, and at the internal os with the cervix. The body of the uterus has a mucous membrane lining of ENDOMETRIUM which is shed about every 28 days. Should an ovum be fertilized, it embeds after 8 days and develops within the uterine cavity. The MYOMETRIUM, which is composed of interlacing spiral muscle fibres, hypertrophies, so growing to accommodate the fetus. The outer covering of the uterus is a fold of peritoneum, the PERIMETRIUM which hangs loosely over the fundus to form the uterovesical pouch between the anterior section of the uterus and the bladder, and the pouch of Douglas between the posterior section of the uterus and the rectum. *Bicornuate u.* a type of congenital malformation in which the uterus has two horns. *U. didelphys* a double uterus resulting from the failure of the two sides to unite during development. *U. unicornus* a uterus with only one horn, the other being underdeveloped.

uvula a small, fleshy mass hanging from the soft palate above the root of the tongue.

V

vaccinate to inoculate with a vaccine in order to procure immunity to a disease. *See* IMMUNITY.

vaccination 1. usually inoculation with the vaccinia virus in order to protect against smallpox. It was given routinely during the second year and again between the ages of 8 and 12 years. 2. where specified, the injection of a particular bacterial vaccine. *See* BACILLE CALMETTE–GUÉRIN.

vaccine a suspension of killed organisms in normal saline. *Attenuated v.* one prepared from living organisms which, through long cultivation, have lost their virulence. *Bacille Calmette–Guérin v.* an attenuated bovine bacillus to give protection from tuberculosis. *Salk v.* one prepared from a strain of poliomyelitis virus.

vacuum aspiration a method used to perform abortions during the first 3 months of pregnancy; also used to remove a hydatidiform mole.

vacuum extractor an apparatus, introduced first in Sweden, for use in suitable cases as an alternative to delivery by obstetric forceps. A metal cup is attached by suction to the fetal scalp, and gentle traction, synchronizing with the uterine contractions, is exerted. *See* Appendix 3, Figure 5.

vagal pertaining to the vagal nerve.

vagina the canal lined with squamous epithelium which leads from the vulva to the cervix uteri. It forms a part of the birth canal. The anterior wall, 6.5–7.5 cm in length, has the urethra and bladder base embedded in it. The posterior wall, 9–10 cm long, is in contact with the perineal body, the rectum and the pouch of Douglas. The lateral walls are in contact with the levator ani muscles.

vaginal pertaining to, or through, the vagina. *V. bleeding, see* ANTEPARTUM HAEMORRHAGE. *V. discharge, see* DISCHARGE. *V. examination* or *examination per vaginam* a means of assessing factors of pregnancy, labour and puerperium and gynaecological conditions by palpation with one or two fingers in the vagina.

vaginismus painful spasms of the muscles of the vagina.

vaginitis inflammation of the vagina. In pregnancy it is commonly due to infection with the fungus *Candida albicans*. This causes considerable irritation and is usually treated with NYSTATIN pessaries or rarely by swabbing with 0.5% aqueous gentian violet solution. Vaginitis due to *Trichomonas vaginalis* is also common. It is characterized by a frothy, intensely irritant, greenish discharge. The woman and her sexual partner are treated with metronidazole (Flagyl).

vagus the 10th cranial nerve, a parasympathetic nerve having a wide distribution in the body and supplying the heart, lungs, liver and part of the alimentary tract.

validation a process of approval of an academic course or award. Within midwifery, the NURSING AND MID-

WIFERY COUNCIL requires institutional approval of all pre-registration programmes, both before commencement and at regular intervals during the agreed period of approval, to ensure maintenance of consistent standards.

validity a term used in research to determine the extent to which a process actually reflects the construct being examined when used for a specific group or purpose.

Valium *See* DIAZEPAM.

Valsalva manoeuvre increase of intra-thoracic pressure by forcible exhalation against the closed glottis. Infants with respiratory distress adopt a partial Valsalva manoeuvre by grunting, thereby maintaining a positive pressure in the chest even during exhalation, i.e. a POSITIVE END-EXPIRATORY PRESSURE (PEEP).

value a measure of worth or efficiency; a quantitative measurement of the activity, concentration, etc., of specific substances. *Normal v's* a range in concentration of specific substances found in normal healthy tissues, secretions, etc.

valve a membranous fold in a canal or passage that prevents backward flow of material passing through it.

valvotomy a surgical operation to increase the lumen of a narrowed valve, e.g. mitral valvotomy to relieve MITRAL STENOSIS.

valvuloplasty plastic repair of a valve, especially a valve of the heart.

vanillylmandelic acid (VMA) an excretory product of the catecholamines, used as a test for adrenaline metabolism. Levels of VMA are raised in cases of adrenal tumours such as PHAEOCHROMOCYTOMA, a benign tumour sometimes diagnosed during pregnancy, when the woman's blood pressure characteristically presents with morning and evening peaks.

The test involves the collection of a 24-hour urine sample; it is used less now than direct estimations of catecholamine levels.

variable in epidemiology any measurement that can have different values. *Dependent v.* a variable which is dependent on the effect of other variables in an epidemiological study. *Independent v.* a variable not influenced by other variables in an epidemiological study but which may be the cause of alterations in these variables.

variance a measure of the variation seen in a set of data.

varicella chickenpox.

varicose swollen or dilated. *V. veins* abnormally distended and tortuous veins, usually those of the leg, due to inefficient valves which permit some back- or cross-flow of blood, particularly in the communicating veins between the superficial and deep veins. They may appear or become troublesome for the first time during pregnancy, when high progesterone levels relax the vessel walls, so permitting further stasis and inefficient venous return. Varicose veins may also develop in the vulva, or the rectum, as HAEMORRHOIDS.

variola smallpox.

varix an enlarged tortuous vein, artery, or lymphatic vessel. pl. *varices*.

vas a vessel. pl. *vasa*. *V. deferens* the tube through which the spermatozoa pass from the testis to be stored in the seminal vesicle to become part of the semen.

vasa praevia the presentation, in front of the fetal head during labour, of the blood vessels of the umbilical cord where they enter the placenta in a velamentous insertion of the cord. When the membranes rupture, bleeding from these vessels may occur, causing severe fetal distress.

vascular relating to, or consisting largely of, vessels.

vasectomy removal of a portion of the VAS DEFERENS through a small incision in the scrotum so that the semen is free of spermatozoa after about 4 months. Other methods of contraception should be continued until three consecutive semen specimens have been clear.

vasoconstrictor causing contraction of blood vessels.

vasodepressor 1. having the effect of lowering the blood pressure through reduction in peripheral resistance. 2. an agent that causes vasodepression.

vasodilator causing dilatation of blood vessels.

vasomotor controlling the muscles of blood vessels, both dilator and constrictor.

vasopressin a pressor agent produced in the pituitary gland. Also known as antidiuretic hormone.

vasopressor 1. stimulating contraction of the muscular tissue of the capillaries and arteries. 2. a vasopressor agent.

vault the part of the fetal skull (excluding the base and face), which contains the cerebral hemispheres. It is made up of the two frontal, two parietal, two temporal and one occipital bone. These bones are separated by membranous sutures which allow moulding of the fetal skull in labour and growth of the brain. *V. cap* a contraceptive device; a bowl-shaped cap which is attached to the vaginal vault by suction to prevent spermatozoa entering the cervix and the subsequent risk of pregnancy. It should be used in conjunction with a spermicidal agent to increase its effectiveness. *V. of the vagina* the upper part of the vagina into which the cervix protrudes.

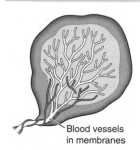

Velamentous Insertion of Cord

Blood vessels in membranes

vegan a vegetarian who excludes from his/her diet all foods of animal origin.

vegetarian a person who eats only food of vegetable origin. *V. diet* one in which no meat is eaten. A *lacto-vegetarian* diet prohibits the intake of meat, poultry, fish and eggs. An *ovo-lacto-vegetarian* diet allows all foods from plants plus eggs, milk and other dairy products. An *ovo-vegetarian* diet allows eggs and foods of plant origin, but prohibits and other dairy products. An *ovo-vegetarian* diet allows eggs and foods of plant origin, but prohibits all animal and dairy products.

vein a vessel carrying blood from the capillaries back to the heart. It has thin walls and a lining endothelium from which the venous valves are formed.

velamentous like a veil. *V. insertion of the umbilical cord* a placenta in which the umbilical cord vessels divide before reaching the placenta. *See also* VASA PREVIA.

vena cava one of the two trunk veins which return the venous blood from the upper and lower parts of the body, respectively, to the right atrium of the heart.

venepuncture the puncture of a vein, usually to obtain blood or administer a drug.

venereal concerning or resulting from sexual intercourse. *V. diseases* SYPHILIS, GONORRHOEA and SOFT CHANCRE.

venesection opening a vein and withdrawing blood to relieve congestion.

ventilation 1. providing fresh air in a room or building. 2. the process of exchange of air between the lungs and ambient air. Pulmonary ventilation refers to the total exchange whereas alveolar ventilation refers to the ventilation of the alveoli where gas exchange with the blood takes place. *Intermittent positive-pressure v. (IPPV)* mechanical ventilation by a machine designed to deliver breathing gas until equilibrium is established between the patient's lungs and the VENTILATOR.

ventilator an apparatus designed to qualify the air that is breathed through it or to intermittently or continuously control pulmonary ventilation; called also respirator.

Ventolin *See* SALBUTAMOL.

ventouse *See* VACUUM EXTRACTOR.

ventricle a small pouch or cavity; applied especially to the lower chambers of the heart, and to the four cavities of the brain.

ventricular septal defect a congenital heart defect in which there is persistent patency of the ventricular septum which allows a flow of blood directly from one ventricle to the other, thereby bypassing the pulmonary circulation and causing cyanosis because of oxygen deficiency.

ventrosuspension an operation. At LAPAROTOMY or laparoscopy the round ligaments are shortened to help antevert a RETROVERTED UTERUS.

venule a minute vein.

vernix caseosa the greasy substance which covers the fetus *in utero*. It is a secretion from the sebaceous glands, together with desquamated cells, which appears at about 30–32 weeks, is abundant at 36–37 weeks, and may remain until term or even past full term.

version turning the fetus *in utero*, to alter a lie or presentation to one which is more favourable. *Cephalic v.* turning the child to make the head present. *External v.* turning the child by manipulation through the abdominal wall. *Internal v.* inserting the hand into the uterus, turning the child with one hand in the uterus and the other on the abdomen. *Podalic v.* turning the child to make the breech present. In practice, external cephalic version is fairly frequently carried out about the 34th week of pregnancy in a case of breech presentation, since vertex delivery is so much more favourable to the child than breech delivery. Internal version is seldom performed, as with good antenatal care the necessity seldom arises. Occasionally, an internal podalic version (followed by a breech extraction) may be performed when a multigravid woman is in labour with an oblique lie of the fetus or in the event of an oblique lie of a second twin.

vertebrae the irregular bones forming the spinal column. They are divided into 7 cervical, 12 thoracic, 5 lumbar, 5 sacral (sacrum) and 4 coccygeal (coccyx) bones. sing. *vertebra*.

vertex an area of the head bounded by the anterior and posterior fontanelles, and laterally by the parietal eminences. *V. presentation* the fetus is so flexed that the vertex lies over the internal os, and is the first part to appear at the vulva. This is the most favourable presentation for delivery.

vertigo giddiness, a temporary dizzy sensation, with loss of equilibrium.

vesica a bladder; usually referring to the urinary bladder; *see* ECTOPIA VESICAE.

vesical relating to the bladder.

vesicle a blister or small sac usually containing fluid.

vesicovaginal pertaining to the bladder and vagina. *V. fistula* an abnormal opening between the bladder and the vagina; a rare complication of prolonged or obstructed labour when the tissues of the bladder are devitalized by prolonged pressure of the fetal head.

vesicular relating to, or containing, vesicles. *V. mole* HYDATIDIFORM MOLE.

vestibule an entrance. The part of the vulva lying between the labia minora.

vestige a remnant of a structure that functioned in a previous stage of species or individual development. *adj. vestigial.*

viable capable of independent life. A term applied to the fetus after 24 weeks of intrauterine life.

Viagra sildenafil citrate, oral drug used to treat erectile dysfunction; increases male ability to achieve and maintain penile erection during sexual stimulation.

vicarious 1. substituted for another; used when one organ functions instead of another. 2. occurring in circumstances where not normally expected. *V. liability* a situation in which the employer is vicariously liable for the torts of the employee during the course of his/her employment, e.g. a health authority is vicariously liable for the torts of a midwife during the course of her employment.

villi fine hair-like processes projecting from a surface. *Chorionic v.* branched processes which develop on the trophoblast, and which dip into the maternal blood of the placental site. *See* PLACENTA *and* CHORIONIC VILLI. *Intestinal v.* minute projections on the intestinal mucosa. Each villus has a blood capillary and a lacteal. They are the sites of absorption of fluids and nutrients.

viraemia the presence of viruses in the blood.

viral caused by or having the nature of a virus.

virgin a girl or woman who has not had sexual intercourse.

virility 1. the state of possessing masculine qualities. 2. male sexual potency.

virus small infective agent which can only grow and reproduce in living cells, and can only be seen with the electron microscope. They are complex and often difficult to culture. They cause, amongst many other diseases: smallpox, poliomyelitis, influenza, rabies, measles and rubella. Viruses cross the placenta and can cause fetal abnormalities, especially during the first trimester of pregnancy.

viscera internal organs in the body cavities, e.g. heart, liver, uterus.

viscid sticky and glutinous.

visual analogue scale a method of quantifying subjective feelings such as pain, sedation, etc. Consists of a line 10 cm long, one end of the line indicating absence of the feeling, e.g. pain, and the other, extreme sensation or pain. The individual marks a point along the line which represents the pain or other sensation he or she is feeling at that time. The distance from the left-hand end of the line to the point is measured and represents a numerical assessment of the pain or other sensation.

visual disturbances during pregnancy may occur in women with severe PRE-ECLAMPSIA or impending ECLAMPSIA, due to retinal and optic nerve oedema.

visualization technique of using imagination and relaxation to create any desired changes in a person's life.

vital relating to or necessary to life. *V. statistics* the records kept of births and deaths among the population, including the causes of death, and the factors which seem to influence their rise and fall.

vitamins essential food substances, minute quantities of which are essential to nutrition and health. Vitamins A, D, E and K are fat-soluble, and B and C water-soluble. *Vitamin A* found in fish liver oils, cream, milk and egg yolk and in vegetables such as carrots, spinach and watercress. Deficiency causes night blindness, failure of growth and lack of resistance to infection. *Vitamin B* this group consists of a number of substances. (*a*) Thiamine (aneurine vitamin B_1) is found in the husks of cereals and yeasts. Deficiency results in neurological symptoms, cardiovascular dysfunction, oedema and reduced intestinal motility. (*b*) Nicotinic acid (niacin) is found in liver, kidney and yeast. Deficiency causes pellagra, where gastrointestinal, skin and mental disturbances occur. (*c*) Riboflavin (B_2) is found in liver, kidney, heart, brewer's yeast, milk, eggs, greens and enriched cereals. Deficiency causes inflammation of the tongue and seborrhoeic dermatitis. (*d*) Cyanocobalamin (B_{12}) and folic acid are both essential for red cell formation. If there is a

deficiency, as may occur due to fetal demands in pregnancy, megaloblastic or macrocytic ANAEMIA may develop. (*e*) Pantothenic acid, pyridoxine (B_6) and biotin are also part of the B complex. *Vitamin C* ascorbic acid. Found in fresh fruits, especially citrus, blackcurrants, tomatoes and rosehips. Deficiency causes scurvy and delays the healing of wounds, probably due to slow formation of collagen. *Vitamin D* found in similar animal sources to vitamin A, but can also be manufactured by skin exposed to sunlight. It is essential for the absorption of calcium and phosphorus. Deficiency causes rickets, osteomalacia and neonatal HYPOCALCAEMIA. Both vitamins are especially necessary during pregnancy and lactation. *Vitamin E* deficiency leads to sterility in rats, but the function in humans is not known. *Vitamin K* is necessary for the formation of PROTHROMBIN. It is found in spinach, cabbage, cauliflower and oats. It is also synthesized in the intestine by bacteria. Deficiency rarely occurs except when the gut is sterile, i.e. when taking a broad-spectrum antibiotic or if HAEMORRHAGIC DISEASE occurs in the first days of life.

volvulus torsion of a loop of intestine, causing obstruction with or without strangulation.

vomiting expulsion of the contents of the stomach through the mouth. *V. of blood* HAEMATEMESIS. *V. in the newborn* this is very common and has many causes. (*a*) Bile-stained vomit without the passage of meconium indicates intestinal obstruction; the sooner after delivery the higher the site. (*b*) Blood-stained vomit may be due to maternal blood swallowed at delivery or ingested from cracked nipples, or to the infant's own blood in cases of HAEM-

ORRHAGIC DISEASE. Maternal and infant blood may be differentiated by SINGER'S TEST. (c) Milk may be vomited owing to various infections (including infections of the urinary tract, GASTROENTERITIS and MENINGITIS), to a relaxed cardia, to feeding problems or to raised intracranial pressure. *V. in pregnancy* (a) occurs in up to 90% of pregnancies, most commonly in the first 3 months but may persist throughout pregnancy. Characterized by nausea, sometimes accompanied by vomiting, often occurring on rising in the morning, but also at other times. There have been many theories as to the cause, but none is as yet proved. (b) HYPEREMESIS GRAVIDARUM. (c) Intercurrent vomiting in pregnancy is often due to PYELONEPHRITIS, other infections and diseases of the gastro-intestinal tract and other severe illnesses. Vomiting in association with hypertension, oedema and protein-uria in late pregnancy may be a serious sign of severe PRE-ECLAMPSIA or impending ECLAMPSIA due to liver oedema and/or haemorrhage. The midwife should consult a doctor about any woman who has persistent vomiting after the 14th week of pregnancy or who, at any time, has KETONURIA. *Projectile v.* this occurs in hypertrophic PYLORIC STENOSIS.

vomitus material vomited.

vulsellum *See* FORCEPS *and* Appendix 3.

vulva the external female genital organs.

vulvectomy excision of the vulva.

vulvitis inflammation of the vulva.

W

'waiter's tip' a characteristic position of forearm and hand with ERB'S PARALYSIS.

warfarin an anticoagulant drug which crosses the placenta so, if used, is confined to the weeks 16–36. The dose given should control the pro-thrombin time to 2.5–3.5 times above normal.

warts an epidermal tumour of viral origin. *Genital w.* spread in pregnancy and may cover the vulva, perineum and anal regions. They can be treated effectively with podophyllin applied locally.

Wassermann reaction a serological test used in the diagnosis of SYPHILIS.

waterbirth a form of care in which the mother chooses to labour and may deliver in water, to achieve relaxation and a degree of pain relief. Portable pools are available to hire or buy for women wishing to have a waterbirth at home or in a maternity unit where no waterbirth facility is provided. Midwives attending these women should have obtained adequate preparation.

weaning detaching or alienating from an accustomed habit or enjoyment. In infant feeding it can be from breast to bottle or cup feeding, from bottle to cup feeding or, more commonly from any type of milk feed to solid food.

webbed connected by a membrane or strand of tissue. *W. hands* or *feet* congenital abnormality in which the digits are not separated from each other. Syndactyly. *W. neck* folds of skin in neck, giving a webbed appearance. Occurs in certain congenital conditions, e.g. Turner's syndrome.

wedlock the state of being married.

weight gain during pregnancy the normal weight gain is about 10–12 kg, though there are appreciable variations. It is accounted for as follows: full-term fetus 3.4 kg, placenta 0.7 kg, liquor amnii 1 kg, uterus 1 kg, blood 1.4 kg, breasts 1 kg and a considerable increase in tissue fluid and fat and protein deposition. The weight gain is about 2.5 kg in the first 20 weeks and 10 kg in the last 20 weeks, so a weekly gain of more than 0.5 kg may indicate occult OEDEMA which occurs as an early sign of PRE-ECLAMPSIA. *W. g. in babies* the neonate loses up to 10% of its birth weight in the first few days of life, but should have regained this by 10–14 days. Subsequently the baby should gain approximately 200 g per week.

Weil's disease spirochaetal jaundice caused by *Leptospira icterohaemor-rhagiae*, transmitted by rat urine and acquired through the skin or infected food or water.

welfare foods nutritious foods sold in clinics at non-profit-making prices.

well woman clinic a 'prophylactic' clinic available to screen women for breast and cervical cancer, anaemia, diabetes and hypertension.

Wernicke's encephalopathy acute haemorrhagic encephalitis, occurring occasionally in severe HYPER-EMESIS GRAVIDARUM as a result of vitamin B$_1$ deficiency.

Wertheim's operation See HYSTER-ECTOMY.

wet-nurse a woman who breastfeeds infants other than her own.

Wharton's jelly connective tissue of the umbilical cord.

whey the fluid part of milk, separated from the curd after the addition of rennet. It is easily digested, as the casein and fat have been removed.

white asphyxia a term formerly used to describe a baby with a low APGAR SCORE where the skin is white due to circulatory collapse. Now called severe asphyxia. See ASPHYXIA NEONATORUM.

white leg See PHLEGMASIA ALBA DOLENS.

white matter, white substance the white nervous tissue, constituting the conducting portion of the brain and spinal cord, composed mostly of myelinated nerve fibres. Grey matter or substance is the term used to describe the tissues composed of unmyelinated fibres.

WHO International Code of Marketing of Breast Milk Substitutes a code developed by the World Health Organization and UNICEF to protect and promote the practice of breast-feeding and to control the marketing of products for artificial feeding, especially in developing countries. Recommendations include: prohibition of advertising/promotion direct to the public; no free samples of breast milk substitutes or any other free gifts, special offers and discounts to be given to mothers; no financial or other rewards to be given to health workers for the purpose of promoting breast milk substitutes; professional information

on breast milk substitutes should contain only scientific and factual data and in no way imply superiority of the product over human breast milk.

whooping cough See PERTUSSIS.

Widal reaction a blood test used in the diagnosis of typhoid and paratyphoid fevers.

Wilson–Mikity syndrome BRONCHO-PULMONARY DYSPLASIA, which is a condition occurring in babies who have been ventilated for long periods or have needed prolonged oxygen therapy.

wolffian bodies two small organs in the embryo, which are the primitive kidneys.

womb the uterus.

World Health Organization (WHO) the specialized agency of the United Nations that is concerned with health on an international level. One of its campaigns was Safe Motherhood for all by the year 2000, since the maternal mortality rate is still very high in many developing countries.

wound a bodily injury caused by physical means, with disruption of the normal continuity of structures. In healing of a wound by first intention, restoration of tissue continuity occurs directly, without granulation; in healing by second intention, wound repair following tissue loss is accomplished by closure of the wound with granulation tissue; healing by third intention occurs when a wound is initially unable to close owing to contamination, and is closed 4–5 days after the injury.

Wrigley's forceps obstetric forceps used for very low forceps deliveries, the aftercoming head of the breech, or at caesarean section. See Appendix 3.

X

X chromosome one of the two sex chromosomes, the other being Y. Female cells carry two X chromosomes (XX) and male cells one X and one Y chromosome (XY). During maturation of the ovum and spermatozoon, one of these is cast off. At fertilization the two remaining determine the sex of the child: X and X, a girl, X and Y, a boy. *See also* TURNER'S SYNDROME *and* KLINEFELTER'S SYNDROME.

X-linked transmitted by genes on the X chromosome; sex-linked.

X-rays RÖNTGEN RAYS. Electromagnetic waves of short wavelength which are capable of penetrating many substances, such as paper, wood and flesh, but are absorbed by lead, platinum or bone.

xiphisternum XIPHOID PROCESS.

xiphoid process a small cartilaginous process at the lower end of the sternum. Also termed xiphisternum and ensiform cartilage. One of the landmarks to which the FUNDUS UTERI is related in the latter weeks of pregnancy.

XO symbol for the karyotype observed in most cases of TURNER'S SYNDROME, in which there is only one sex chromosome, an X chromosome.

Xylocaine *See* LIDOCAINE (LIGNOCAINE) HYDROCHLORIDE.

XYY syndrome a rare condition in males in which there is an extra Y chromosome, making a total of 47 in each body cell. Often the affected males are very tall, and liable to exhibit aggressive and antisocial behaviour.

Y

Y chromosome one of the two sex chromosomes, which, united with X is found in the cells of males.

yaws a non-venereal treponemal infection found widely in tropical areas. Local lesions resemble those of SYPHILIS and serological tests for syphilis are positive.

yeast a species of fungi which reproduce by budding. They produce fermentation in malt and fruit juices, producing alcohol, as in beer and wine. THRUSH is due to infection by the yeast-like fungus *Candida albicans*.

yin and yang two complementary principles of Chinese philosophy incorporated into traditional Chinese medicine. Yin is feminine, dark, negative; yang is masculine, bright and positive. Yin–yang balance and har-

mony denotes optimum health and well-being.

yoga Indian philosophical approach to health and well-being, involving breathing, relaxation and exercise. Some forms are suitable for pregnant women.

yolk sac one of the two spaces which occurs in the inner cell mass of the trophoblast (the other space being the amniotic cavity). It is surrounded by entodermal cells, whereas the amniotic cavity is surrounded by ectodermal cells and between the two is an intervening layer of mesoderm. The embryo is formed from the area where the three tissues, ectoderm, mesoderm and entoderm lie in apposition.

Yutopar *See* RITODRINE HYDROCHLORIDE.

Z

zero the symbol 0. Nought. The point in any thermometric scale at which the measuring of temperature starts. In the Celsius thermometer, zero is the melting point of ice. In the Fahrenheit thermometer, zero is 32° below the melting of ice. *See* FAHRENHEIT *and* CELSIUS.

zidovudine antiviral drug used to retard the process of AIDS. Also known as azidothymidine or AZT.

zinc a trace element that is the component of several enzymes. It is found in red meat, shellfish, liver, peas, lentils, beans and rice. A severe deficiency of zinc can retard growth in children, cause a low sperm count in men and retard wound healing.

zona pellucida the transparent, noncellular, secreted layer surrounding an OVUM. SPERM release the enzymes which allow penetration of the zona pellucida but only one will enter the ovum at the time of fertilization.

Zovirax *See* ACICLOVIR.

zygote the fertilized OVUM prior to SEGMENTATION.

zygote intrafallopian transfer (ZIFT) infertility treatment in which ovulation is stimulated artificially, oocytes are harvested using ultrasounddirected follicle aspiration (UDFA) transvaginally or at laparoscopy and transferred at laparoscopy into the midampullary section of the fallopian tube, once fertilization has taken place.

Appendices

Appendix 1
Apgar Score

Sign	Score		
	0	1	2
Colour	Blue to pale	Body pink, limbs blue	Pink
Respiratory effort	Absent	Irregular gasps	Strong cry
Heart rate	Absent	Less than 100/minute	Over 100/minute
Muscle tone	Limp	Some flexion of limbs	Strong active movements
Reflex irritability	Nil	Grimace or sneeze	Cry

Apgar score 8–10: normal.
Apgar score 5–8: mild asphyxia.
Apgar score 4 or below: severe asphyxia.
See also Appendix 7.

Appendix 2
Normal Blood and Urine Values and Tests

Values given below should be used as a guide only. It is extremely likely that values for normal or reference ranges will vary between laboratories. This variation will usually now be minimal due to national and international standardization. However, certain parameters, particularly enzymes, may show considerable variation, depending on assay conditions and units of measurement. Some laboratories may report values using 'traditional' units as opposed to SI units, which may have a very significant effect on the numeric value of a result.

Before taking samples for laboratory analysis, it is advisable to check whether any preparations of the patient, or special timing or conditions for handling the sample are necessary. These may vary between laboratories.

It is *essential* that the reference ranges for the laboratory providing the analysis are used to evaluate results of tests.

Specimens should be collected at appropriate times and under appropriate conditions into the correct containers.

Specimens and request forms must be adequately labelled with:

- patient's name,
- number or date of birth,
- location,
- date and time of specimen.

Failure to comply may result in serious errors in diagnosis and management.

Specimens required for common tests
Note that the colour coding of blood sample bottles is not standardized, and care should be taken to use the correct specimen preservatives. Separate specimens may not be required for each test. Care should be taken to avoid contamination of samples with preservatives from other bottles.

Pathology departments usually contain different laboratories: *B*iochemistry (may be called Chemical Pathology), *H*aematology, Blood *T*ransfusion, *M*icrobiology, Histopathology. Location of tests may vary between establishments.

Laboratory	Note	Test/reason	Mother sample	size	Baby sample	size
T/H		ABO group + Rh factor	clotted/EDTA	6 ml	clotted/EDTA	1 ml
B		Abuse drug screen (urine)	MSU	20 ml	MSU	2 ml
B	1	AFP/Bart's/Leeds	clotted	6 ml		
T/H		Antibodies	clotted/EDTA	6 ml	clotted/EDTA	1 ml
B		Blood sugar	fluoride oxalate	2 ml	fluoride oxalate	1 ml
H/B		Chromosomes	heparinized	4 ml	heparinized	2 ml
H		Clotting studies	citrate	3 ml	citrate	1 ml
H		Ferritin	clotted	6 ml	clotted	2 ml
H		Folate (RBC)	EDTA	3 ml		
H		Folate (serum)	clotted	6 ml		
T/H	1	Fragile X	EDTA	3 ml	EDTA	2 ml
H	2	Full blood count (FBC)	EDTA	3 ml	EDTA	1 ml
H		Genotype/electrophoresis	EDTA	3 ml	EDTA	1 ml
H		Haemoglobin (Hb)	EDTA	2 ml	EDTA	1 ml
B	4	HbA1c	EDTA	2 ml		
M	4	HBsAg	clotted	6 ml	clotted	2 ml
M	4	HIV	clotted	6 ml	clotted	2 ml

Laboratory	Note	Test/reason	Mother		Baby	
			sample	size	sample	size
B	3	Liver function test	clotted	6 ml	heparinized	2 ml
B		Pregnancy test (blood)	clotted	2 ml		
M		Pregnancy test (urine)	MSU	20 ml		
M		Rubella immunity	clotted	6 ml	clotted	2 ml
B	3	Thyroid function test	clotted	6 ml	heparinized	2 ml
M		Toxoplasmosis	clotted	6 ml	clotted	2 ml
M		TPHA	clotted	6 ml	clotted	2 ml
B	5	U & E	clotted	6 ml	heparinized	2 ml
B		Urate	clotted	6 ml	heparinized	2 ml
M		VDRL	clotted	6 ml	clotted	2 ml
H	6	Vitamin B$_{12}$	clotted	6 ml		

Notes
1. May not be routinely available or subject to local practice – check with laboratory.
2. Sample must go to laboratory immediately.
3. Note local reference ranges.
4. May need preliminary patient counselling.
5. Sample should reach laboratory in < 3 hours for potassium.
6. Vitamin B$_{12}$ falls throughout pregnancy.

Blood

	Units	Mother Non-pregnant	Mother Pregnant	Baby	Baby age	Comments
Red cells (erythrocytes/RBC)	$\times 10^{12}/l$	4–5		6–6.5 / 4–5	Birth / 4 weeks	
Glucose (fasting)	mmol/l	3.3–5.3	3.3–6.1	1.0–6.0		
Haemoglobin	g/dl	12–15		12.2–24 / 12.2–22	Birth / 1 week	Check local units
Packed cell volume (PCV haematocrit)	l/l	0.42–0.50		0.52–0.58 / 0.46–0.54	Day 1 / 2 weeks	Check local units
Reticulocytes	$\times 10^{9}/l$	20–100		100–300 / 5–23	Day 1 / Day 7	
Leucocytes	$\times 10^{9}/l$	4.0–11.0	4.0–15.0	5–19		
neutrophils	$\times 10^{9}/l$	2.5–7.5				
lymphocytes	$\times 10^{9}/l$	1.8–3.5				
monocytes	$\times 10^{9}/l$	0.2–0.8				
eosinophils	$\times 10^{9}/l$	0.04–0.4				
basophils	$\times 10^{9}/l$	0.0–0.1				
Platelets	$\times 10^{9}/l$	150–400				
pH		7.35–7.45		7.35–7.45		
P_{CO_2}	kPa	4.7–6.0				
Standard bicarbonate	mmol/l	24.0–32.0				Check local units

Plasma/serum						
Albumin	g/l	36–52	22–44	28–40		Check local ranges
Alanine transaminase AlT/SGPT	IU/l	5–35				Check local ranges
Aspartate transaminase AsT/SGOT	IU/l	5–35				See charts below
Bilirubin	μmol/l	<17	<17	<200	<10 days	
				<40	>10 days	
Calcium	mmol/l	2.1–2.6	2.2–2.4	1.9–2.9		
Chloride	mmol/l	95–105		96–106		
Cholesterol	mmol/l	3.6–6.7	5.4–7.8	2.1–4.1		
Creatinine	μmol/l	60–120		9–62	2 weeks–	
Ferritin	μg/l	14–40		90–640	6 months	
Folate	μg/l	1.7–10				
Magnesium	mmol/l	0.8–1.0		0.6–1.6		
Osmolality	mOsm/kg	285–295		280–305		
Phosphate	mmol/l	0.8–1.4	0.8–1.5	1.3–2.7		
Potassium	mmol/l	3.8–5.0	50–70	4.0–6.0		Elevated by haemolysis
Protein (total)	g/l	62–75		50–65		
Sodium	mmol/l	135–145	elevated	136–143		
Thyroid-binding globulin TBG	variable	variable				Check local units
Thyroid-stimulating hormone TSH	mU/l	0.5–4.7		<0.5–8.0		
Thyroxine (free) FT4	pmol/l	9–25		15–30	1–3 days	
Thyroxine (total) TT4	nmol/l	50–140	72–206	140–300	1–4 weeks	
				125–200		
Triiodothyronine (free) FT3	pmol/l	3–9	3–9	3–9		

	Units	Mother		Baby	Baby age	Comments
		Non-pregnant	Pregnant			
Plasma/serum *continued*						
Triiodothyronine (total) TT3	nmol/l	0.9–3.0				
TT4/TBG ratio			reduced			Check local units
Urate	mmol/l	0.09–0.36	0.15–0.52	0.12–0.34		
Urea	mmol/l	2.5–5.8	2.3–5.0	3.4–8.4		
Vitamin B₁₂	ng/l	179–1132	reduced			Falls until term
Red cell						
Folate	µg/l	125–800				
Glucose-6-phosphate dehydrogenase (G6PD)	IU/g Hb	4.6–13.5		4.6–13.5		Elevated by reticulocytosis
Urine						
Calcium	mmol/24 h	2.5–7.5				
Creatinine	mmol/24 h	9–17				
Calcium:creatinine ratio				<1.2		

	Units	Mother		Baby	Baby age	Comments
		Non-pregnant	Pregnant			
Creatinine clearance	ml/min	80–130	80–140	40–1400		Consider with serum
Osmolality	mOsm/kg	>600		25–125		
Potassium	mmol/24 h	25–125				
Protein	g/24 h	<0.15		<0.05		Must be fresh sample
Reducing substances		negative		negative		Diet dependent
Sodium	mmol/24 h	27–290		40–210		
CSF						
Glucose	mmol/l	2.5–4.5		2.5–5.0		Relates to blood glucose
Protein	g/l	0.15–0.40		0.15–0.50		
Stool						
Reducing substances				negative		Must be fresh sample

Values given are intended as a guide. Local units and reference ranges should always be used in preference to those shown. Where ranges are not shown, the same values as given for *non-pregnant mother* apply.

289

Appendix 3
Obstetric Instruments

FIGURE 1. Cross-section of a Copeland fetal skin electrode.

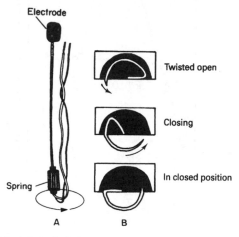

A, Copeland electrode; B, Cross-section of a Copeland electrode.

FIGURE 2. Instruments for artificial rupture of the membranes.

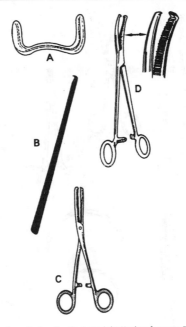

A, Sims' speculum; B, Amnihook; C, straight Kocher forceps; D, curved Kocher forceps.

FIGURE 3. Instruments for perineal repair.

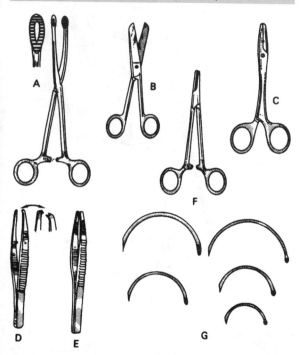

A, Sponge-holding forceps; B, blunt-ended scissors; C, needle holder; D, toothed dissecting forceps; E, non-toothed dissecting forceps; F, small Spencer Wells artery forceps; G, needles: left, round-bodied Nos. 8 and 12; right, cutting, Nos. 6, 8 and 12, Atraumatic needle 40 mm on Dexon suture now commonly used.

FIGURE 4. Obstetric forceps.

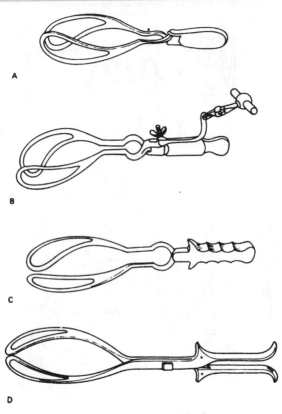

A, Wrigley's; B, axis-traction; C, Anderson's; D, Kjelland's.

FIGURE 5. Malmström vacuum extractor, showing the vacuum pump and three sizes of cup; chain and handle, and components of the extraction pump.

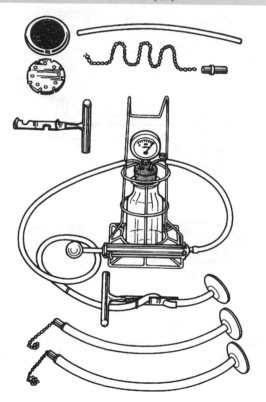

FIGURE 6. Various specula.

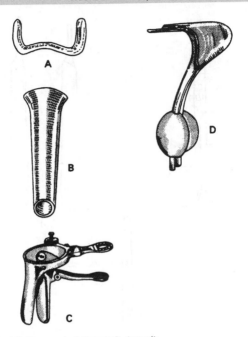

A, Sims'; B, Fergusson's; C, Cusco's; D, Auvard's.

FIGURE 7. Instruments for caesarean section.

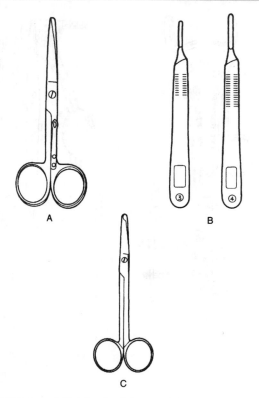

A, Nurse's scissors; B, Blade handles; C, Spencer stitch scissors.

FIGURE 7. Instruments for caesarean section (*continued*).

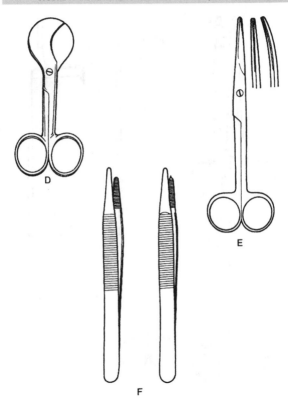

D, Umbilical scissors; E, Mayo scissors; F, plain and toothed Bonney dissecting forceps.

FIGURE 7. Instruments for caesarean section (*continued*).

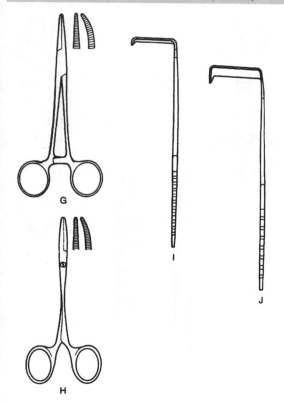

G, Moynihan artery forceps; H, Spencer Wells forceps; I, Langenbeck retractor; J, Morris retractor.

FIGURE 7. Instruments for caesarean section (*continued*).

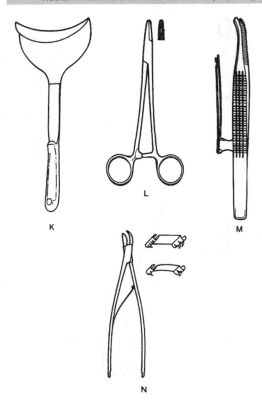

K, Doyen retractor; L, Mayo needle holder; M, Childe approximating forceps; N, Michel clips.

FIGURE 7. Instruments for caesarean section (*continued*).

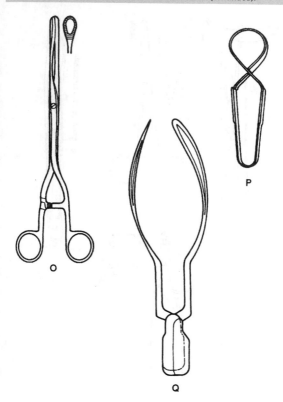

O, Rampley sponge-holding forceps; P, Backhaus H cross action towel clips; Q, Wrigley's forceps.

FIGURE 7. Instruments for caesarean section (*continued*).

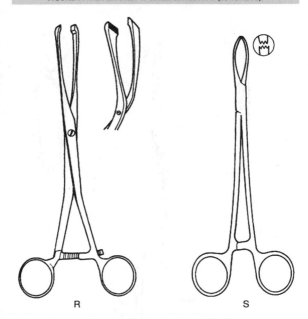

R, Green Armytage forceps; S, Littlewood tissue-holding forceps.

FIGURE 7. Instruments for caesarean section (*continued*).

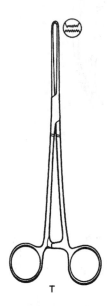

T

T, Stiles forceps.

Appendix 4
Identification of Fetal Position on Examination *per vaginam*

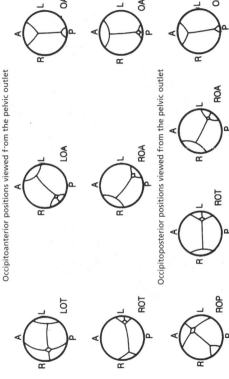

Occipitoanterior positions viewed from the pelvic outlet

Occipitoposterior positions viewed from the pelvic outlet

Identifying the position of the fetus on vaginal examination by identifying the position of the sutures and fontanelles in relation to the pelvis

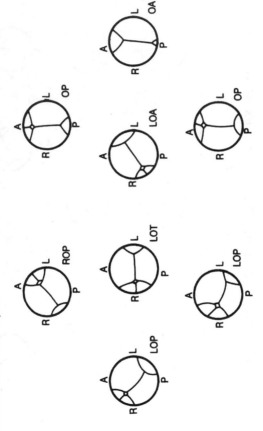

Appendix 5
Normal Labour: Cervicogram; Partogram; Cardiotocograph Recordings

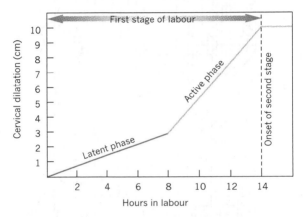

A cervicogram. (Reproduced from Sweet B.R. 1997 *Mayes' Midwifery – a Textbook for Midwives* with permission, Mosby)

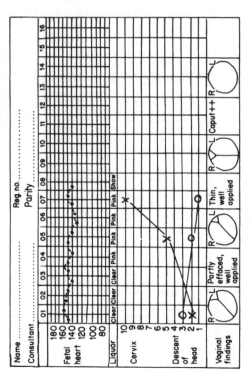

Diagram of a partogram.

306

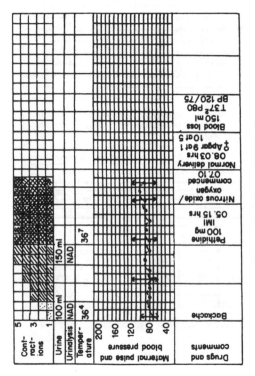

Diagram of a partogram *(continued)*.

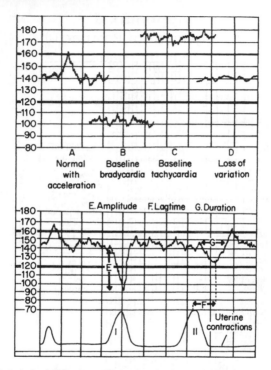

1. Early deceleration (type 1 dip); II. late deceleration (type 2 dip)

Cardiotocograph recordings.

Appendix 6
Management of Postpartum Haemorrhage

(*See also* dictionary entry for POSTPARTUM HAEMORRHAGE.)

Aims of management:

1. to help the uterus to contract firmly;
2. to deliver the placenta if still *in situ*;
3. to arrest haemorrhage as soon as possible and reduce shock.

Action:

- Call skilled obstetrician or emergency obstetric unit if available.
- If bleeding is uterine, give oxytocic drug, e.g. ergometrine 0.5 mg intravenously or Syntometrine 1 ml intramuscularly.
- Massage uterine fundus via abdomen to encourage contraction.
- Empty bladder, catheterize if necessary; examine vagina for lacerations.
- When uterus well contracted attempt controlled cord traction to deliver placenta.
- Prepare equipment for oxytocic intravenous infusion and manual removal of placenta; take blood for cross-matching.
- In rare cases, bimanual compression of non-contracted uterus can save life.
- In isolated areas midwife may have to perform MANUAL REMOVAL OF PLACENTA.

Appendix 7
Neonatal Resuscitation

Asphyxia neonatorum should be anticipated if there are any signs of fetal hypoxia in labour. The midwife should check and prepare resuscitation equipment and alert the paediatrician. At delivery the midwife should:

- note the time;
- aspirate mucus from the baby's naso- and oropharynx;
- cut the cord;
- dry and wrap the baby warmly;
- place the baby under a radiant heater on the equipment, in a supine position with the head slightly lower and extended;
- assess the Apgar score at one minute (*see* Appendix 1).

Apgar score 8–10: no further treatment needed.

Apgar score 5–8: mild asphyxia:

- call paediatrician;
- give oxygen by intermittent positive pressure ventilation via bag and mask, or mouth to mouth/nose resuscitation;
- stimulate the baby gently;
- administer naloxone 0.01 mg/kg body weight if mother had pethidine.

Apgar score below 5: severe asphyxia:

- summon paediatrician urgently;
- clear airways gently;
- give oxygen (max pressure 30 cmH$_2$O) by IPPV at 30 times/minute;
- or intubate with endotracheal tube if trained to do so;
- check heart rate;
- apply cardiac massage if less than 40 beats per minute at 100–120 times per minute;
- assist with administration of drugs as appropriate.

Appendix 8
Conversion Charts

Conversion of babies' weights (lb, oz to g).

oz	0	1	2	3	4	5	6	7	8	9	10	11	12	13	14	15
lb																
0		28	57	85	113	142	170	198	227	255	283	312	340	368	397	425
1	454	482	510	539	567	595	624	652	680	709	737	765	794	822	850	879
2	907	935	964	992	1020	1049	1077	1105	1134	1162	1190	1219	1247	1275	1304	1332
3	1360	1389	1418	1446	1475	1503	1531	1560	1588	1616	1645	1673	1701	1730	1758	1786
4	1815	1843	1871	1900	1928	1956	1985	2013	2041	2070	2098	2126	2155	2183	2211	2240
5	2268	2296	2325	2353	2381	2410	2438	2466	2495	2523	2551	2580	2608	2636	2655	2683
6	2721	2750	2778	2806	2835	2863	2891	2920	2948	2976	3005	3033	3061	3090	3118	3146
7	3175	3203	3231	3260	3288	3316	3345	3373	3401	3430	3458	3486	3515	3543	3571	3600
8	3628	3656	3685	3713	3741	3770	3798	3826	3855	3883	3911	3940	3968	3996	4025	4053
9	4081	4110	4138	4166	4195	4223	4251	4280	4308	4336	4355	4383	4421	4450	4468	4506
10	4535	4563	4591	4620	4648	4676	4705	4733	4761	4790	4818	4846	4875	4903	4931	4960

In making this conversion it is generally sufficient to use the nearest round figure, e.g. $5\frac{1}{2}$ lb = 2495 g, rounded to 2.5 kg.

WEIGHT   HEIGHT

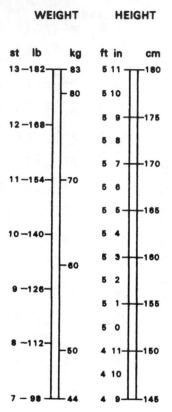

Weight and height conversion charts for antenatal women.

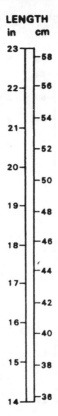

LENGTH

in   cm

Linear equivalents for lengths of babies.

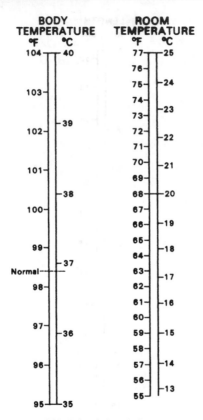

Celsius/Fahrenheit equivalents.

Appendix 9
SI Units
(Système International d'Unités)

Metric system for scientific measurements. The unit of weight is the gram (g), of length the metre (m) and of capacity the litre (l).

Measurements smaller than a unit

Prefix	Symbol	Meaning	Example
deci	d	1 tenth	dl = 1 tenth of a litre
centi	c	1 hundredth	cm = 1 hundredth of a metre
milli	m	1 thousandth	ml = 1 thousandth of a litre
micro	μ	1 millionth	μg = 1 millionth of a gram

Multiples of units

Prefix	Symbol	Meaning	Example
deca	da	10	da l = 10 litres
hecto	h	100	hg = 100 grams
kilo	k	1000	kg = 1000 grams
mega	M	1 million	MJ = 1 million joules

Mass

Calculation of drug doses is vitally important, especially with neonates, when the dose is given according to the weight of the baby. The following equivalents may be useful:

1 kilogram (kg) = 1000 grams (g)
1 gram (g) = 1000 milligrams (mg)
1 milligram (mg) = 1000 micrograms (μg)
1 microgram (μg) = 1000 nanograms (ng)
1 nanogram (ng) = 1000 picograms

Index notation

One unit is used for very large or small quantities but the numbers may involve many zeros and be clumsy to read or write, with the risk of inaccuracies. The 'index' is a small raised number to multiply the products of 10. For example:

$100 = 10 \times 10$ $= \text{index } 10^2$
$10\,000 = 10 \times 10 \times 10 \times 10$ $= \text{index } 10^4$

When fractions of a unit are used the index has a minus sign to represent the number of times the unit should be divided by 10. For example:

$0.1 = \frac{1}{10}$ $= \text{index } 10^{-1}$
$0.01 = \frac{1}{100}$ $= \text{index } 10^{-2}$

Index notation is now used in pathology reports. For example:

	Old value	*Index notation*
Total white blood count	5000–10 000 mm³	5–10.0 × 10⁹/l
Red cell count	4.5 million/mm³	4.5 × 10¹²/l

Appendix 10
Features of Preterm and Small for Gestational Age Babies

	Preterm	Small for gestational age
Skin	Reddish pink with lanugo	Grey or yellowish from meconium, dry, sometimes cracked
Length	Proportionate to weight	Proportionate to gestation, i.e. long for weight
Head	Cranial bones soft	Cranial bones hard, unyielding
Face	Eyes closed; peaceful expression	Eyes often open; worried expression
Ear pinna	Soft, remains folded	Resistant to folding
Breast size	Tissue less than 1 cm diameter	Palpable tissue, 1 cm diameter +
Abdomen	May be prominent	Often scaphoid
Behaviour	Weak cry, inactive; no attempt to suck/swallow; flaccid limbs abducted; lies in 'frog' position	Stronger, more mature cry; hungry sucking; swallows; lively, active, good muscle tone

Appendix 11
Limits of Serum Bilirubin Levels in Neonates

Kernicterus may occur where the levels of unconjugated bilirubin exceed the following levels, depending on gestation:

Under 27 weeks	250 μmol/l
28–30 weeks	280 μmol/l
31–34 weeks	310 μmol/l
35–38 weeks	350 μmol/l
30+ weeks	380 μmol/l

Appendix 12
Social Security Benefits

Benefit	Details	Amount per week (2002)
Child Benefit	Weekly payment to parent or guardian for each child under 16; not affected by income or savings	First child £15.75 Each other child £10.55
Disability Living Allowance	For those who have needed help with care or *mobility* for more than 3 months and likely to need help for at least 6 months more; not dependent on NI contributions, savings or Income Support income	Higher rate £56.25 Middle rate £37.65 Lower rate £14.90
Family Credit	For those whose income is below specified level; not dependent on NI contributions but may be affected by savings	Variable according to income of household, number of children and ages, number of hours worked or if child under 11 is cared for by registered childminder
Incapacity Benefit	Paid from 34/40 to 2/52 postnatal to women unable to obtain SMP or MA	Short-term lower rate £53.50 Short-term higher rate £63.25

Benefit	Details	Amount per week (2002)	
Income Support	Non-contributory for those not in full-time work whose income is insufficient for needs; usually eligible for other benefits	Couple Single parent up to Dependent child	£84.65 £53.95 £33.50
Maternity Allowance (MA)	Paid for 18 weeks to employed women unable to obtain SMP	Standard rate	£75.00
NHS Dental Care	Free during pregnancy and for one year after EDD	According to costs	
NHS Prescriptions	Free during pregnancy and for one year after EDD; free for under-16s	According to costs	
Social Fund	Discretionary one-off payment to low income families whose needs are not met by other benefits	Sure Start Maternity Grant	£500
Statutory Maternity Pay (SMP)	Paid by employer for 18 weeks to women employed for minimum 26 weeks by 15th week before EDD; commences between 29/40 and 1/52 postnatal; requires MatB1 form to claim	Higher rate 90% of average earnings Lower rate	£75

Appendix 13
Useful Addresses and Resources

Association for Improvements in Maternity Services (AIMS), 163 Liverpool Road, London N1 0RF

Association of Medical Research Charities, 29–35 Farringdon Road, London EC1M 3JB
www.armc.org.uk

Association of Radical Midwives, c/o Haringey Women's Centre, 40 Turnpike Lane, London N5 1PB

British Association of Counselling, 37a Sheep Street, Rugby, Warwicks CV21 3BX

British Medical Association, BMA House, 179 Tavistock Square, London WC1H 9JP

British National Formulary (drug information)
www.bnf.org

Childline, Royal Mail Building, Studd Street, London N1 0QW

Cochrane Foundation (Electronic publication of high quality professional health research evidence)
www.update-software.com

Complementary Maternity Forum, c/o Denise Tiran, University of Greenwich, Mansion Site, Avery Hill Road, Eltham, London SE9 2PQ
M.D.Tiran@gre.ac.uk

Department of Health (England), Richmond House, 79 Whitehall, London SW1A 2NS
www.doh.gov.uk

Family Planning Association, Margaret Pyke House, 27–35 Mortimer Street, London W1N 7RJ

Foresight (Preconception Care), The Old Vicarage, Church Lane, Witley, Godalming, Surrey GU8 5PN

Foundation for the Study of Infant Deaths, 14 Halkin Street, London SW1 7DP

Health Education Authority, Hamilton House, Mabledon Place, London WC1H 9TX
www.hea.org.uk

Index medicus (includes full listing of journal abbreviations used for Index Medicus)
www.medscape.com

International Confederation of Midwives, 10 Barley Mow Passage, Chiswick, London W4 4PH

King's Fund, 11–13 Cavendish Square, London W1M 0AN
www.kingsfund.org.uk

Medicines Control Agency, Market Towers, 1 Nine Elms Lane, London SW8 5NQ

MIDIRS (Midwives' Information and Resource Service), 9 Elmdale Road, Clifton, Bristol BS12 2LQ
www.midirs.org

MIND (National Association for Mental Health), 15–19 Broadway, London E15 4BQ
www.mind.org.uk

MIRIAD (Midwifery Research Database), National Perinatal Epidemiology Unit, John Radcliffe Hospital, Headington Lane, Oxford OX2 6HE

Miscarriage Association, c/o Clayton Hospital, Northgate, Wakefield, West Yorkshire WF1 3JS

National Association for Maternal and Child Welfare, 1st Floor, 40–42 Osnaburgh Street, London NW1 3ND

National Childbirth Trust, Alexandra House, Oldham Terrace, Acton, London W3 6NH
www.nctpregnancyandbabycare.com

National Council for One Parent Families, 255 Kentish Town Road, London NW5 6NH

National Institute for Clinical Excellence (NICE), 90 Long Acre, London W3 6PH
www.nice.org.uk

National Society for Prevention of Cruelty to Children (NSPCC), 67 Curtain Road, London EC2A 3NH
www.nspcc.org.uk

Nursing and Midwifery Council, 23 Portland Place, London W1N 3AF
www.nmc-uk.org

Office for National Statistics (ONS), 1 Drummond Gate, London SW1V 2QQ
www.statistics.gov.uk

Pregnancy Advisory Service, 13 Charlotte Street, London W1P 3DG
Prince of Wales Foundation for Integrated Health (formerly Foundation for Integrated Medicine), 12 Chillingworth Road, London N7 8QJ
www.fimed.org.uk
PubMed (National Library of Medicine's free search service for contemporary professional research and review papers)
www.ncbi.nlm.nih.gov/entrez
Research Council for Complementary Medicine, 60 Great Ormond Street, London WC1N 3JF
www.rccm.org.uk
Royal College of Midwives, 15 Mansfield Street, London W1M 0BE
www.rcm.org.uk
Royal College of Nursing, 20 Cavendish Square, London W1M 0AB
www.rcn.org.uk
Royal College of Obstetricians and Gynaecologists, 27 Sussex Place, Regent's Park, London NW1 4RG
Safe Motherhood Initiative
www.safemotherhood.org
Society to Support Home Confinements, Lydgate, Wolsingham, County Durham DL13 3HA
Stillbirth and Neonatal Death Society (SANDS), 28 Portland Place, London W1N 4DE
www.uk-sands.org
Twins and Multiple Birth Association (TAMBA), 54 Broad Lane, Hampton, Middlesex W12 3BG
Wellbeing (formerly Birthright), 27 Sussex Place, Regent's Park, London NW1 4RG

Appendix 14
Immunization and Vaccination Schedule for Children

Age due	Immunization	
2 months	Poliomyelitis Diphtheria Whooping cough	Tetanus Meningitis C Hib
3 months	Poliomyelitis Diphtheria Whooping cough	Tetanus Meningitis C Hib
4 months	Poliomyelitis Diphtheria Whooping cough	Tetanus Meningitis C Hib
12–15 months	Measles Mumps Rubella	
Preschool	Poliomyelitis Diphtheria Whooping cough	(booster)
10–14 years	BCG	
School leavers	Poliomyelitis Diphtheria Tetanus	(booster)

Appendix 15
Nursing and Midwifery Council Documents Relevant to Midwives

The Nursing and Midwifery Council (NMC) replaced the United Kingdom Central Council for Nursing, Midwifery and Health Visiting (UKCC), and the four National Boards, in April 2002. The majority of documents originally produced by the UKCC have been updated and are listed below. Further information is available (and documents can be downloaded) on the NMC's website: http://www.nmc-uk.org.

- Complaints about Professional Conduct, 2002
- Code of Professional Conduct, 2002
- Guidelines for the Administration of Medicines, 2002
- Guidelines for Records and Record Keeping, 2002
- Midwives' Rules and Code of Practice, 1998
- Nurses and Midwives Working Outside the NHS, 2002
- Practitioner–Client Relationships and the Prevention of Abuse, 2002
- Professional Advice from the NMC, 2002
- Reporting Misconduct – Information for Employers, 2002
- Reporting Unfitness to Practise – Information for Employers, 2002
- Requirements for Pre-registration Midwifery Programmes
- Standards for the Preparation of Teachers of Nursing and Midwifery, 2002
- Standards for Specialist Education and Practice, 2001
- Supporting Nurses and Midwives Through Lifelong Learning, 2002

Appendix 16
Abbreviations

ACH	aftercoming head (of breech)
ACTH	adrenocorticotrophic hormone
ADH	antidiuretic hormone
AF	artificial feeding
AFP	alpha-fetoprotein
AID	artificial insemination by donor
AIDS	acquired immune deficiency syndrome
AIH	artificial insemination by husband
AN (C)	antenatal (clinic)
AP	anteroposterior
AP(E)L	accreditation of prior (experiential) learning
APH	antepartum haemorrhage
ARM	artificial rupture of membranes
ASD	atrial septal defect
BBA	born before arrival (of the midwife)
BCG	bacille Calmette–Guérin
bd	twice daily
BF	breastfeeding
BFI	Baby Friendly Initiative
BLISS	Baby Life Support System
BMA	British Medical Association
BMI	body mass index
BMR	basal metabolic rate
BP	blood pressure
BPD	biparietal diameter
BSD	bisacromial diameter
C	Celsius
Ca	calcium
CAT	computed axial tomography
CATS	credit accumulation and transfer system
CCT	controlled cord traction
CDH	congenital dislocation of the hips

CESDI	Confidential Enquiry into Stillbirth and Deaths in Infancy
CHD	congenital heart disease
CIP	continuous inflating pressure
CNP	continuous negative pressure
CNS	central nervous system
COSHH	Control of Substances Hazardous to Health
CPAP	continuous positive airways pressure
CPD	cephalopelvic disproportion
CRL	crown–rump length
CSF	cerebrospinal fluid
CSM	Committee on Safety of Medicines
CSU	catheter specimen of urine
CT	computed tomography
CTG	cardiotocograph
CVS	1. chorionic villus sampling. 2. cardiovascular system
Cx	cervix
D & C	dilatation and curettage
D & V	diarrhoea and vomiting
DH	Department of Health
DHA	district health authority
DIC	disseminated intravascular coagulation
Dip	Diploma
DMA	directly managed unit
DNA	1. did not attend. 2. deoxyribonucleic acid
DSS	Department of Social Security
DTA	deep transverse arrest
DVT	deep venous thrombosis
E_1	oestrone (estrone)
E_2	oestradiol (estradiol) 17β
E_3	oestriol (estriol)
EBM	expressed breast milk
ECG	electrocardiogram
ECT	electroconvulsive treatment/therapy
ECV	external cephalic version
EDD	expected date of delivery
EEG	electroencephalogram
EPA	examination *per abdomen*
EPV	examination *per vaginam*
ERPC	evacuation of retained products of conception

ESR	erythrocyte sedimentation rate
EUA	examination under anaesthetic
F	Fahrenheit
FAS	fetal alcohol syndrome
FBS	fetal blood sampling
Fe	iron
FH (HR)	fetal heart (heard and regular)
FIGO	International Federation of GynEcology and Obstetrics
FRCGP	Fellow of the Royal College of General Practitioners
FRCOG	Fellow of the Royal College of Obstetricians and Gynaecologists
FSH (RF)	follicle-stimulating hormone (releasing factor)
g	gram
G	gravida
GIFT	gamete intrafallopian transfer
GIT	gastrointestinal tract
GMC	General Medical Council
GP (O)	general practitioner (obstetrician)
G6PD	glucose-6-phosphate dehydrogenase
GTT	glucose tolerance test
H	hydrogen
HAI	hospital-acquired infection
Hb	haemoglobin
HCG	human chorionic gonadotrophin
HCl	hydrochloric acid
HEA	Health Education Authority
HELLP	Haemolysis, Elevated Liver proteins and Low Platelets
Hg	mercury
HIV	human immunodeficiency virus
HPL	human placental lactogen
HPV	human papilloma virus
HV (A)	Health Visitor (s' Association)
HVS	high vaginal swab
ICM	International Confederation of Midwives
ICN	International Council of Nurses
ICP	intracranial pressure
ICSH	interstitial cell stimulating hormone
ICSI	intracytoplasmic sperm injection
ICU/ITU	intensive care unit/intensive therapy unit

Ig	immunoglobulin
IM	intramuscular
IMV	intermittent mandatory ventilation
IPPV	intermittent positive pressure ventilation
IUCD	intrauterine contraceptive device
IUD	intrauterine death
IUGR	intrauterine growth retardation
IV (I)	intravenous (infusion)
IVF	*in vitro* fertilization
IVH	intraventricular haemorrhage
IVP/IVU	intravenous pyelogram/urogram
J	joule
K	potassium
k	kilo
kcal	kilocalorie
kJ	kilojoule
LA	local authority
LBW	low birth weight
LFD	light for dates
LFT	liver function tests
LH	luteinizing hormone
LMA	left mentoanterior
LML	left mentolateral
LMP	1. left mentoposterior. 2. last menstrual period
LOA	left occipitoanterior
LOL	left occipitolateral
LOP	left occipitoposterior
LOT	left occipitotransverse
LP	lumbar puncture
LSA	1. local supervising authority. 2. left sacroanterior
LSCS	lower segment caesarean section
LSL	left sacrolateral
LSP	left sacroposterior
L/S	ratio lecithin sphingomyelin ratio
m	milli, meta
M	mega
MAFF	Ministry of Agriculture, Fisheries and Food
MAOI	monoamine oxidase inhibitor
MCA	maternity care assistant

MCH	mean corpuscular haemoglobin
MCHC	mean corpuscular haemoglobin concentration
MCV	mean corpuscular volume
ml	millilitre
mm	millimetre
mmol	millimole
MOH	Medical Officer of Health
MRC	Medical Research Council
MRCOG	Member of the Royal College of Obstetricians and Gynaecologists
MRI	magnetic resonance imaging
MRSA	methicillin-resistant *Staphylococcus aureus*
MSAC	Maternity Services Advisory Committee
MSH	melanocyte-stimulating hormone
MSU	midstream specimen of urine
Na	sodium
NAD	nothing abnormal detected
NAI	non-accidental injury
NBFD	Neville Barnes forceps delivery
ND	normal delivery
NHS	National Health Service
NICE	National Institute for Clinical Excellence
NMC	Nursing and Midwifery Council
NND	neonatal death
NNU	neonatal unit
NSAID	non-steroidal anti-inflammatory drug
NSU	non-specific urethritis
NTD	neural tube defect
O	oxygen
OA	occipitoanterior
ODA	operating department assistant
OL	occipitolateral
OP	occipitoposterior
OPD	outpatient department
OT	occipitotransverse
OTC	over-the-counter (drugs)
P	1. phosphorus. 2. para, parity
P	probability
Pa	pascal

PA	*per abdomen*
PaO$_2$	partial pressure of oxygen in arterial blood
PAP	Papanicolau (smear)
PAPP	pregnancy associated plasma proteins
PCG	primary care group
PCO$_2$	partial pressure of carbon dioxide
PCT	primary care trust
PCV	packed cell volume
PEEP	positive end-expiratory pressure
PG	prostaglandin
pg	picogram
PGCE (A)	Postgraduate Certificate in Education (of Adults)
pH	acid–alkali balance
PID	pelvic inflammatory disease
PIH	pregnancy-induced hypertension
PKU	phenylketonuria
PM	post mortem
PMR	perinatal mortality rate
PO$_2$	partial pressure of oxygen
POP	persistent occipitoposterior
PPH	postpartum haemorrhage
PPR	Price precipitation reaction
PR	*per rectum*
PREP	post-registration education and practice
prn	as required, when necessary
PUO	pyrexia of unknown origin
PV	*per vaginam*
Q	quadrant
QAA	Quality Assurance Agency
qd	every day
qds	four times a day
qh	every hour
qid	four times daily
qqh	every four hours
RBC	red blood cell/count
RCGP	Royal College of General Practitioners
RCM	Royal College of Midwives
RCN	Royal College of Nurses
RCOG	Royal College of Obstetricians and Gynaecologists

RCT	randomized controlled trial
RDS	respiratory distress syndrome
R(G)N	Registered (General) Nurse
Rh	Rhesus (factor)
RM	Registered Midwife
RMA	right menotanterior
RML	right mentolateral
RMP	right mentoposterior
RNA	ribonucleic acid
ROA	right occipitoanterior
ROL	right occipitolateral
ROP	right occipitoposterior
RPCF	Reiter's protein complement fixation
RSA	right sacroanterior
RSL	right sacrolateral
RSP	right sacroposterior
Rx	treatment
S	sulphur
SB	stillbirth
SBR	serum bilirubin
SC	subcutaneous
SCBU	special care baby unit
SFD	small for dates
SGOT	serum glutamate oxaloacetate transaminase
SGPT	serum glutamate pyruvate transaminase
SI	Système International d'Unités
SIDS	sudden infant death syndrome
SMP	Statutory Maternity Pay
SPD	symphysis pubis diastasis/discomfort
SRM	spontaneous rupture of membranes
SSP	Statutory Sick Pay
STI/STD	sexually transmitted infection/disease
SVD	spontaneous vaginal delivery
TBA	1. traditional birth attendant. 2. to be advised
TBC	to be confirmed
TCM	traditional Chinese medicine
tds	three times daily
TENS	transcutaneous electrical nerve stimulation
TORCH	toxoplasmosis, rubella, cytomegalovirus, herpes

TPHA	*Treponema pallidum* haemagglutination
TPN	total parenteral nutrition
TSH	thyroid-stimulating hormone
TTA/TTO	to take away/to take out
U & E	urea and electrolyte (estimations)
UNICEF	United Nations International Children's Emergency Fund
URTI	upper respiratory tract infection
US (S)	ultrasound (scan)
UTI	urinary tract infection
VDRL	Venereal Disease Research Laboratory
VE	vaginal examination
VMA	vanillylmandelic acid
WBC	white blood cell/count
WHO	World Health Organization
WR	Wassermann reaction
ZIFT	zygote intrafallopian transfer